WOMEN'S BODIES

WOMEN'S BODIES

A Social History of Women's Encounter With Health, Ill-Health, and Medicine

Edward Shorter

With a New Introduction by the Author

Transaction Publishers
New Brunswick (U.S.A.) and London (U.K.)

New material this edition copyright © 1991 by Transaction Publishers, New Brunswick,
New Jersey 08903
Originally published in 1982 by Basic Books, Inc., as *A History of Women's Bodies.*

Library of Congress Catalog Number: 89-20672
ISBN: 0-88738-848-5
Printed in the United States of America

Library of Congress Cataloging-in-Publication Data
Shorter, Edward.
   Women's bodies / by Edward Shorter ; with a new introduction by the author.
      p.   cm.
   Reprint. Originally published: New York : Basic Books, c1982.
   ISBN 0-88738-848-5
   1. Obstetrics—History. 2. Childbirth—History. 3. Women—Physiology—
History. 4. Sex customs—History. I. Title.
   RG51.S48   1990
   362.1'98'009—dc20   89-20672
                                                                        CIP

CONTENTS

PART THREE

OTHER PHYSICAL DIFFERENCES BETWEEN

MEN AND WOMEN

LIST OF TABLES

INTRODUCTION TO THE TRANSACTION EDITION

SINCE I WROTE this book in 1982, there has been a great interest in the history of women's physical experience with their bodies. Some of this writing has speculated about body images and what difference they make to more deeply felt senses of femininity and masculinity. Other writers have dealt with health and disease issues. Both streams are part of the great curiosity about women and their history that has helped to characterize the new field of "the social history of medicine." This book represents a contribution to that field, although I should be pleased if regular historians of medicine, social historians, and general readers find it of interest as well.

After I finished *Women's Bodies* in 1982, I went on to learn quite a bit more about medicine. In fact, I went to medical school, or at least did all the courses—and passed all the exams—in the first year and a half of a medical program. I also spent much time observing family doctors in their practice. A history of the doctor-patient relationship that I put my hand to was partly shaped by the experience.[1] Still later, I spent a period of time observing in a hospital neurology service and an office practice, in preparation for taking on a history of "nervous diseases."[2] So, I believe there is some advantage for historians in staying in touch with bedside realities.

During the last decade I have also become interested in the application of science to medicine over the past fifty years. The marriage of the

[1]Edward Shorter, *Bedside Manners: The Troubled History of Doctors and Patients* (New York: Simon and Schuster, 1985).

[2]See, for example, Edward Shorter, "Women and Jews in a Private Nervous Clinic in Late Nineteenth-Century Vienna," *Medical History*, 33 (1989), 149–183.

one to the other has produced a therapeutics which, in contrast to much of the medicine described in *Women's Bodies*, really has made a major difference in health care. This story has a social dimension, one greatly tied up in the flight of Jewish physicians and scientists from Central Europe to the United States in the years after 1933.[3] Although verging on contemporary history, great sagas such as this belong still to the "social history of medicine."

I am describing my intellectual meanderings not because readers necessarily have a burning interest in the subject, but to make the point that the history of women's experience with obstetrics and gynecology—which in a narrow sense is what *Women's Bodies* is about—has offered a springboard to a number of themes that I have found intensely challenging. There is a cornucopia of subjects, embracing the history of the doctor-patient relationship, the history of actual disease and death, and the history of medical practice and of fashions in therapy, which is now pressing to spill forth. I think it likely that many other writers in coming years will help pry it open.

Since 1982 several specific themes in this book have come in for discussion:

The Course of Maternal Mortality Since 1870

This apparently rather technical subject has turned out to be quite important as a test of the quality of the medical care of women. I argue here that the number of maternal deaths in childbirth fell sharply after the 1880s with the introduction of aseptic procedures and the understanding of germs as the mechanism of "puerperal fever." This decrease suggests that the new lessons doctors learned in medical school about washing their hands and cleansing their instruments were being put into practice, to the benefit of women. If this lower maternal mortality does not show up in official statistics on the number of maternal deaths in childbirth per 1,000 deliveries, it is, I believe, because of a simultaneous rise in the mortality from abortion (abortion deaths are also counted as "maternal").

Now, this hypothesis has been flatly contradicted by Irvine Loudon, who places confidence in the official statistics and dismisses the

---

[3]Edward Shorter, *The Health Century* (New York: Doubleday, 1987).

"rising abortion mortality" argument.[4] The implication of his interpretation is that doctors and midwives, although they knew better,
continued to be criminally irresponsible in their management of
deliveries, infecting mothers in the course of routine pelvic exams and
intervening unnecessarily in the normal process of labor. There is no
point in my pounding the podium here and insisting that I am right.
Only further research will resolve this issue.[5]

The History of the Birth Experience

I argue here that women who, on an average, gave birth six times in
their lives and who in each delivery ran a not inconsiderable risk of
dying, did not always greet the birth experience joyously. Since 1982
several new studies have appeared that refine and enhance this picture.
Jacques Gélis's magisterial work on childbearing in early modern
France gives much precious detail.[6] Several scholars have described
childbearing in American history, not always in the sense of this book.[7]
And Judith Schneid Lewis has written a well-documented study not
just of childbirth, but of the changing context of family life among the
British aristocracy.[8] It is true that *Women's Bodies* offers a harrowing
account of the traditional experience of normal birth and of the
management of obstetrical complications. But I have seen little in the
subsequent literature to convince me that I am wrong.

---

[4]Irvine Loudon, "Deaths in Childbed from the Eighteenth Century to 1935," *Medical History*, 30 (1986), 1–41, esp. pp. 3 and 26. I responded to Dr. Loudon's arguments in a paper, "The Supposed 'Failure of Maternal Mortality to Decline': A Case of British Exceptionalism?" for a conference on "Infant, Child, and Maternal Mortality" at the University of Liverpool in 1988. This paper, and Dr. Loudon's reply to it, will be included in the forthcoming proceedings of that conference, edited by Robert Lee.

[5]But see Angus McLaren and Arlene Tigar McLaren, "Discoveries and Dissimulations: The Impact of Abortion Deaths on Maternal Mortality in British Columbia," *BC Studies*, 64 (Winter 1984–85), 3–26, esp. tab. 4, p.12, who also find a decline in full-term maternal deaths in late nineteenth century Vancouver and a rise in abortion mortality. See also Ulf Högberg, *Maternal Mortality in Sweden* (Umeå, Sweden: Umeå University Medical Dissertations, New Series, No. 156, 1985).

[6]Jacques Gélis, *L'Arbre et le fruit: La naissance dans l'Occident moderne, XVI–XIX siècle* (Paris: Fayard, 1984).

[7]Catherine M. Scholten, *Childbearing in American Society: 1650–1850* (New York: New York University Press, 1985), and Judith Walzer Leavitt, *Brought to Bed: Childbearing in America, 1750–1950* (New York: Oxford University Press, 1986).

[8]Judith Schneid Lewis, *In the Family Way: Childbearing in the British Aristocracy, 1760–1860* (New Brunswick, NJ: Rutgers University Press, 1986).

The "Traditional" Midwife: Good or Bad?

Women's Bodies argues that the best of the traditional midwives, those organized in urban guilds, were probably superior to the best male surgeons of the day, but that the average village midwife, following traditional rules for conducting a delivery, often implicated her clients in an obstetrical disaster. The thesis has not been received in all circles with hosannas, but I think it substantially true.[9] We must not, however, forget that late in the eighteenth century a great change occurred. The body's physiological mechanism of labor and delivery was discovered, and medical doctrines began to circulate that emphasized noninterference in this normal process.[10] Simultaneously, formal training programs for midwives were established on the continent of Europe. The midwives who emerged from these programs, generally younger women enthusiastic about their new learning, were very competent indeed.[11]

The Role of Abortion in Birth Control

This book offers information about the role of herbs and of mechanical procedures for abortion. Several other writers have now amplified our information about the former. Angus McLaren has assembled a detailed account of abortifacient drugs used in early modern England.[12] We also know more about the use of these drugs in the ancient world.[13] It is clear that women historically have often been able to procure relatively safe abortions with teas brewed from local herbs, which is of interest because it means that these women were able to take control

[9]One realistic study substantially confirming this is Hilary Marland, M. J. van Lieburg, and G. J. Kloosterman, eds., *"Mother and Child Were Saved": The Memoirs (1693–1740) of the Frisian Midwife Catharina Schrader*, Eng. trans. and annotations by Hilary Marland (Amsterdam: Rodopi, 1987; Dutch ed., 1984) For a more upbeat assessment of the traditional midwife, see Jean Towler and Joan Bramall, *Midwives in History and Society* (London: Croom Helm, 1986).

[10]See Edward Shorter, "The Management of Normal Deliveries and the Generation of William Hunter," in William F. Bynum and Roy Porter, eds., *William Hunter and the Eighteenth-Century Medical World* (Cambridge: Cambridge University Press, 1985), pp. 371–384.

[11]See Jacques Gélis, *La Sage-femme ou le médecin: Une nouvelle conception de la vie* (Paris: Fayard, 1988). A riveting contemporary document is Christa Hämmerle, ed., *Maria Horner: Aus dem Leben einer Hebamme* (Vienna: Hermann Böhlau, 1985).

[12]Angus McLaren, *Reproductive Rituals: The Perception of Fertility in England from the Sixteenth Century to the Nineteenth Century* (London: Methuen, 1984), pp. 89–112.

[13]See Achim Keller, *Die Abortiva in der römischen Kaiserzeit* (Stuttgart: Deutscher Apotheker Verlag, 1988).

of their fertility in their own hands. It is therefore useful to see the medications for abortion that have reappeared in our own time as the latest chapter in a centuries-old tradition of female-initiated abortion, rather than as a sudden new departure in women's ability to govern their own destinies.

Images of the Body and How the Culture Changes Them

There is emerging a fascinating new subject of what one might call "body history." Bryan S. Turner offers the best overview.[14] The theme has several dimensions:

First, whether attitudes to the body have been transformed from the supposed free-and-easy casualness of the Middle Ages to the nervous repression of "bourgeois society," or the reverse! Here the battle lines have been clearly drawn. Norbert Elias is associated with the view that medieval people accepted tolerantly the physicalness of their own and others' bodies. The "process of civilization" therefore entails, according to him, repressing one's sexuality and physiology with a series of mannerly constraints.[15] It is interesting that Hans Peter Duerr has tackled this thesis head-on, declaring Elias wrong on virtually every point. The process, says Duerr, went in the opposite direction: from repressed and shamed medieval men and women to a modern population far more comfortable with sex and body use.[16]

Both these authors talk about men and women. The second issue in the "body" debate, however, concerns women alone and addresses the history of the psychiatric disorder, *anorexia nervosa*. Anorexia, in this sense, is the deliberate refusal of food in the belief that one is too fat, a belief not modified by subsequent weight loss. Is the disorder as old as time, or a product of nineteenth- and twentieth-century cultural changes about the way women are "supposed" to look? Rudolph M. Bell believes that anorexia nervosa may already be identified in the behavior of a number of medieval saints, and that there is really little

[14]Bryan S. Turner, *The Body and Society: Explorations in Social Theory* (Oxford: Basil Blackwell, 1984).

[15]Norbert Elias, *Über den Prozess der Zivilisation* (Basel, 1939); 2nd ed.: *Über den Prozess der Zivilisation: Soziogenetische und psychogenetische Untersuchungen*: vol. 1:*Wandlungen des Verhaltens in den weltlichen Oberschichten des Abendlandes*; vol. 2: *Wandlungen der Gesellschaft: Entwurf zu einer Theorie der Zivilisation* (Berne: Verlag Francke, 1969; pb. ed. Frankfurt/M.: Suhrkamp, 1976). Eng. trans: *The Civilizing Process* (Oxford: Oxford University Press, 1978).

[16]Hans Peter Duerr, *Der Mythos vom Zivilisationsprozess*, vol. 1: *Nacktheit und Scham* (Frankfurt/M.: Suhrkamp, 1988).

new under the sun here.[17] Not so, counters Joan Jacobs Brumberg. Although various "fasting girls" run back over the centuries, the disease anorexia nervosa is the product of a certain style of nineteenth-century family life and of medical diagnosis.[18] My own views weigh in more on Brumberg's side, but much more research on the rich case literature needs to be done.[19]

A third issue in "body history" addresses the social valuation placed upon female bodily functions. *Women's Bodies* argues, of course, that they were scorned and feared. And the considerable historical literature on this theme since 1982 has not contradicted this view.[20] But by the late nineteenth century such medical specialties as neurology and gynecology had become riven with conflicting evaluations of women's bodies, one school deeming women totally (and pathologically) different from men, another finding only minor differences in the architecture of the nervous system and accepting women and their complaints as equivalent to men and theirs.[21] The whole subject of how doctors have looked at women has been the subject of caricature and awaits serious researchers.[22]

A final theme in body history concerns the mind-body relationship. One might ask how the body makes the mind sick, which historically is as much a "men's history" question, in the form of such diseases as alcoholism and neurosyphilis. Or one might ask how disturbances of the mind affect the body. It is true that men as well develop "conversion disorders," physical symptoms that are psychogenic in nature. But the great bulk of such disorders, called "hysteria" in the past, has affected women. Whether this is because of the social roles women have been forced to adopt, because of a preference among women for "body language" in conveying psychological distress, or because of other, undiscovered factors is not clear. In any event, there

---

[17]Rudolph M. Bell, *Holy Anorexia* (Chicago: University of Chicago Press, 1985).

[18]Joan Jacobs Brumberg, *Fasting Girls: The Emergence of Anorexia Nervosa as a Modern Disease* (Cambridge: Harvard University Press, 1988).

[19]Edward Shorter, "The First Great Increase in Anorexia Nervosa," *Journal of Social History*, 21 (1987), 69–96. A major recent contribution is Walter Vandereycken and Ron van Deth, *Vom Fastenwunder zur Magersucht: Anorexia Nervosa historisch betrachtet* (Münster: Regensberg and Biermann, 1988).

[20]Much of this writing is highly polemical and adds little to our knowledge of women's real lives. See, however, Jocelyne Livi, *Vapeurs de femmes: Essai historique sur quelques fantasmes médicaux et philosophiques* (Paris: Navarin, 1984).

[21]For a preliminary attempt to disentangle some of these themes, see Edward Shorter, "Medizinische Theorien spezifisch weiblicher Nervenkrankheiten im Wandel," in Alfons Labish and Reinhard Spree, eds., *Medizinische Deutungsmacht im sozialen Wandel* (Bonn: Psychiatrie-Verlag, 1989), pp. 171–180.

[22]An egregious though widely read caricature is Barbara Ehrenreich and Deirdre English, *For Her Own Good: 150 Years of the Experts' Advice to Women* (Garden City: Anchor Books, 1979).

is nothing in *Women's Bodies* on hysteria and the subject is currently a research interest of mine.[23]

Thus the issues considered in this book may lead many readers, just as they have led me, to a further consideration of how women's physical experience historically has affected the whole constellation of values that represents womanliness, and the constellation of power relationships that binds men and women together.

One final word. In its initial edition, this book was called *A History of Women's Bodies*. Some reviewers took umbrage at the title, deeming it lurid. Indeed as I state in the first sentence of the introduction, it *is* lurid, but deliberately so. I had wanted to call attention to the fact that this whole subject has an independent validity of its own. The present title reflects more precisely the contents of the book. But the point remains that this is a subject whose history is of immense interest and importance. The current volume represents only a small step in telling the story.

Edward Shorter
December 1989
Toronto, Canada

---

[23]See, for example, Edward Shorter, "Paralysis: The Rise and Fall of a 'Hysterical' Symptom," *Journal of Social History*, 19 (1986), 549–582.

PART ONE

WOMEN, MEN, AND BODIES

CHAPTER 1

Men, Women, and Sex

THROUGHOUT much of this book, I shall describe the harm done to women by sexual activity over which they had no control. "No control?" wonders the twentieth-century reader. In our own time, a married woman who dislikes her husband's advances can leave the marriage, and an unmarried woman is usually able to avoid a man's embraces if she so wishes. But today we have the "modern"—even the "post-modern"—family, and things are very different from two hundred years ago, when the traditional husband's "conjugal rights" meant that the married woman could not in fact refuse intercourse.

Put yourself in the shoes of the typical housewife who lived in a small town or village then. Neither she nor anyone else had any idea when the "safe" period for a woman was; and for her, any sexual act could mean pregnancy. She was obliged to sleep with her husband whenever *he* wanted. And in the luck of the draw, she would become pregnant seven or eight times, bearing an average of six live children. Most of these children were unwelcome to her, for if one single theme may be said to hold my story together, it is the danger to every aspect of her health that this ceaseless childbearing meant.

The first issue thus becomes men. What was going on in the minds of husbands to make them subject their wives to these endless births?

Men over Women

A male unconcern for the welfare of women lay in the nature of traditional marriage. Two decades of research in the history of the family has now clearly established that the assumptions of traditional marriage differed radically from those of modern marriage.[1] Unlike the twentieth century, when the point of matrimony is generally thought to be the emotional gratifications of romance and companionship, people in earlier times married for reasons of "lineage": a man needed a wife to help him run the farm or to provide male children to whom he could pass along the patrimony. There was little emotional contact between man and wife; and in fact, men saw other men as their main "spiritual companions" and thus formed the basis of what Lionel Tiger has called "male bonding."[2] Women, in their turn, did not even imagine that their husbands might somehow "understand" them, and saw as their main allies other women. This was the basis of "female bonding." Thus, with both men and women seeking their major sentimental allies outside the family, power relations inside were jarringly unequal. The woman had the status of "chief servant of her sons and of the farmhands," to quote one observer of Brittany.[3] And the man was the "master of his little kingdom," or *Herr im Hause,* as the Germans said.

I should like to make several points about family life then, and call the reader's attention to the anecdotal nature of the evidence that follows. Although one would like firm statistics on such things as wife beating, they are simply not to be had. I have worked for many years in the sources, and what follows is my general impression of relations between men and women—"anecdotal" to be sure, but I am convinced that it is nonetheless accurate.

The husband's overtowering supremacy appears in many rituals of daily life. At table, the closer one sat to the father's chair, the more status one had. In the farm kitchens of the Sauerland, the farmer would be at the head of the table, the other men sitting next to him on the bench against the wall, male children at the end. The women sat on stools across the table. A guest would usurp not the father's place at the head, but the mother's, and she and all the other females would bump down one place. An alternative arrangement would be for all the men to be seated at table, first the father, then the retired grandfather, then his unmarried brother, then the sons in order of their age, with the women all *standing.*[4] Or, as in Vaud Canton, the father might eat alone, served separately by his wife. "Nobody dares raise his voice in the father's presence."[5]

So overawing was the authority of men that in Languedoc a wife would not open the door to searchers from the police when her husband was away, lest she dishonor his authority. His wife would call him "mister" (*notre homme*) and fall silent in the presence of a guest.[6] In the Limousin a wife would not accompany her husband to the market, would not "stand at his side during civil or religious ceremonies," and would address him with the polite *vous*. The husband would not refer to her directly, would never say, "My wife did such-and-such," but, "The woman of this house did such-and-such."[7] French peasant proverbs demonstrate that a man was boss by virtue of his gender:

- "A rooster no larger than your fist will get the best of a hen as large as a stove." (Lower Brittany)
- "A woman who doesn't fear her husband doesn't fear God." (Catalogne)
- "As a man you're strong as plaster if of your wife you aren't the master." (Languedoc)[8]

A woman ethnographer who lived in a German village just before the First World War reported how intensely the "subordination of the woman" was drummed into a young bride's head right from the beginning of her marriage. She would find herself in a strange, already established household, where her mother-in-law and all the relatives were constantly inspecting her. Her new husband sharply criticizes her work, and she starts to get the impression that his good will depends not on her qualities as a woman but on her ability as a farm worker. . . . The custom is that a wife does not go out on her own, even if she pays for it out of her own money. It is like pulling teeth to persuade him to let her go on a small trip or a pilgrimage. He, for his part, goes out every Sunday afternoon with his neighbors to the tavern, and often spends the afternoon or evening there during the week."[9] Actual authority in a particular marriage would depend more on the characters of the individual man and woman; but custom stipulated that affection and intimacy were unimportant in negotiating the pitfalls of married life. The man was master.[10]

Moreover, the average husband in small towns and villages would beat his wife. Legally his right to do so was unclear, yet he certainly was responsible for his wife's actions—a responsibility in which was implicit the power to correct her physically.[11] As a practical matter, wife beating was universal. Midwives saw a lot of domestic violence simply because they were so close to the family circle. Midwife Lisbeth Burger told of one husband who kept strongly urging his wife to get an abortion. She kept refusing.

He: "Why don't you just go into town like everyone else and see the abortionist. Otherwise I'm leaving you."
She: "No. If I'm really pregnant, then our child has a right to live and I won't touch it."

He: "You dare to say that in my face! You dare disobey me! Who's the boss around here, you or me?"

Then "in a blind rage he grabbed her by the hair and started kicking her," saying, " 'By God, I'll show you what's what around here.' "[12] Burger's account implies that this kind of marital scene occurred frequently in her practice.

The doctors, too, saw many beaten women. Eduard Dann in Danzig thought the reason that working-class wives did not drink brandy was that they suffered from the consequences of their husbands' drinking— "terrible beatings," among other things.[13] The obstetrical literature often mentions in passing that a beating was the cause of a woman's miscarriage. Thus in Fischhausen, in 1765, the medical examiner asked a woman who had miscarried:

"Did your husband strike you on that Tuesday?"

"He gave me a slap on the head, and then I went out of the room and when I came back in again he tore my dress off."[14]

Johann Storch of Gotha, investigating the cause of a maternal death in 1724, found that the mother had a broken rib, probably caused by a kick from her husband sometime during the pregnancy. (Storch thought that the broken rib had made the placenta grow fast to the womb, thus killing her in childbirth.)[15]

These stories go on and on. The doctors were not particularly distressed by wife beating, but mentioned it casually along with other medical details.

The proverbs and jokes, which are a culture's very core, assumed that a husband would normally use force to correct his wife. In peasant France:

- "Good or bad, the horse gets the spur. Good or bad, the wife gets the stick." (Provence)
- "If your wife gets an attack of nerves, the best medicine is a good thrashing." (Provence)
- Question: "What do mules and women have in common"? Answer: "A good beating makes them both better." (Catalogne)[16]

Here is a joke from a seventeenth-century German collection of humor:

"A man beats his wife so badly that he has to call both the doctor and the apothecary, paying them twice."

"Paying them twice"?

"Once for this time and once for the next!"[17]

These jokes and proverbs represent situations that were familiar to the men who told them and passed them on. If wife beating had not been widespread among the common people, the sayings would have been meaningless to them.

Along with a husband's overt brutality to a wife went his apparent lack of concern over her illnesses, deliveries, and death. The point is important, for if men were uncaring at these crises, they would also be indifferent in general to a wife's physical welfare. In an earlier book, I argued that the peasant's stolidity in the face of a wife's death betokened a lack of grief and an equal lack of attachment.*[18] Critics of this viewpoint have maintained that men really felt bereaved, yet expressed their grief in ways unfamiliar to us.† Here I should like, therefore, to present several other indexes of male unconcern that may not be easy to explain away.

One is the ubiquity of folk sayings about how much more farmers valued their livestock than their wives:

> *If the cow kicks off, mighty cross.*
> *If the wife kicks off, no big loss.* (Hesse)[22]
>
> *Got a dead wife? No big deal*
> *Got a dead horse? How you squeal.* (Franconia)[23]

The underlying logic of these sayings is that farm animals were expensive, whereas a wife could easily be replaced with a new bride who would bring another dowry to the farm. Hence while the loss of a horse was a blow, the death of a wife definitely carried with it a silver lining.

Contemporary observers, moreover, confirm the cool emotional calculus that lay behind these proverbs. Jacques Cambry wrote of Brittany in the 1790s, "If the horse and the wife of a peasant fall sick simultaneously, he will call the blacksmith, but let nature act upon his wife, who will suffer without complaining."[24] A priest in the Marne region wrote in 1777, "The peasants of the parish worry more about their cows when they birth their calves than about their wives when they have babies."[25] When Rudolf Dohrn was teaching obstetrics in Königsberg, he said, "A country doctor from Lithuania told me that the death of a wife in childbirth meant little to the peasant. When a cow dies, it is very painful to the peasant, but another wife he'll get easily."[26]

The indifference of men to the physical welfare of women is most striking in regard to childbirth. As we shall see later, child bearing was a woman's event, occurring within the women's culture; a man's primary concern was to see a living heir brought forth. Midwife Burger was called urgently to the bedside of a mother in labor. "I knew there was no

---

* Segalen remarks on what a deliverance a wife's loss was for a husband;[19] and the wives felt more or less the same about their husbands.[20]

† Several French ethnographers believe that grief at the departure of loved ones in traditional society was just as intense as in modern times, only expressed in different ways. See, for example, Francoise Loux's discussion of infant deaths.[21]

rush," she later wrote, "but I try to please when it's a young mother."

The peasant farmer awaited her. "It has to be a male child," he said, "an heir for the farm."

"And if it's a girl?" Burger asked.

"Then the devil take her," the farmer said.[27]

Surgeon Max Thorek was delivering an immigrant woman around the turn of the century in the slums of Chicago. "I had just begun to work, when a sound made me look up.

"Against the closed kitchen door stood the husband—about two hundred and fifty pounds of flesh, blood, and irascibility. In one hand he held a long thick old-fashioned iron stove poker. In the other a half-gallon pot filled with boiling coffee.

"All right, you go ahead," he shouted. "But I watch. If anything happen to my woman, I keel you."

It turned out to be a healthy baby boy. "The father relaxed. He began to cry, to pray, to laugh. All his other children were girls. Now he had a son."[28] Thus the sex of the infant was crucially important for fathers, especially when it came to a boy who would carry on the family name. The rest was secondary.

We know that it was secondary because many traditional husbands showed themselves loath to pay the cost of a trained midwife or doctor. They felt the neighbors' help was good enough. Thus a Soissons doctor said in 1775: "The fathers for their part contribute by their negligence to the multitude of obstetric disasters. Just as tight, or tighter, with the purse than city dwellers, they pay close attention to the slightest expense. They neglect nothing in the care of their livestock, but in terms of interests that are much closer to the hearthside, they act with stupid immobility: the successful delivery of their pregnant wives has definitely second place."[29] Wrote Dr. Flügel of the Frankenwald a century later, "There is very little attention paid to childbirth, in that not only many poor but also well-to-do dispense with a midwife in order to save money, letting their own wives give birth as best they can. Through such parsimony I have in the last few years been witness to several maternal deaths."[30] Maria Bidlingmaier said of rural Württemberg at the beginning of the twentieth century: "When something goes wrong in childbirth, first the experience and knowledge of the village crones is sought out. The doctor is far away, and the peasant shies away from the expense of paying him."[31] Midwife Burger frequently encountered these misers. She needed help in one protracted labor:

"Hey, farmer, have you finally called the doctor?"

"Aw, what are you talking about. Nature needs time. You have to know how to wait," he said.

"No," she replied. "Waiting's not going to do it. I'm telling you some-thing's wrong with your wife. Send for the doctor!"

"It takes time," he said again. "In the stable you can easily spend three whole nights waiting. My God what a racket you womenfolk make."

The story goes on and on in this vein. There's a thunderstorm. The farmer insists the doctor will charge even more if he has to come in bad weather. The wife dies.[32]

Beneath this male torpor lay a massive indifference to the sufferings of wives which is the antithesis of "modern" family sentiment. This indifference appears in a number of traditional practices, themselves far less repugnant than the preceding stories, yet equally telling. A middle-class London woman gave birth on 21 April 1770 and came down a few days later with a post-delivery infection, which had a nasty odor. This went on for several weeks. As Dr. Charles White tells us, the husband refused to go into his wife's sickroom, leaving her with the other women, "upon account of the excessive heat and offensive smell which it afforded."[33] So we may imagine the scene: the wife lying ill for weeks, the other women clustering about, the husband virtually refusing to see her because he didn't like the smell. The doctor did not comment on the husband's absence as unusual.

I am not trying to cast the husbands of traditional society as fiends but want merely to show what an unbridgeable sentimental distance sepa-rated them from their wives. Under these circumstances it is unrealistic to think that men would abstain from intercourse in order to save women from the physical consequences of repeated childbearing.

The Quality of Intercourse

A modern hypothesis might be that the sex was so satisfying that women were willing to overlook its disadvantages. But no, intercourse in the traditional family was brief and brutal, and there is little evidence that women derived much pleasure from it.

The main characteristic of the sexuality of traditional men is its ruthless impetuosity. When a man desired his wife, he would take her—that was all there was to it. It fell, for example, always to the man to initiate intercourse. Limousin peasants expressed this idea in the "rooster-hen" metaphors they used for sexual relations: "When the hen hunts out the rooster, love isn't worth beans."[34]

Impetuousness appears in men's refusal to abstain from intercourse during the mother's lying-in period. Stories abound of husbands mounting their wives just after they had delivered, heedless of the doctor's pleas.

Sex too soon after delivery can give the mother an infection. Thus, we are not surprised to learn that, a couple of days after a smooth delivery, Frau Stengel had a slight fever and some bleeding. "Something is wrong here," thought midwife Burger.

"Did you get out of bed yesterday, Frau Stengel," she asked.

"Oh no, no that." The woman looked embarrassed. Burger kept pressing her until the truth came out.

"It's just that . . . my husband was . . . with me."

"That scoundrel, that wretch," cried Burger. And gave him an earful. "What's a wife there for?" responded the husband.[35]

This happened often among the common people, despite custom's prescribing much longer waits.*

Nor is this impetuosity some particularly brutal "peasant" quality. The seventeenth-century Virginia gentleman William Byrd was given to taking his wife on the spur of the moment—for example, on the billiard table—and often referred in his diary to having "rogered" her or "given her a flourish." Perhaps Mrs. Byrd liked this. Yet historian Michael Zuckerman's view is that Byrd thought of sex as a regular body function, unconnected to romantic ardor. It "was marked by only the most perfunctory exhibitions of human connectedness or emotional intensity. Except on the rarest occasions, Byrd scarcely seemed to notice his wife's response to him."[37]

A collection of sexual folksongs from pre-Christian Latvia gives some notion of the images traditional men had in mind as they cohabited with their wives. These songs brim over with force and violence:

> Run and hide in osiers, twot,
> 'Cause here your suitors come!
> Hirsute Hank, Testicle Tom
> and Indrick the Dick himself.

> Daddy grinds and grinds mommy
> As if he wants to grind her down.
> He rests a little in-between,
> Then he starts to grind again.

> Canter, blackie, tra-la-la!
> Tomorrow we hit Riga.
> We'll kidnap young broads
> And drill into old hags.

> Gramps goes to tend cattle
> He puts a chisel in his bag.
> When he encounters a black spot
> He chisels a hole in it.[38]

* According to Hungarian custom, marital relations should recommence at the earliest in fourteen days and later among "the more intelligent class."[36]

Blasting, drilling, and chiseling at women—this is not the language of tenderness. Also, when men were to be on their best behavior, they had to be reminded not to fart during intercourse. How do you act if you want to conceive a child during sex? The Finns had various rules, such as wearing clean underwear and having sex in bright daylight. But if you don't want a child that lisps, don't fart, they said.[39] It would be interesting to know if the women were as flatulent, but I doubt it.

To the extent that couples departed at all from the "missionary position," they seem to have done so largely at the man's urging and for his benefit. Among the Latvian songs describing oral-genital sex—from both male and female viewpoints, the least common theme is a married woman expressing pleasure at her husband's performing cunnilingus upon her.[40] A typical song of this genre:

> *Eat, eat, Trina,*
> *Take big bites!*
> *Our smokehouse still has*
> *Food of three kinds:*
> *Smoked partridge and snipe*
> *And an old man's pecker.*[41]

There are a number of references to the wives of peasants performing fellatio or masturbating them. A Finnish proverb suggests, for example, that after withdrawing his penis in *coitus interruptus,* a man should poke it into his wife's mouth.[42] I found fewer references to men masturbating their wives. (Dr. G. H. Fielitz, however, seems to have encountered one such example of sexual mutuality in his practice, though he disapproved of it. He was called to a difficult delivery and asked himself afterward what might have caused the problem. "Because the woman's entire physiognomy was rather suspect to me, and there was no need to keep her calm, I lured from her with various questions the confession [that she masturbated], only with the difference that she did not do this herself, but that her husband did it to her."[43])

The best measure of men's impetuosity is the extent to which women had the right to say no. If a married woman could not refuse sex, she would be vulnerable indeed to her husband's desire. Does it sound as though Madame Dubost, at the age of forty-nine, had the right to refuse sex to Monsieur Dubost? She appeared at Lyon's Hôtel Dieu, in July of 1812 with an extensive cervical cancer, bleeding and smelling awful. However her immediate problem was that she was pregnant, for despite her "advanced sarcoma," Monsieur Dubost had insisted upon intercourse. On 16 September she miscarried, and died shortly afterward.[44] The wife of a wealthy burgher of Valognes suffered a continuous hemorrhage during pregnancy, and sent for Guillaume de la Motte, a man midwife. De la

Motte examined her, then turned to the husband and made him promise to abstain from sex for the remainder of the pregnancy. "They were the prettiest promises in the world, but immediately forgotten.[45] Does it sound as though this woman had the right to avoid intercourse?

Few women did, not even when they had a grim pelvic condition (see pages 22–25) where the bones have grown too small for the infant's head to pass. Other women had hideous forceps deliveries, and were themselves mutilated and bedridden for months, only to become pregnant again! One hapless woman, who died in August 1797 while giving birth to her sixth child, had an unusually small pelvis. "Each delivery was very difficult. In the second she was delivered with forceps, in the fifth, when an arm was the presenting part, I delivered her with an arduous turning."[46] The remarkable thing is that she kept getting pregnant. Because she felt the "joy of sex"? Or because her husband insisted on sleeping with her?

Thus we see the reality of "conjugal duties," a euphemism for the *task* of intercourse. The obligation existed on both sides. According to old German law, a husband who had refused his wife sex would lose the use of her dowry. She, however, in refusing *him* sex would find her dowry confiscated and herself totally penniless.[47] We may ask how often husbands among the common folk refused to sleep with their wives. Probably not often. Moreover, in cohabiting with their wives they risked nothing. Much of this book, however, will detail what the women had to lose when they had sex with their husbands.

Did Women Enjoy Sex before 1900?

This question can be approached from two radically opposed points of view—the man's and the woman's. As far as traditional men are concerned, women were raging volcanos of desire. The view that women need to have orgasm in order to conceive goes back to the second-century Greek physician Galen.[48] After Saint Augustine, in the fifth century, Christian doctrine was to glare suspiciously on the sensuality of both sexes. But after the late Middle Ages, the Catholic Church mistrusted the woman in particular, "the most dangerous of all the serpents."[49] Classic medical views of the uterus reinforced this image of women's devouring sexuality. One writer said in 1597 that "the uterus has naturally an incredible desire to conceive and to procreate. Thus it is anxious to have virile semen, desirous of taking it, drawing it in, sucking it, and retaining it."[50] As these views filtered down, the message was: women are furnaces of carnality, who time and again will lead men to perdition, if given a chance.

The point of much brutal male sexual behavior was to deny women this chance. Because the flame of female sexuality could snuff out a man's spirit, women had sexually to be broken and controlled. "Of women's unnatural, insatiable lust," said Robert Burton in 1621, "what country, what village doth not complain."[51] The French proverbs present women as "devourers of males." Martine Segalen interprets a whole series of proverbs, comparing supine women and upright trees, to mean that both are equally fearful challenges for a man: he never knows how much force it will take to get the woman under control or the tree felled. Another series of proverbs presents women as sexually insatiable:

· "Satisfying a woman is like confessing to the devil." (Limousin)
· "You can't satisfy everyone and your wife too." (Picardy)[52]

Thus the underlying male rationale for this ramrod impetuosity in sexual matters was to shatter a woman's natural sexual force before it could get the best of a man.

How about women? How did they feel about sex?

One preliminary point. Evidence on the subject of female sexuality, among middle-class and aristocratic women, starts to accumulate during the eighteenth and early nineteenth centuries, precisely at the time when modern attitudes toward family life, which value emotional expressiveness among women, begin to appear among these classes.[53] So we must be on guard against taking these new sexual attitudes as in any way "traditional." At this time as well, a sort of premarital "sexual revolution" was accomplished among unmarried young women from the lower classes, in which sex before marriage began to be seen as an extension of personal happiness rather than as a way to "get a man" (or as a form of rape).[54]

The people who interest us, however, are those vast numbers of married women from the popular classes who lived before the twentieth century. What was their "traditional" sexual response? Some bits of evidence, such as Emmanuel Le Roy Ladurie's study of a medieval French village, seem to go against my case.[55] Yet I believe the overwhelming body of evidence suggests that, for married women in the past, sex was a burden to be dutifully, resentfully borne throughout life rather than a source of joy.

The sexually *least* inhibited population in Western society seems to have been the pre-Christian Latvians. The evidence on them is limited, yet it's the best evidence available for any historical population, because thousands of their "sex songs" survive. In some of them, to be sure, women do come across as avid for intercourse:

The gals say doing the wash:
We get only pants—empty pants.
Wish we'd get those nuts
That repose in these pants.

I whirl the laundry club
High above my head,
As I launder a guy's pants.
Wish I only had the club
That sits in those pants. [56]

Although we don't know whether married or unmarried women are speaking, these verses, designed to be sung at village festivals, do convey female enthusiasm.

Yet the majority of the sex songs that were apparently sung by women reflect dread at male brutality or the desire to use sex as a medium of exchange:

My mother says she gave me
To one who has compassion.
What kind of compassion is that?
He stabs a dirk into my stomach.

Marry me to anybody, mama,
Just don't marry me to a blacksmith.
A smith feels women ruthlessly
Using his black fingers. [57]

There may have been some difference in the sexual response of unmarried and married women, as the following suggests:

When I was a young maiden,
I lit my fire with my pussy;
Now I'm old and unable to light
With a lighter made of steel. [58]

Some of the Latvian songs hint that women regarded their sexuality more as a means to an external end rather than as an end in itself:

I got a small but deep box
At the tip of my belly;
Whoever will feed my head,
May unlock the box.

My drunkard husband wants to screw,
Why should I—without my share?
Gimme half a pint of brandy,
Screw, turning me around. [59]

A final theme in these Latvian songs is the physical revulsion many women felt for unkempt rustic men:

> *I was straining out of love*
> *To make kiss-kiss with Johnny.*
> *Every time I'd offer my lips,*
> *I'd notice lice on Johnny.*
> *Never mind those damn lice,*
> *I just couldn't stand the snot.* [60]

This theme of physical revulsion surfaces time and again in the world we have lost. In May 1693, de la Motte counseled two women who were unable to lubricate when their spouses wanted sex. His analysis was that "the sword was too big for the scabbard," but it is more likely that the women simply were not aroused. He advised them to lubricate their fingers with oil and manually to dilate their vaginas, which they did successfully.[61] This male midwife made casual references to women who "vomit during coitus"—a symptom he ascribed to some anatomical relationship between the stomach and the uterus.[62] As he treated none of these complaints as remarkable, they may well have been common.

When in the 1930s, Margaret Hagood interviewed women in the rural South of the United States, she got responses reminiscent of these seventeenth-century French peasants. One woman "has always hated" sex but "has never let her husband get the upper hand of her." Even when first married she would say, "Take your hands off me," if she thought sex too frequent. "Now since she has arthritis, which makes intercourse painful, he tries to be as considerate as possible and holds off as long as he can—usually two or three weeks." Another, older, woman said that "she supposes she is now like other women after the menopause—that is, she knows what is going on, but she feels nothing (a commonly held notion)." "I never enjoyed it one bit," said a third.[63]

Salient in this revulsion against sex was fear of pregnancy. In 1925, Marie Stopes said of one of the women whom she interviewed in her birth control clinic in London, "She could hardly bear to hear an amiable note in her husband's voice for fear it should lead to sex indulgence, when she was at the mercy of his all too unreliable 'self control.' "[64] Emma Goldman, a noted radical intellectual, recalled the immigrant women she delivered in New York in the 1890s when she was a midwife, "During their labor pains some women would hurl anathema on God and man, especially their husbands. 'Take him away,' one of my patients cried, 'don't let the brute come near me—I'll kill him!' "[65]

In fact, the predominant attitude toward sexuality among peasant and working-class women before the twentieth century—and afterward, in isolated communities—seems to have been quiet resignation. Lisbeth Burger's patients thought that "it was a sin to refuse him sex."[66] And Marta Wohlgemuth, a young German doctoral student who lived in several

Badenese villages just before the First World War, described the role of "Sunday afternoons" in the sexual subordination of the farm wife. The farmer is at the bar: "The farmer's wife remains at home. Tired from the week's work she sleeps a bit; then she does some knitting or reads in the Sunday religious magazines or in the Bible, and thus comes to the quiet submission which one sees so often on the faces of these women. . . . Revolt against the husband seldom occurs, and if so she regrets it, because for her it is a religious commandment that she practice obedience and self-effacement." It is for her similarly a religious commandment that "every year she bring a new child into the world."[67] Maria Bidling-maier, who around the same time was observing life in other villages, confirmed the passive acceptance of sex which lay behind this docility. "The wife feels it as a burden to be married, although as a young woman she was robust and full of life. From this arises often a quiet bitterness toward her husband, who dominates her physically and exploits her pow-ers. Already in the first year she is expecting. . . . Birth follows birth. . . .

"Under the pressure of her first years of marriage the wife drifts toward a quiet resignation to her fate. Some become unfeeling, hard, and inaccessi-ble to all sentiment, interested only in gain. Others seek 'refuge and shelter' in the will of the Lord and His guidance."[68]

Some of the working-class English women who responded, just before the First World War, to a Women's Co-operative Guild questionnaire, said they saw sex "only as a duty." "I submitted as a duty," wrote one woman in explaining why she had six children, "knowing there is much unfaithfulness on the part of the husband where families are limited." Another was explicitly anti-erotic: "I do wish there could be some limit to the time when a woman is expected to have a child. I often think women are really worse off than beasts. . . . If the woman does not feel well she must not say so, as a man has such a lot of ways of punishing a woman if she does not give in to him."[69]

There is no shortage of quotes from around the turn of the century suggesting that married women dislike marital relations. The point I wish to make, however, is that this "Victorian" prudery and passivity are a continuation of negative female feelings about sex that reach far back into time, rather than being a creation of the nineteenth century.

This material is anecdotal and sketchy, but it helps to set the stage for the hard realities to come. Traditional women were sexually cowed and emotionally brutalized by men. They found it impossible to escape intercourse, and sought solace for its unpleasant consequences only in the company of other women. Not until women solved the problems of abortion, contraception, and safe childbirth, discussed elsewhere in this book, would they be able to relax about marital sexuality.

CHAPTER 2

The Architecture of the Body

IT WOULD MAKE a fascinating chapter if the structure of women's bones and the shape of their internal organs had changed greatly over the years. But they have not. The architecture of both men's and women's bodies is largely hammered into place by genetics. In four important ways, however, changes in the body's shape over the years have affected the lives of women: women have become taller and heavier; they have overcome their traditional inequality in access to food; their pelvises are no longer misshapen by a disorder called "rickets"; and they have stopped wearing corsets, although this is the least significant of these changes. Thus, the actual physical structure of the female body has something of a history.

Women Grow Bigger

That men are bigger than women has had relatively little to do with determining male dominance historically, for in the past—when male supremacy triumphed absolutely—women were much closer to men in physical size than they are now. How people grow, when considered in the aggregate, is largely a function of how well they eat. And the height and weight of women has gone up in some eras as their diets improved, down at other times as their diets worsened. The details of this story have been largely lost, because before the nineteenth century, nobody made the necessary physical measurements on samples of sufficient size. Yet two points may be made:

1. Women probably grew smaller between the fourteenth and the eighteenth centuries as the general downturn in Europe's economy over that time meant that they got less to eat. This point will be demonstrated in a moment.
2. A long-term increase in women's physical size seems to have begun at some point late in the eighteenth or early in the nineteenth century; it has come to an end only in the 1960s.

There are, to my knowledge, no direct physical measurements on large numbers of women from earlier times. What suggests that average body size might have diminished at the end of the Middle Ages and during the Early Modern period is the apparently later age at which they began menstruating, for it seems to be true—again for women as a whole— that the better they eat, the earlier they start getting their period.* The age of first menstruation, or "menarche," is heavily influenced by heredity, disease, and race as well as by diet. But historically the only factor among these likely to have changed greatly is diet.

A long period of scarcity settled over Western society at the end of the Middle Ages, apparently affecting women by increasing the average age at which puberty began. The later women begin menstruating, the smaller they will probably be; the earlier the onset of puberty, the larger their ultimate body size.[3] Hence, an increase in the age at menarche in the fourteenth to the eighteenth centuries probably means that the average seventeenth-century woman was less sturdy than her eleventh-century or her ancient Roman counterpart.

In Classical Greece and Rome, and during the Middle Ages, women seem to have started menstruating at about thirteen or fourteen. The sources assume that twelve is the earliest menarche ever happened, and few writers mention puberty arriving later than fifteen. Two scholars who have reviewed all the available documents write of the late Middle Ages, "There is no evidence that the retardation of age at menarche evidenced at the end of the eighteenth century had yet begun."[4]

Then, in the seventeenth and the eighteenth centuries, the average age of menarche seems to have climbed to sixteen, and even beyond. One author said in 1610 of the area around Innsbruck, "The peasant girls of this County in general menstruate much later than the daughters

---

* Rose Frisch has argued that better diets, leading to an increase in the amount of fat stored in girls' bodies, have been responsible for earlier ages of menarche;[1] this thesis has, however, had several critics.[2]

of the townsfolk or the aristocracy, and seldom before their seventeenth, eighteenth or even twentieth year. . . . The townsfolk have usually born several children before the peasant girls have yet menstruated. The cause seems to be that the inhabitants of the town consume more fat food and drink and so their bodies become soft, weak and fat and come early to menstruation."[5] We might regard these figures a touch suspiciously, because seventeen as an *average* age for beginning puberty would be high indeed. But in plenty of historical situations the average woman did not begin menstruating before sixteen. Whether sixteen or seventeen, the implication of these statistics is that in the past the average adolescent would have spent more than half her teen-age years in a prepubescent state.

At some point late in the eighteenth or early in the nineteenth century, a massive decline occurred in the age at puberty—a decline that lasted until the 1960s. In France, for example, the average age at menarche seems to have declined as follows:

1750–1799	15.9
1800–1849	15.5
1850–1899	15.1
1900–1950	13.9[6]

Similar declines occurred elsewhere, to go by less complete data: from 16 in Norway in 1840 to 13.3 near the Second World War; from 15.6 in Sweden in 1886 to a little less than 13 in 1970.[7] Most women today, probably as in ancient times, reach puberty around twelve and a half or thirteen.[8]*

I dwell upon the onset of menstruation only because it seems to indicate how big and strong women ultimately become.† The figures on the "secular" increase in people's height and weight over the last hundred years are well known to specialists, and I shall not repeat them here. But keep in mind that in the 1830s the average Belgian woman was only about 5 feet 2 inches tall and weighed around 121 pounds. By the 1970s her American counterpart would be 2 inches taller and 20 pounds heavier.[11]

Women's Disparity in Diet Disappears

Obviously people are eating better in our time. But I want to make the point that under the regime of the traditional family—before the

---

* Note that the decline in menarcheal age seems now to be coming to an end.[9]
† Increasing age at menopause would be another such indicator.[10]

advent of the routine chivalry in relations between men and women of "modern" family life—women ate less well than men. Before I document this point, however, I wish to give the reader a general sense of what everyone ate. Much is known of the history of diet, so merely by way of illustration let us look at the daily regimen of a comparatively well-nourished area, the Margraviate of Hochberg, in 1783:

- Breakfast. "Most of the inhabitants have a thick bread soup, to which not infrequently are added leftover dried beans, peas and lentils."
- Midday meal. "Mostly of green or dried vegetables, or of bread-dishes, dumplings in soup, all kinds of potatoes, cooked, dried or fresh fruit."
- Dinner. "A soup of dried potatoes with salt, or sour milk, or a salad prepared with whatever is around, even potatoes, and moistened with nutoil. On holidays bacon is added to the salad."

Hochbergers, like many others in pre-industrial Europe, would wash their meals down with water and coffee, occasionally with wine. Most families had a pig or two and, after the annual slaughter, salted away some pork to last for the year, eating it for lunch once or twice a week. "Seldom" did Hochbergers eat beef, veal never.[12] These facts are all familiar to historical demographers. They mean that, after the eighteenth century, starvation was rarely seen, for the potato and the rye loaf provided gross calories. And such a diet meant that one could expect *some* variety, as opposed to the endless round of "bread soup" which was the hallmark of truly backward areas. But within this diet grave deficiencies in protein and other nutrients might nonetheless prevail.

Of interest to us, however, is that within this minimally adequate diet women came off considerably worse than men, for they got less meat, when meat was available, and smaller portions of everything. The rules of the game in the village said—whether this was true or not—that men's work was physically harder than women's, and that men needed more food. How much more? In the seventeenth century, Faroe Islanders, who divided up the food from a central bowl rather than passing it around, "gave the men twice as much as the women." The household book of a Norwegian pastor said in 1772 that when the Christmas rye loaves were baked, those of the men weighed 1,350 grams; those of the women, 900 grams.[13]

Different spaces for socializing meant that men would not necessarily take all their food at home. Around Sigmaringen the men would go to the tavern for their evening meal, the women and children contenting themselves, "year in and year out, with a miserable water soup."[14] Until the twentieth century, men in Provence would gather daily, or weekly on Sundays, for a self-cooked meal in a kind of men's club called a *chambrette*. Provisions would be taken from family larders at home, "despite the mouths remaining to be fed. The family meal is usually quite modest, a simple crêpe, of which the family father takes the greatest part for his *chambrette*."[15]

Yet most men ate at home, where a strict table order determined that they would receive the lion's share. Thus, a vintner's family in Baden, who bought their meat at the butcher's, made "one pound do for six. After the wife has carved the meat, the peasant father makes use of his privilege of taking the largest and best piece. After him come the sons, then the daughters, and finally the wife herself."[16] How much remained for her, *out of a pound?* When the food was portioned out in Norwegian peasant families before the First World War, "the men received most, the women least." Custom agreed in the village of Alta that "wives should receive less food and should do without when things are short." Most Norwegians who responded to a survey about folk customs and beliefs agreed that "women needed less than men." And in some districts it was "thought polite" for women to eat less. In Sandeid and Rogaland one could slander a woman by saying, "She eats as much as a man."[17]

Female servants suffered as well (so did male servants, but there were many more live-in female domestics). When the plate was passed around, they would receive it last, getting the pieces with the maggots, in those areas where the family would salt away pork for the whole year. One young woman said, "Once I had fifteen maggots on my plate." After the First World War another female servant in one of those big peasant farms accidentally let the plate go the wrong way, so that the other servants helped themselves first to the good pieces. "You should have heard the uproar the family made," she said. They refused to eat the maggoty pieces.[18]

Giving father more was also a working-class as well as a peasant, tradition. Thus, Dr. Edward Smith in 1863: "The remark was constantly made to me that 'the husband wins the bread, and must have the best food.' . . . The labourer eats meat and bacon almost daily, whilst his wife and children may eat it but once a week, and both himself and his household believe that course to be necessary, to enable him to perform his labour."[19] A German recalled how he ate as a child in a weaver's family in the 1840s. In addition to potatoes, "sometimes there would be a herring, which they would send me to fetch. My father would take half of it and give the other half to my mother, which she would then divide with us children. If you didn't get enough, well, there was plenty of salt left in the saltshaker to eat."[20] Another German worker said, "I eat butter, the wife and the kids, they eat margarine."[21] It is evident that these workers were living at a considerably higher level than the peasants.

Yet within both kinds of household the same rule prevailed: the men got more.

Of course, the women, who prepared the food, could sneak all the bread soup they wanted. This inequality obtained only when protein- and fat-rich foods like meat and fish were apportioned—which would be brought in one piece to the table and divided for all to see. The consequences of this inequality would appear not in such areas as body size, where men were probably closer to women than they are today, but in relative ability to resist infection or in the levels of physical energy. A powerful factor explaining gender differences in these domains would be differences in nutrition.

Childhood Rickets: A Scourge of Adult Women

The shapes of women's bodies have changed in one significant way over the years. Now women have an overwhelming chance of growing up with straight bones, properly curved backs, and large, roomy pelvises. Before the Second World War, a significant proportion of lower-class European women, and of black women in the United States, did not grow up straight and tall owing to the childhood disease of rickets, which happens when the bones don't harden properly.

Let me make clear right at the beginning that rickets was especially a problem for women, even though male infants got it, too. Only women give birth, so the pelvic deformities accompanying rickets would matter greatly only to them. The problem is that bones that grow crooked in the first years of life may never straighten out. Here is how rickets begins:

- At about four months, soft patches of defective bone tissues, called "craniotabes," appear in the child's skull, creating a sort of squarish head and a high, bulbous brow.
- At six months, a string of swellings appears on the chest around the sternum, where the bone meets the cartilage. They were called the "rickety rosary"; and a mother, when she saw them, feared her child was doomed. In fact, the child was not, unless for other reasons. But the rickety rosary has always been a hallmark of the disease.
- At twelve months, the long bones of the arms swell out at the wrists, because the growth plates in them are splayed out by the weight of the child's body as he or she crawls about on hands and knees.[22]
- At various points other changes may or may not appear, such as swollen bellies, delayed teething, or bow legs.[23]

These problems, as I have said, afflicted both male and female infants. But only women deliver children. To give birth easily, one's pelvic bones must be large enough to accommodate the child's head. Rickets twists the pelvis, and women who have had the disease as infants may experience difficulty in labor.

So fearful were women of the consequences of these growth deformities that, as Percivall Willughby reported: "The wild Irish women do break the pubic bones of the female infant, so soon as it is born. And I have heard some wandering Irish women affirm the same to be true, and that they have ways to keep these bones from uniting. It is for certain that they be easily, and soon, delivered. And I have observed that many wanderers of that nation have had a waddling and lamish gesture in their going."[24] If, in fact, Irish mothers did try to shatter the pubic bones of their girl children, so as to let them give birth easily later, it shows what a matter of anxiety were these questions of the body's architecture for the women's culture.

Rickets is caused by the failure of the bones to get enough calcium and phosphorus. Here's how it works: Calcium fits between the individual bone cells after it combines with phosphorus, and makes them hard. If calcium fails to be absorbed into the matrix of the bones, they will bend and bow when weight is put upon them. The problem in rickets is not that children don't get enough calcium in their diets, for sufficient amounts almost always come in with the milk. It is rather that children can't absorb the calcium they take in. What permits the absorption of calcium and phosphorus in the intestine is vitamin D. And infants with rickets usually are not getting enough vitamin D. One does not have to obtain it from dietary sources, for only egg yolk and fatty fish have much anyway. Most vitamin D is synthesized in the skin by exposure to sunlight; thus, rickets is a "sun deficiency," rather than a "nutritional deficiency," disease. If, however, a child has too little sunlight, cod liver oil will still prevent rickets.

Readers will thus understand that rickets is not a problem in sunny climes* (unless children are kept indoors along with women in purdah in India) or when children play outside in the winter. But when parents believe—as did so many traditional Europeans—that exposure to "drafts" causes colds, and that it is dangerous to take infants outside in the cold air, the door is opened wide to rickets. "In every case of rickets which has come under our observation," wrote London's James R. Smyth in 1843, the child had been "excluded in a greater or less degree from the due influence of the sun."[27]† Many parents in Lodève left the infant "in its room, rarely clean and swaddled in humid rags. . . . Children

---

* According to an executive of the California State Board of Health in 1920, "Rickets is so negligible in California that the Board has never attempted to amass statistics of any sort on the disease"[25]; and August Hirsch noted how rarely it was seen in Africa and Asia.[26]

† Smyth also mentioned other "causes," such as damp habitation.

rarely leave the house and do not get any sun during the winter. . . .
Soon the fruits of this conduct appear. The child does not walk like
the others. Its limbs are deformed. The parents blame ghosts, a fall, too
much fat in the milk."[28]

Of the child-rearing practices that kept children from the sun, most
hurtful was "swaddling," in which the infant is wrapped mummylike
in a long linen bandage and kept in it for the first half-year of life. In
the little town of Montereau, for example, parents swaddled. We are
thus not surprised to learn in Dr. Olivet's 1819 "Medical Topography"
that rickets was "almost universal." It would appear about the fifth month.
At twelve months the children showed no interest in walking and, even
at two years, had trouble doing so. Their dentition was slow and irregular.
Even at the age of fifteen years, many of the girls had deformed spines
and backbones.[29] Dr. Olivet does not tell us about their pelvic bones,
but there is little chance that they remained unaffected.

What I have just described is the traditional pattern of rickets. It is
associated more with a certain set of childbearing practices than with
any given environment. And it is as old as time. One student of the
Middle Paleolithic era found that "every Neanderthal child skull studied
so far shows signs compatible with severe rickets."[30]* Viking skeletons
from the fifteenth century in Greenland showed many rickety changes,
such as twisted spines and narrow pelvises, in a population of women
whose average height was only four feet nine inches. One female pelvis
was so narrow that the woman was "incapable of giving birth." A second
had a twisted spine and a very flat pelvis and presumably would have
been unable to deliver spontaneously.[32] Rickets is "the scrofula of the
cold countries," wrote one French doctor in the eighteenth century. This
says a lot, considering how common nonrespiratory tuberculosis, or "scrofula," was among children.[33]

This traditional pattern was to be found in countryside and city alike,
wherever sunlight was inadequate for children in the first two years of
life.† Many references to rickets may be found in the old "medical topographies." It was amazingly widespread in some areas, unknown in
others. Rickets abounded, for example, in Bayonne, Hof, Lubljana, London, Lyon, Memel, Regensburg, and Stettin.[36] Thus, Dr. W. Fordyce,
writing in 1773: "I speak within the bounds of truth when I assert that
there must be near 20,000 children in London and Westminster and the
suburbs ill at this moment of the hectic fever, attended with tun-bellies,

---

* But according to H. Grimm, other disorders could have been responsible for the bone
lesions.[31]

† Paleopathologists have a special inclination to believe that rickets is primarily an urban,
industrial disease.[34] See however, the numerous references to rickets in the writings of
small-town and rural doctors.[35]

swelled wrists and ankles, or crooked limbs."[37] Although one cannot make a quantitative estimate, rickets was clearly omnipresent in traditional Europe.

Then in the nineteenth century, as old-style child-rearing practices changed, rickets ceased to be associated with fear of cold and swaddling.* It started to become a disease of the industrial environment, a result not of keeping children inside for health reasons but of keeping them in factories, schools, and cities where the rays of the sun were blotted out by soot and smoke (for rickets can also affect children later in life). In mid-nineteenth century Vienna rickets was so common in factory children that one writer thought it should be called not the "English disease" but the "Viennese disease."[41] Its geography in late nineteenth century Britain mapped the course of the Industrial Revolution, "accumulating in large towns and thickly peopled districts, especially where industrial pursuits are carried on." There was little in rural areas. A survey of English doctors in the 1880s found it mainly in the "great industrial districts of Lancashire, Yorkshire, Cheshire, Derbyshire and Nottingham," in the Black Country, the mining and industrial regions of South Wales, and in London.[42]† A 1932 report on Bradford, center of the worsted trade, said, "Adult women are apt to be small and stunted. . . . At one time rickets was extremely prevalent; it has decreased steadily during the past 20 years and there are now few marked cases of rickets." But of course those women who twenty years ago had had infantile rickets were now giving birth. "There is an impression at the Ante-Natal Clinics that small and flat pelves are relatively common."[43] This observation held true for many other places.

By the first quarter of the twentieth century, when systematic medical surveys were being done, rickets was astonishingly prevalent. Among eight hundred children treated at Boston's Infants' Hospital in 1898, 80 percent "showed more or less marked evidence of rickets."[44] Of sixteen hundred Manchester children under two seen in 1933, over one quarter demonstrated clinical signs of rickets.[45] In Dortmund in 1921, 43 percent of children ages two to ten had rickets in some form, active or healed; in Berlin, 60 percent.[46] Among children of Polish Jews in East London, "about 80 percent" had rickets.[47]

---

* Several medical topographies for cities comment on a decline of rickets early in the nineteenth century, before the atmospheric pollution of the industrial revolution began. Johann Jakob Rambach associated it directly with new child-rearing styles ("cleanliness" in particular).[38] Dr. Wunderlich in Sulz also thought its decline was due to more bathing of children. Bathing in and of itself would not have influenced the frequency of the disease; yet it is a sign of new child-rearing methods.[39] Dr. Franz Álois Stelzig thought that the decline of rickets in Prague might have been owing to smallpox vaccination.[40]

† Tyne, Tees, and the coast of Durham were also mentioned. Note that only severe rickets was being reported.

I trust the reader will see why I have dwelt so long upon this childhood disease: it deformed women and made them vulnerable to some of the dangers of childbirth I shall shortly describe.[48] Of one hundred tall women booked for delivery at the Aberdeen Maternity Hospital in Scotland in the late 1940s, only seven had "flat" pelvises, the anatomical hallmark of rickets. Of one hundred short women, thirty-four had flat pelvises. Many of those smaller women had probably been attacked by rickets.[49] (As children they may simultaneously have been deficient in vitamin C, with the result that growth of their long bones was stunted.)

How often did girls recover from their rickets by the time they passed into womanhood? William Smellie, who was among the first to associate infantile rickets with pelvic anomalies in adults, felt that just about all victims would suffer later. "Most of those who have been rickety in their infancy, whether they continue little and deformed, or, recovering of that disease, grow up to be tall stately women, are commonly narrow and distorted in the pelvis: and consequently subject to tedious and difficult labours."[50]* Is this judgment too extreme? The view today is that if the rickets has not healed by a child's second year, there are likely to be later troubles.† But severe, prolonged rickets is rarely seen today. In eighteenth-century France, where it was common, children often didn't heal "until the fifth or sixth year. Those who have not yet recovered at that age ordinarily remain incapacitated and deformed for the rest of their lives. . . . Girls who are rickety until eight or nine will ordinarily have a very narrow pelvis."[53]

Women whose rickets had been mild would—if they later had any pelvic contraction at all—probably end up with a "flat" or a "rachitic-flat" pelvis, in which the back wall grows too close to the front (anatomically, in these cases the sacrum slips down and forward, so that the sacral "promontory" is too close to the pubic bone). A flat pelvis meant that the child's head might have some difficulty "engaging," or slipping into the pelvis; but once it was inside, the rest of the birth would progress smoothly.

Women with more severe rickets might end up with a "generally contracted" or a "generally contracted-flat" pelvis in which the entire pelvis— not just the front-to-back diameter—was too small. In these cases the bottom of the pelvis might resemble a funnel, because the side walls had grown too closely together (anatomically, the pubic arch becomes

* Other authors had previously mentioned a connection between rickets, contracted pelvises, and difficult deliveries;[51] but Smellie's work became far better known.

† Harold E. Harrison says, "If the diagnosis is not made until the second year of life or later, significant deformities may have developed and healing is so slow that these deformities may progress."[52]

narrower and the distance between the "ischial tuberosities" lessens). In the generally contracted pelvis, not only might the infant's head have trouble slipping into the top of the pelvis (the "pelvic inlet"), but the rest of its passage through the pelvis would be laborious as well.[54]

In statistics from twelve German maternity clinics at the end of the nineteenth century, the distribution for these various kinds of pelvic contraction was:

---

25 percent generally contracted
15 percent generally contracted-flat
33 percent simple flat
25 percent rachitic flat*

---

100 percent[56]

---

* A distinction between "flat" and "rachitic-flat" is probably meaningless, for rickets was likely the cause of most of the former as well as of the latter. "Among the large number of flat pelves at the Northwestern University Medical School," wrote Joseph DeLee, "not one could be found that did not at the same time show positive evidences of rachitis." Similarly, most "generally contracted" pelvises were probably rachitic in origin, the other causes of pelvic deformity—such as accidents, hip dislocations, and other bone diseases—being relatively seldom. Today, for example, when rickets has virtually been abolished, only about 5 percent of all women have pelvic contractions severe enough to interfere with the course of labor.[55]

Keep in mind, of course, that many areas had no rickets at all, and there the women would have normal pelvises. Thus in Chambéry in the 1780s, women had "pelvises which are large and well shaped"; this was an area where swaddling was dying out.[57] In Eschwege, where swaddling lasted only three months, "women are well formed; abnormal pelvises rarely occur, and never in a degree which would make Caesarean section necessary upon a live mother."[58] Around 1930 in Iowa contracted pelvises were rare.[59] And so forth. I do not wish to create the impression that all women everywhere were subject in huge proportion to these deformities.

Yet many women were. Of 8,000 deliveries in Florence between 1883 and 1895, 18 percent were complicated by pelvic deformity.[60] Of 275 mothers in the Giessen Clinic, 20 percent had pelvic contractions.[61] Of 6,400 white women who gave birth at the Johns Hopkins Hospital from 1896 to 1924, 14 percent had contracted pelvises of some degree (of black women, 43 percent).[62]* Franz von Winckel concluded in 1905, on the basis of a number of reports, that in perhaps 14 to 20 percent of all births there was some pelvic contraction, severe in 3 to 5 percent.[63]

It seems to me likely that before the 1920s, when vitamin D was finally isolated and the mechanism of rickets understood,† one lower-class, urban woman in four was likely to have had pelvic bones sufficiently misshapen to cause a delay in labor. (This subject is more fully developed in chapter 5.) Whether it would have been a significant delay, whether she would therefore have to undergo a dangerous obstetrical operation, whether she would become infected or run any of a dozen other risks, are questions for later chapters. I want here simply to emphasize that behind these arid statistics on "pelvic anomalies" lies a world of suffering that we have largely forgotten about. "On 23 March 1660," wrote Willughby, "I was called to a young woman who had been three days in labor, and the midwives knew not how to deliver her." He reached in his hand to bring the child out, "but through the ill position of the bones and the greatness of the child, squeezed in a lump together, I could not move it or get my hand to the upper part of the head."

"She was of a low stature, and the birth-place was narrow and in those places, ill framed." In fact, Willughby finally succeeded, and the woman survived. But he noted: "This woman, in her infancy, was afflicted with the rickets."[65]

Corsets: A Bit of Debunking

Although the corset has been paid endless attention in the "history of fashion," two essential points have been missed: (1) outside of the aristocracy and urban middle classes, very few women ever wore corsets; (2) whether they wore them does not much matter from the viewpoint of their health because the corset was essentially innocuous.

The general reader may not realize what devastating consequences the corset was once thought to have had for women's bodies. According to one historian of the nineteenth century, "in no other age throughout history was . . . the female body so concealed and disfigured by clothing"—a reference mainly to the corset.[66] Samuel Thomas Soemmerring, foremost in a long line of physicians who have thundered against the device, thought corsets responsible for spinal deformities, tuberculosis, all kinds of internal bleeding, fainting, diarrhea, anal prolapse, and so

---

* This percentage is a minimum, because the hospital began routinely measuring the pelvic outlet only after two thousand admissions.
† Cod-liver oil was first used therapeutically against rickets in 1824.[64]

on.[67] A Danish doctor wrote in 1931, "We no longer see corset liver as often as before on the autopsy table, and then only among older women."[68] So if the conventional wisdom is in agreement about any aspect of the architecture of the body, it is that corsets crippled and deformed countless generations of women. In this section I aim to debunk that view.

The "lacing in" of women's garments began around the eleventh or the twelfth century, with the discovery of body "form" among aristocratic women. By the fourteenth century, according to Paul Diepgen, a kind of corset had become obligatory in upper-class dress.[69] At some point— the exact chronology being still indistinct—tight lacing began to trickle down to "middle-class" women in small towns. The general triumph of the corset was then briefly interrupted by the "classical" modes at the end of the eighteenth century, the desire to dress freely and flowingly as it was imagined the ancient Greeks had once done. But in the 1820s and 1830s the corset again became fashionable, and would endure until the first decade of the twentieth century, when new notions about bodily freedom suddenly swept it away forever.

Thus, there is no doubt that corsets were routinely worn by girls and women in the better classes of Europe's big cities. Lawrence Stone gives fulsome details from the lives of the well-to-do in eighteenth-century England.[70] Doctors in places like Cologne, Memel, and Berlin all indicated the corset as a source of every evil imaginable from constipation to cancer.[71] A young lady's toilette in early nineteenth-century Vienna would consist of "rising at 9:00 A.M., her body already flabby and enervated by an excessive stay in the soft featherbed. . . . Scarcely is the girl up than she proceeds to squeeze her chest and abdomen, which during the night had been freed from their servile bonds, anew into the pincers of a tyrannical corset."[72] All this is well known, having been the meat and drink of a certain kind of social history for many years.

It is less well known, but also true, that corsets were much beloved of small-town notables in nineteenth-century Europe and America. John S. and Robin M. Haller have documented how widespread was "corsetitis" among the kind of American lady who could afford a maid.[73] Of women in the little town of Schwandorf, it was said in 1799 that "if they were on horseback, their armored corsets and their many thick skirts would make them sooner resemble heavily armed cavalrymen than members of the female sex."[74] Bourgeois women in little "burghs" like Weiden and Gmünd in Germany, and Mantes in France, also decked themselves out in corsets.[75]*

But there the corset stops. As nearly as I can tell from the sources, it was not worn by women of the common people except on holidays, and

* The whalebone corset appeared, for example, in Mantes around 1830.[76]

rarely then. Soemmerring himself said that "among the lower orders of the villages and small towns, and especially where heavy work and terrible loads keep one from getting too fat . . . how many lovely female forms does one see, and never a corset!"[77] (He thought that corsets deformed the skeleton, rather than holding it straight, as they were intended to do.) A historian of eighteenth-century Vaud Canton has found no evidence that "the women of the people" there wore corsets.[78] Jean-Marie Munaret noted in 1862 that French peasants "do not wear them at all."[79] And both of the female doctoral students who studied peasants in German villages just before the First World War said it was custom that women wore them either not at all or only on holidays.[80]* Thus, whatever devastating effects corsets may have had upon the upper 5 percent of the population, they played no role in the health of the bottom 95 percent.

But it is now unclear whether corsets were harmful even to that upper crust of well-to-do women. The doctors of the time thought corsets responsible for all kinds of symptoms. But just because the women had particular symptoms does not mean the corset was responsible. As you will see in chapter 9, doctors shoved the blame for anemia onto the corset, yet a majority of anemic women almost certainly never wore them. Much of the famous "physical" evidence indicting corsets—such as supposedly "crushed rib cases," internal organs folded in half, and mangled intestines—turns out to be fanciful or improbable in light of our current knowledge of anatomy. After doing an autopsy on a woman and finding "spleen and kidneys intensely congested and enlarged, brain membranes intensely congested . . . an apoplectic spot on the surface of the right hemisphere with some effusion of lymph," Dr. W. H. Sheehy in 1871 attributed her death to "tight-lacing."[82] The death sounds much like meningitis, and Dr. Sheehy obviously did not know what he was talking about. Other doctors dwelt upon supposed deformities of the rib cage found at autopsy, and were evidently unaware of the wide variation possible in the bones of the thorax. In fact, the only injury that can reliably be attributed to tight lacing is "hiatus hernia," in which a portion of the stomach slides up into the lower chest. The other symptoms were probably all either coincidence or the work of overactive medical imaginations.†

---

* Maria Bidlingmaier said of one village, "The peasant wife shuns the corset, and the young women wear it mainly on Sundays."[81]

† Gerhart S. Schwarz wrote of Soemmerring (see page 28), "That his conclusions were emotionally conditioned or flavored becomes apparent through his failure to ascribe to the corset the only disease which has withstood the test of time, hiatus hernia. Soemmerring discovered this condition, yet when it came to his own discovery he disregarded the corset as etiology."[83] There was also an exchange in the *New England Journal of Medicine* on "Soemmerring's Syndrome," about which Dr. Schwarz had the last word, pooh-poohing the entire notion.[84]

Thus, the architecture of the body turns out to have something of a history—not quite the same one as previous historians have thought, who overlooked rickets and concentrated instead upon the relatively unimportant corset. But a history nonetheless unfolds, in which women become taller, heavier, and better proportioned. Those questions are, however, among the least interesting of those that occupy us in this book. What *happened* to women as they gave birth or faced disease is far more intriguing, and it is to this aspect of the story that I now turn.

PART TWO

A HISTORY OF
THE BIRTH
EXPERIENCE

CHAPTER 3

Traditional Births: Women Take Charge

BEFORE 1900 the overwhelming majority of mothers in Europe and North America were assisted in birth by other women—usually midwives, but sometimes neighbors or village "grannies." Just as three quarters of all births in the developing world today are attended by midwives,[1] so in the traditional epoch of Western society doctors were absent from the normal birthing scene, except in upper middle class Anglo-Saxon homes. The competence of those early midwives is therefore crucial in chronicling the experience of the average woman.

There are two sharply opposing viewpoints. *Engagé* scholars in the women's movement see the midwives of the past as a great boon to womankind. One such scholar writes, "It seems that throughout most of history medical men had no advantages to offer parturient women over the services of a midwife."[2] According to one student of colonial New England, "As much as possible midwives managed deliveries by letting nature do the work" (although she concedes that they "examined the cervix . . . from time to time").[3]

The male author of the first midwives' manual, Eucharius Rösslin, presented in 1513, however, a more uncomplimentary assessment:

I'm talking about the midwives all
Whose heads are empty as a hall,

And through their dreadful negligence
Cause babies' deaths devoid of sense.
So thus we see far and about
Official murder, there's no doubt.[4]

Rösslin's contemptuous dismissal could be matched by dozens and dozens of other unfavorable opinions about the midwives, coming from all over Europe and Britain until virtually the beginning of the twentieth century.[5] I shall forbear quoting them because the whole question of the midwives' competence in normal deliveries (as opposed to obstetric emergencies) has been misleadingly posed.

Rather than asking, in absolute terms, how good the midwives were, we should ask how closely they conformed to the standard of the best medical knowledge available at the time. The question whether they were better or worse than the typical male doctor resolves little, because with the exception of several celebrated individuals, doctors then did not do deliveries. But if it turns out that the midwives fell far short of the knowledge they might be expected to have had, we—with our four hundred year hindsight—may find them wanting.

"Urban" versus "Traditional" Midwives

Before perhaps 1800 midwives must be sharply divided into two groups: the "urban" midwives, highly qualified and supervised by a corps of their peers; and the "traditional" midwives, practicing in small towns and villages without training or supervision. These traditional birth attendants scarcely deserve the name "midwife" at all, for rarely did they practice full-time; they had little sense of professional élan, found themselves at a complete loss in dealing with any emergency, and were usually elderly, impoverished women without other means of support. Because their entire knowledge was acquired by trial and error, or by "osmosis" from the collective lore of the local women's culture, the label "traditional" is apt. They did things the way things had always been done, and without necessarily understanding why. For none of these reasons, however, would they necessarily have poorly managed normal deliveries.

In contrast, the urban midwives tapped a body of formal learning that had been passed on from antiquity, though scarcely augmented since then. Even if they generally did not read midwifery textbooks or attend academic lectures, they were nonetheless subject to the close discipline of other women within a professional setting;[6] they could call upon such expertise as these other women possessed during emergencies; and they generally had the social status of minor city officials—a completely different situation, in other words, from that of the traditional midwives in smaller communities.

It was in Germany that these urban midwives enjoyed fullest autonomy. Typically the midwife corps would be headed by a "mother superior" (*Obfrau*), over whom neither the local doctor nor the town council had any legal power. Under her control would be a handful of female "midwife inspectors" who were available if the salaried town midwives ran into emergencies. The mother superior served on an honorary basis, but the other midwives were paid partially—or fully—by the city. And their number was limited. Each regular midwife had the right to take on a trainee, who sometimes would wait ten or twenty years before a regular position opened. Upon retirement these midwives would be pensioned off.[7]

Although exact arrangements varied from city to city, the whole affair was run by women themselves. Thus in Nürnberg in 1652 midwifery personnel consisted of: seven "honorable ladies," who were "mostly widows from the town élite," and whose job it was to organize alms and to give emergency advice; eight "supervisory midwives" whose specific task, the record says, was to give enemas but who obviously helped in difficult deliveries; and twenty regular midwives. All these women were sworn in annually in a little city hall ceremony that involved signing the town register, after which they were feted with "wine, bread and cookies."[8]

In Nürnberg the midwives governed themselves until 1755, when they became administratively subordinated to the *collegio medico.*[9] The Frankfurt midwife ordinance of 1573 stipulated that the midwifery exam was to be conducted by the "supervising matrons."[10] A 1653 ordinance in Leipzig said that the mayor's wife was to appoint and examine the midwives.[11] In Munich the midwives were supervised by other women until at least 1716 (fifty years later, the "court barber-surgeon" was appointed supervisor).[12] So even though it was occasionally stipulated that in case of trouble the midwife had to call in a doctor—as in Heilbronn at the end of the fifteenth century—the women were normally on their own.[13]

These independent corps of German midwives reach far back into the Middle Ages. In 1298 we encounter in Coblence a reference to "Frau Aleyt," midwife in the Nonnengasse, who was a "full citizen" (*Burger*); this was a dignified appellation.[14] In 1355 a new settlement outside the walls of Frankfurt petitioned the city council to "leave open the gates of the old city, where the midwives live," at night so that if a woman went into labor, someone could reach her.[15] In 1427, records in the Swiss town of Baden refer for the first time to an official midwife; two years later the town bought a special chair for giving birth.[16]

Elsewhere midwife autonomy existed, too, though it was less sweeping. In Bruges, for example, a municipal ordinance said in 1551 that in emergencies the midwives should consult with doctors or with other women; it set, moreover, a standard of competency so high that the city had trouble getting midwives.[17] The midwives of Breton towns had in the eighteenth century an elaborate hierarchy of qualifications; and although male surgeons examined a potential midwife for admittance to the trade, an apprenticeship with another woman was nonetheless the entry card.[18] And so on. I wish not to write an institutional history of midwives, but merely to point out that, in many European cities, female birth attendants had high professional standards imposed by *other women*.

One might argue that these urban midwives were even more competent than the best doctors of the epoch. Keep in mind that almost until the beginning of the eighteenth century obstetrics slumbered in the thousand-year doze that had commenced with the end of classical civilization. Aside from a few useful emergency techniques, which I shall discuss in following chapters, nothing of use in normal delivery had been added to scientific knowledge since ancient Rome. For the average doctor, obstetrics was a defiling activity, and textbook knowledge was still contaminated with useless mumbo-jumbo about "the chambers of the uterus" and "how the fetus aids in its own delivery." These urban midwives, by contrast, could rely on the practical experience of centuries, transmitted not by vague "old wives' tales" but by a professional guild. Although I do not want here to enlarge overly about problems in delivery, we might remember that—long before the subject was mentioned in medical books—these urban midwives had procedures for handling an umbilical cord that was born before the baby.[19] And they demonstrably used ergot to energize a torpid uterus before the medical profession discovered the drug (see chapter 8).

Moreover, they refused to communicate their knowledge to the doctors. A Heilbronn ordinance at the end of the fifteenth century rapped midwives on the knuckles, saying, "If you should be called before the local Herr Physicians Doctors to be asked and examined about your trade, you should not resist but be respectful, and give the correct information on the basis of your experience."[20] Late in the eighteenth century, Dr. Friedrich Osiander found himself stranded in a village and wanted an enema syringe to apply to some sick infant. After a reluctant midwife had finally dredged a syringe up, he turned to her and asked about her obstetrical work: "But she let show that her trade consisted of secrets which she was not disposed to reveal."[21] Dr. Goldschmidt encountered a similar silence years later: "The local grannies . . . consider it advisable to give the doctor no insight into their techniques for delivery. And they normally have such influence that the mothers, too, preserve a deep silence about the midwives' means of accelerating labor and managing the lying-in period."[22] By this time the doctors no longer really needed to know the midwives' techniques because medicine had advanced far beyond the "state of the art" that prevailed in the sixteenth or the seventeenth century, when the midwives had ruled the roost. The point is that these midwives felt that they had special knowledge which would be of great good to their patients, and which, moreover, should remain a secret women kept to themselves.

Unlike the urban midwives, before 1800 the traditional midwives in the countryside did fall below the standard of implementing the "best knowledge available." I shall in the following chapter show exactly in what ways, but here I want to describe the women. They corresponded more closely to the caricature of the murderous crones that has come down to us in medical literature. A Silesian doctor, writing in 1802, sets the stage: "It's country fair time, and a number of old women are hanging around the merchants' stands, filling their baskets with laxative pills, uterus drops, easy-labor drops, tranquilizers and so forth. Who are they? Midwives, doing doctor duty." Let us say, the writer continued, that these midwives are called to a mother in labor: "They carry on their backs a heavy birthing stool, which also doubles as a potty chair. . . . If the cervix is even slightly dilated, the mother has to climb onto the chair immediately." Her vagina is then smeared with "stinking oils, labor creams, marjoram, saffron and brandy one after the other."[23] This scene conveys a major theme in our analysis of the traditional midwives: that a "normal" labor without complications in traditional Europe was accompanied by the most active interventions imaginable on the midwife's part.

Unlike the sophisticated urban midwives, these rural women were ignorant of anatomy. Horror stories abound of them mistaking one part for another. Percivall Willughby relates that Goodwife Ann Frith of Derby, having in 1646 "a hard and long labor, was much haled and pulled by her midwife, who hoped, through much tugging, quickly to deliver her. So that the lips of the vulva were greatly swelled, and turned outward, and became discoloured, with sundry colours.

"The midwife, supposing these swellings to be part of the afterbirth, thrust her fingers into them; forthwith the blood spurted on the midwife's face, and ran down her gorget." Thereupon Willughby was sent for.[24]

Willughby relates another tale of a midwife who, called to a supposed labor, "thrust her hand into [the mother's body], took hold of she knew not what, and endeavoured violently to pull it away." She was unsuccessful, so Willughby was sent for and found, "instead of a child, a swelled, cancerous tumour in the womb, that tortured this woman with terrible shootings and stinging pains." She died several months later.[25] There are, to be fair, some tales of doctors too who confused uterine cancer or ovarian tumors with pregnancy, but there are many more for the traditional midwives, who had no basic knowledge of anatomy and pathology.

The great flaw in the rural and small-town midwives was their lack of training. A 1739 report on the Ansbach area found only thirty of two hundred to be "trained and certified." Of course, the report continued, there were reasons for this situation: the pay was so bad that no competent woman should take on the work, and often the godparents of the infant failed to tip.[26] But for whatever reason, in formal terms, these traditional midwives were "untrained."

What they knew instead was a "blind routine" handed down from generation to generation, to use Dr. Berthelot's phrase.[27] A recent French scholar speaks of a "climate of ritual and of resistance to new ideas" prevailing among the midwives.[28] Dr. Anne Amable Augier du Fot, who practiced medicine around Soissons, wrote in 1775 that the rural midwives were "guided by a murderous routine, denuded of any understanding, and ridden with prejudices as hurtful as they are numerous. Their lackings are grave, even fatal, for almost all of them begin to practice the art of midwifery without knowing anything, without having learned anything."[29] "Midwives who have got their knowledge from their mothers and grandmothers," wrote J. B. Gebel, "seldom let themselves be recruited in our midwife school. They are convinced that their wisdom requires no further accretions." They do things "mechanically," he said, "as their great-great grandmothers two hundred years ago did them."[30]

So when we talk about the midwives' "ignorance," we must keep in mind that it was only from the viewpoint of the practitioners of scientific medicine that midwives were unlearned. They themselves believed that their inherited lore was completely valid, and that in situations where it failed to suffice, probably God's will had carried the mother away.

Regulating the Midwives

Aware of these shortcomings in the traditional midwives, the various governments of Europe began, from the thirteenth century onward, to put those who were not already professionally organized under some kind of supervision. And while I do not intend to chronicle this legislation, I should like to give the reader an overview because of the heavy impact of these new laws on women through the ages.

The pattern of events falls roughly into three stages:

- Initial church and municipal laws regulating the moral and religious side of midwifery were laid down in the fifteenth and the sixteenth centuries.
- Legislation making the doctors the examiners and supervisors of the midwives started generally to appear in the seventeenth century.
- Training schools for midwives began to be established in the eighteenth century.

Let's first consider this "moral" side of midwifery. The Church's main concern was that the midwives administer emergency baptism according to the correct formulas, if they thought the infant was not going to survive the passage into the outside world. Accordingly, the Trier Synod of 1277 stipulated that priests were to instruct lay women in the words of emergency baptism; and another church synod stated in 1310 that midwives should perform such baptisms.[31] The first formal midwife oath to have survived dates from Regensburg in 1452. It made the midwives promise, among other things, to deliver all women "whether rich or poor" except for Jews; to bring any woman they may find doing deliveries unlawfully in front of the female board of supervisors; not to drink too much; and not to leave one woman in labor in order to deliver another who can pay more.[32] The City of Aachen had a similar oath, the 1527 version of which specified in addition that the midwife was to report all "secret births" to the authorities as an anti-infanticide measure.[33] A 1544 church ordinance for Hildensen instructed the midwives to "pray repeatedly" if the infant's arrival were delayed.[34] Clearly, this early supervision did little to improve the quality of the actual care the midwife supplied the mother.

Medical supervision began generally in the seventeenth century. As doctors slowly came to understand more than the midwives about the anatomy of the pelvis and the mechanism of labor, they began to examine midwife candidates and to supervise those in practice. The first ordinance of this nature of which I am aware is Zurich's in 1554, assigning doctors to teach midwives. In 1554, it will be recalled, Jakob Rüff of Zurich published his midwifery textbook, the first practical manual since classical antiquity (Eucharius Rösslin's earlier text of 1513 was notably vague in its instructions).[35] Much later other communities started to instruct their doctors to train and supervise midwives: Amsterdam in 1668, Darmstadt in 1669, parts of Bavaria in 1699, and so forth.[36] By the beginning of the eighteenth century, humane and pronatalist considerations had largely replaced the earlier moral and religious reasons for controlling the midwives. Schwäbisch-Hall's 1706 ordinance, which appointed physicians as supervisors of midwifery, said, "Every Christian authority should attempt to see that women are cared for as well as possible before, during, and after giving birth. Therefore intelligent, conscientious, and experienced persons are to be appointed [to the office of midwife]."[37]

Elsewhere in Europe and Britain similar efforts were underway. Paris's first midwife ordinance dates from 1560.[38] A 1617 church synod required midwives in the Angers area to swear an oath.[39] And France received its first nationwide regulations on midwifery in 1726 and 1730, though the decrees remained in many places a dead letter.[40] Not until the French Revolution did France receive a systematic nationwide program for training and appointing midwives.

In England such controls as existed were even less effective. Local bishops acquired the power to examine midwives, among other medical personnel, in 1512. And by 1567 it is clear that church authorities were regularly administering oaths to candidates, as one Eleanor Pead in the diocese of Canterbury swore not to use "any kind of sorcerie or incantation in the time of travail of any woman," and to baptize only with plain water. But in the judgment of Jean Donnison, the foremost student of the history of English midwifery, many women remained unlicensed. The whole business was gradually forgotten during the eighteenth century, and there was no national regulation of any kind in England until 1902.[41] The Obstetrical Society of London began giving a diploma to midwives in 1872; but before that time, aside from a couple of unimportant training programs in London maternity hospitals, there was virtually no medical instruction of midwives.[42]

For completeness, let me conclude this rather dull chronicle by mentioning that in the American colonies only New York City showed much interest in regularizing midwife practice. In 1716 its common council obliged aspirants to swear they would "help any woman in labor, whether poor or rich," that they would not "suffer any woman's child to be murdered or hurt," and that they would "not administer any medicine to produce miscarriage."[43] (These anti-abortion provisions were fairly standard in midwife oaths everywhere.) Elsewhere in the New World laissez-faire obstetrics prevailed.

Small-town and country midwives began to lose the appellation "traditional" once formal training programs were established for them. Contrary to a popularly accepted myth, the "male medical doctors" did not attempt to keep scientific knowledge out of the midwives' hands. In fact, the doctors desperately tried to persuade them to acquire it. The first step was encouraging midwives to bone up on anatomy by requiring them to attend autopsies occasionally. For example, Duke Julius of Braunschweig-Wolfenbüttel instructed, in 1573, his court doctors to do post-mortems on all dead new mothers in the presence of the local midwives, so that "in the future other women who are afflicted with similar dangerous and painful burdens, illnesses and problems may be helped."[44] The midwife ordinances of Frankfurt, Paris, and numerous other communities also insisted that midwives learn from autopsy findings.[45] But the mid-wives apparently were put off by the Latin and Greek anatomical terms, since they knew only the vernacular words, and pulled back from this kind of exercise.[46] (I myself found the nomenclature a bit alienating when I began "gross anatomy," and can imagine what these early midwives must have thought about the *testes muliebris* upon looking into the abdomen.)

Obviously the only way midwives could realistically be medically quali-fied was to send them to school for a few weeks or months, preferably to a school situated in a maternity hospital. The first such school seems to have been established in 1589 in Munich; the second in Paris with the reconstruction of the maternity ward of the Hôtel Dieu in 1618.* Then for a long time no further programs were set up. A new wave of foundations, starting with the establishment of a midwifery school in 1737 in Strasbourg, occurred in the eighteenth century.[49] Würzburg orga-nized a school in 1739, Berlin in 1751, Neuötting in 1767, Basel in 1771, Coblence in 1772, to name just a few.[50]

The French began a little later; but a 1759 government edict, combined with a famous grand tour of France and the Low Countries on the part of a highly skilled midwife, Madame du Coudray, gave impetus to the founding of a number of courses for midwives.[51] Of actual schools, with buildings and beds, there was as yet little sight outside of Paris.

Thus, by 1800, Central Europe started to be supplied with medically trained midwives; in France only some of the cities were. In the Anglo-Saxon world there were virtually none trained formally; there were only the traditional sort.

The Midwives toward 1800: A Balance Sheet

Let me attempt to draw some kind of balance sheet on these women, who were practicing for the most part in small towns and villages through-out Europe.

First, a profile. What kind of women were they? Here are some of those active around 1760 in the Baden districts of Rötteln and Sausenberg:

· Verena Küsterin, age seventy-four, in office twenty-four years; "is praised by all and is very skillful and experienced"; she had delivered 558 infants.

---

* Heinrich Fasbender says Munich's was first; [47] but the training of midwives was doubtless conducted in the Hôtel Dieu before the seventeenth century. Marcel Fosseyeux mentions the reconstruction of the maternity ward in 1618 and prints a list of the hospital's chief midwives in the seventeenth and eighteenth centuries.[48]

- Other midwives in nearby villages were similarly praised by the author of the report, Doctor G. V. Jägerschmidt.
- One, age sixty-five and in office for eighteen years, was reported as having "a good reputation but is weak because of her age."
- The most negative report Dr. Jägerschmidt made was on one "gossipy in her official capacity, but good."[52]

Typically midwives were, in fact, elderly women. A study of the Nieder-lausitz in the 1790s found only 3 percent younger than 40.[53]

Despite the doctors' horror stories, it would be a mistake to consider these village midwives as dangerous know-nothings. As we shall see, most births progressed normally. The only special qualities needed to bring them to a happy conclusion were *judgment* about what constitutes an abnormality, and *patience*, which means the willingness to withstand both the entreaties of the mother and the relatives to end the birth swiftly, as well as the urgency of one's own commitments. And when someone like Dr. Jägerschmidt speaks of the local midwives as "good," this is probably what is meant.

In addition to their elderliness and experience, rural midwives were marked by their great poverty. Except in certain areas, to be discussed in a moment, most midwives seem to have been driven by want into the job. Alois Valenta in Ljubljana, who had taught over sixty midwifery courses through the years, knew from experience that only "the poorest peasant women" ever applied.[54] The staff of the midwifery school in Calau believed that peasants generally regarded midwifery as dishonorable, and suited only for women who "possessed no further feeling for honor and shame," and who had chosen this job "only to confess to the world their desperation at not making a livelihood in a more honorable way."[55]

Why were no women save the aged and the desperate to be had? The midwives' work was so hard that few wanted to do it. In the village of Oppin, for example, the local midwife had "in addition to delivering the mother, to stay up all night with her until the infant was baptized, to wash out the diapers and swaddling clothes, to invite the guests to the baptismal feast, and to change the infant daily until the mother's churching, at least three weeks. For all this the midwife gets eight groschen. That's eight groschen!" No wonder, concluded the author, so few women are willing to become midwives.[56]

In a minority of communities, however, the midwife apparently was something of a notable personage, a "social authority" (*Vertrauensperson*), as one observer put it. And that seems to be because, in those communities, she was elected by the local women. Look at the following contrast. In the Kiel area a "majority of candidates in the midwives' school were women whom want had driven into the occupation, women who had a sick husband or an ailing father to support; out of love for the job virtually no one applied." How different were things in Hesse, wrote Rudolf Dohrn, who had run the midwives school in both regions. "In these villages the election is announced by the reeve with the churchbell, and each mother has to confirm her choice with her signature, often with comments added. . . . The midwife's election is seen in some villages as an important act of state."[57] In the northeast of France, particularly Lorraine, local custom had the midwives elected, as opposed to the rest of the country, where local assemblies or local notables appointed them. In Lorraine candidates were generally older women, presumably because local mothers preferred the experience they imagined that age conferred.[58] We know little about exactly what those elections entailed, but probably the victors did not belong to the wretched of the earth.

I don't mean to contrast too starkly the "priestess" versus the "aged hag" theories of how one became a traditional midwife. It's likely that the local women always had some say, else they would have complained mightily if the midwife later made mistakes. Similarly, given the moral tasks imposed on birth attendants, the local clergy doubtless spoke up, too. The 1748 ordinance applying to Cologne's outlying villages was probably typical. A candidate would first apply to the local pastor. He would ensure that she didn't suffer from insanity, was not a heretic, and did not practice witchcraft. Then he would convene the "most pious and honorable women" of the place and poll them. Then the Cologne public health doctor and several colleagues would examine the candidate, after which she would be sworn in and her "test results" sent to the local authorities.[59]

I dwell upon these complex and now long-forgotten procedures only because who the midwife was, and how she was chosen, mattered tremendously to the women of the community, who are the real subjects of our story. The local midwife served them as a general practitioner. She must have loomed as large in their eyes as the pastor. Whether she had been trained and could be counted reliable were therefore crucial.

Into this balance sheet on midwives around 1800, we must enter some debits, some dark sides.

First, even though Western Europe was starting to be laced with midwife schools, the schools themselves had considerable difficulty getting teachable candidates. Some teachers, starting to encounter a new breed of midwife, complained that the candidates were too young and inexperienced. Knowing mainly their local patois, "they scarcely understand French. How can you make them comprehend that the oblique diameters of the pelvis extend from the sacro-iliac symphysis to the ilio-pectineal eminence?" Once graduated, the writer continued, they were cautious to a fault, "inactive when they should intervene"[60]—probably because they had been so intimidated by all this scientific medicine.

The more traditional candidates appeared too elderly and unmalleable. "Aging, decrepit, and fragile crones are sent to midwife school, women who have already attended some births and who harbor ineradicably pernicious prejudices and superstitions. . . . All of our effort and work avails nothing; we finally send them back, and the village has wasted six to eight thalers."[61] Complaints of this sort abound in the literature and reflect nothing so much as the head-on clash of two kinds of knowledge: traditional and scientific. The village women were gripped powerfully by the former, for it was all they knew. The doctors, of course, were horribly impatient with "patient sensibilities" and "native folkways" and with anything smacking of superstition and custom. And so the lessons of the schools were brusquely taught and quickly forgotten.

Yet even if the schools' graduates were good, nothing obliged them to settle in the countryside, where the midwife's life was laborious and unremunerative. They preferred to go to the cities. Trained midwives "could scarcely earn bread crusts" in the villages outlying Hamburg, and settled there "only if it is promised them that they can transfer to the city after a couple of years."[62] Toward 1870 in Finland over three fourths of the regular midwives lived in towns, because "the peasants were not in general willing to pay even the modest fees claimed by the midwives."[63]

That was the seat of the problem. As we saw in the first chapter, the male peasants did not think it important to have a trained person at their wives' deliveries. Thus it was that the grannies persisted right alongside the midwives in the nineteenth century in the Limousin, and into the twentieth century in the Sologne region.[64] As late as 1900 in the Königsberg area, more than half of all rural deliveries were attended by grannies, not by midwives.[65] In eighteenth-century Brittany, "the licensed midwives who live in cities are scarce and too expensive for the peasants. They ask twelve livres to travel two miles to do a delivery, and it is necessary to drive them back and forth. The majority of peasants prefer a granny, or death."[66] Simpler for the peasants around Memel was to let some "old, experienced woman" or even the husband himself do the delivery.[67] Marcelle Bouteiller tells of a family of eleven children toward 1900 near Bayonne, all of them delivered by the husband.[68]

Thus, even if trained midwives were available, village women would not necessarily be delivered by them. But after 1800 they were increasingly available. In Rügen Island, armed with their "Stein birthing chairs" and their enema syringes, they were said to be "not bad."[69]* Especially in the cities their numbers were increasing. Since the middle of the eigh-

* They had been trained by doctors and licensed by the college of hygiene in Griefswald.

teenth century Frankfurt midwives had become so up to date that "they go around talking about the axis of the pelvis."[70] And so on. These testimonies could be multiplied many times.

The important point, however, is that this training was saving mothers' lives. By 1835 almost all the Danzig midwives had graduated from the local training school, "so that for a long time there have been no stories of deliveries botched up by them."[71] Whereas giving birth in Glarus before 1780 meant, according to Dr. Johann Gottfried Ebel, a veritable massacre of the innocents: "for the last twenty years the doctors have been circulating instructions about the birthing stool and now far fewer women become sacrifices of sheer ignorance. During these two decades only four new mothers have died in Glarus and in the neighboring communities."[72]

An index of improvements in urban midwifery is the general decline in the maternal death rate *in cities* which set in during the last half of the eighteenth century. I shall present the evidence in chapter 5 but call here the reader's attention to the undoubted link between the better education of midwives and the mother's improving chances of surviving her delivery.

To recapitulate, the answer to the question, were the midwives any good?, has three parts. First, the urban midwives before 1750 or so were probably better than the doctors and represented the best practice of the time in terms of the knowledge then available. Second, the traditional midwives before 1750—and thereafter to the extent that they remained untrained—probably had the judgment and the patience that go with experience but were unable to handle any obstetric emergency. Also, as we shall see in the next chapter, in even normal deliveries they fiddled and meddled harmfully, unaware that they were doing harm. Third, the trained midwives who started to come from state-sponsored midwife schools after 1750 were highly proficient, did not indulge in the pernicious practices of the traditional midwives in managing a normal delivery, and knew when to call in a doctor. Unfortunately, they were found mainly in the cities of continental Europe.

CHAPTER 4

A Typical Birth Then

PEOPLE TODAY have a romanticized and generally false picture of the typical birth in traditional times. We imagine somehow that the "wise woman" who did midwifery in the village sat with her hands gently folded waiting for the child to be born, after which the neighbors all did some kind of women's dance around the new mother. At every step, we are told, Nature is left to take her course, and "intervention" is absent. Thus, according to one widely cited account, "Childbirth was part of the natural order of things." Women approached it "instinctively and without fear" and did not experience "what we call pain in childbirth." The author believes that midwives were "reluctant to tamper with the process for fear of creating an unnatural situation which might cause pain . . . to the birthing mother."[1] Even specialists in obstetrics today have accepted this fantasy as a true account. According to one august medical body, "In the past, women gave birth to their children at home. There, among family and friends, they were not 'patients' and childbirth was not an 'illness.' It was a natural process."[2]

These descriptions are highly misleading. While it is true that the typical birth occurred at home, and that neighbors would cluster about the bedside, it is untrue that people regarded birth as a "natural process" and abstained from intervention. The typical mother was in fact harassed by meddlers and officious interveners from the moment she realized she was pregnant until she finally received her ritual "cleansing" a month after giving birth.

This chapter takes the average woman of times past through a typical normal pregnancy. We begin with the "antenatal care" thrust upon her and conclude with her lying in a steaming featherbed after her birth attendants have pulled out the afterbirth. At every step, those around her felt compelled to take a hand in Nature's work, *except* on those occasions when a little "intervention" might have been welcome to the mother.

Antenatal Care

"Antenatal" care today means basically that the mother's doctor will measure her pelvis to see if it's large enough for an easy delivery, and monitor her every few weeks for the rises in blood pressure, the swelling of the tissues, or the deposits in the urine which might signal the onset of convulsions. In traditional Europe nobody understood the scientific basis for this variety of prenatal care; and none of it, of course, was done. Instead, mothers received pre-birth care of quite a different sort.

First, they had to take precautions against a whole armada of threats from the supernatural, from those dark forces which, most of our ancestors believed, hovered constantly at the threshold. Thus, in parts of Lorraine people thought that if the mother "curses, blasphemes, or swears at someone, her child will be born a monster." Villagers there believed implicitly in "maternal impressions," thinking that the mother would communicate to the infant whatever startled her during pregnancy. So pregnant women "went outdoors as little as possible" to avoid potentially startling encounters. Nor did they "leave home between sundown and sunrise." If, for example, a mother looked at the moon, people thought her child would become "a lunatic or a sleepwalker."[3] Around Nürtingen in Württemberg it was thought that if a mother was startled as a dog jumped up, her child would have "dog feet." Mothers there would always go out of the way of deformed people, for similar reasons.[4] In the Rhön area a pregnant woman would never agree to be godmother of a newborn, "else one of the two children—the born or the unborn—will die."[5]

These fables could be multiplied for pages. Pregnant women had to roll the washtub out of the room in a certain way, avoid cats, and be careful to touch themselves in particular spots to prevent birthmarks. The rules in which they were enmeshed amounted to a special variety of "antenatal care," the purpose of which—then as now—was to produce a healthy, unblemished infant. But these rules were highly restrictive and, in addition to filling the mother with uneasiness about the forces of darkness that lurk about birth, curtailed her daily activities.

A much more direct form of intervention in pregnancy came from the practice of bleeding, or "venesection" as it is known medically. You open a vein with a scalpel and let a pint or two of blood run out, on the theory that illness is caused by a plethora of blood. Some readers may blink at seeing this called folk-medicine practice, because therapeutic bleeding was also standard in academic medicine before the middle of the nineteenth century. Indeed, doctors of the past have been fulsomely roasted in the orthodox feminist literature for having bled their patients in normal pregnancies.* What is not understood, however, is that bleeding was far more widely practiced in peasant medicine.

A noblewoman in Normandy sent for Guillaume de la Motte, on 13 March 1697, to bleed her. She was in her ninth month. De la Motte thought she didn't need to be bled at all, "but she insisted absolutely and I was obliged to obey." "The majority of women," he wrote, "are so alert to this supposed necessity, by a tradition that passes among them from one to the next, that they believe they risk a dangerous delivery if they are not bled at midterm."[8] Until the end of the eighteenth century, women in the small Austrian town of St. Pölten wanted "without fail to be bled at least once in their pregnancy; many wanted a good portion of blood to be drained off even two or three times because they thought that otherwise the child would drown in blood at delivery."[9]† A Vienna doctor said in 1800 that "previously it had been customary that without exception every pregnant woman would undertake to be bled at least three times, in the fifth, the seventh, and the last month, in order to avoid a hemorrhage and to prevent the child from growing too large."[11] Even in the 1860s bleeding still thrived in Upper Bavaria:

The female peasants would consider it a sinful act of negligence if they omitted being bled during pregnancy. So in some barbers' shops [Baderstube] in which venesection records are kept . . . hundredweights of mostly healthy blood are still drawn every year. And in addition to this shop, several other barbers' shops exist in the same county, though less frequented.[12]

When barber-surgeons did not do the bleeding, midwives did. Even at the beginning of the twentieth century, sixteen of the twenty-eight midwives in Fischhausen County continued to bleed with "cupping glasses,"

---

* Denunciations of this sort are expressed by Barbara Ehrenreich and Deirdre English,[6] who also contend that the doctors did away with Europe's midwives by having them executed as witches.[7]

† This source also said that unmarried pregnant women wanted to be bled "to achieve the opposed result" (i.e., an abortion).[10]

because "the older people are so accustomed to being bled" that if the midwives did not do it, less qualified persons would.[13]

Thus, pregnant women would have themselves bled as part of a folk tradition of venesection that had existed since time out of mind, probably having sunk into popular culture from the Hippocratic medicine of ancient times. It was because everybody demanded venesection as a tonic—and certainly as folk medicine—that pregnant women, too, wanted it.

In the matter of diet, which today figures so largely in prenatal care, little special consideration was accorded to the traditional woman. We now know that pregnant women do best when they gain about twenty to twenty-five pounds, and when they are able to add to their diet significantly increased amounts of protein, iron, calcium and other vitamins and minerals. Nobody in the world we have lost knew anything about vitamins and minerals. Yet mothers probably did feel a need to eat more, if we may infer that some collective sense of undernutrition lies behind the erroneous folklore about "tooth decay in pregnancy" (in Norway and Germany people generally believed that "every child costs the mother a tooth").[14] To what extent, therefore, did traditional mothers eat better during pregnancy? The answer seems to be, Not at all.

To be sure, custom sometimes said a mother's food cravings should be indulged.[15] In Germany, village law often expressly stipulated pregnant women's food privileges—a sign either of general male solicitude, or of such a lack of familial interest in maternal diets that the community as a whole found it necessary to legislate on the subject. These rules provided that pregnant women could pick fruit and grapes wherever they wanted; that their husbands or servants could violate the strict hunting rules and bag game for the wife; that even where fishing was forbidden "on forfeit of an eye," pregnant women could go and fish for themselves.[16] It is unclear how much difference these special exemptions made over the course of pregnancy.

But even when the community went along with free cherries or whatever, we are still not in the presence of a collective willingness to shift the basic distribution of food at table from men to pregnant women. A doctor in Franconia described "the most complete indifference" to the diets of pregnant women, who ate only "legumes, weak bread dishes, and water or bad beer." Even though in the Périgord region better-off women during pregnancy got such delicacies as pork and vegetable stew twice daily, or eggs and fruit, the poorer women received a diet "scarcely better than that of the livestock," as one doctor put it.[17] A systematic investigation of rural Norwegians in the twentieth century concluded that "no importance at all is attached to special nutrition for the pregnant."[18] And a German village study from 1900 found pregnant

women so desperate that they were willing to snatch potatoes from the
pig's trough. That may be a special case, the author said, "but even for
later years there is evidence that pregnant women were not permitted
to take from the family's store of preserves, even if they were rotting.
Even today many women who grew up in that period secretly buy fruit."[19]
The point is that, before the twentieth century, most pregnant women
did not receive any special dietary consideration. If in other areas of
prenatal care their peasant healers and medical advisers intervened too
officiously, in this domain little was done.

Similarly, traditional peasants granted their pregnant wives no special
dispensations from work. When today we encourage the pregnant to lead
normal, physically active lives until the onset of labor, we speak in the
context of tennis, office work, or gardening. "Normal physical activity"
for Europe's traditional populations meant back-breaking field work, and
it is significant that pregnant women received no relief from it. In Württemberg's Wangen area, "women pay no attention to their pregnant condition," said Dr. Zengerle, "and do heavy lifting and carrying just like
the men."[20] Labor pains surprised one Wolsfeld mother as she was loading
hay. Because she had to stop working, her husband became irritated and
told her, "At least you could have waited until we were finished."[21]
And, in truth, most rural women worked not just through most of the
pregnancy but until the onset of labor. Only 3 of 65 women polled in
two Baden villages about 1911 said that they stopped work earlier; most
worked "right up to the last minute."[22] In a Württemberg village only
11 of the 108 mothers questioned around the same time said they were
able to "take it easy" during pregnancy. Three fourths of them "did
field work right until the end."[23] According to Dr. Louis Caradec, labor
pains often caught women in Brittany's Finistère department by surprise
in the fields: "They have to go to the nearest neighbor's house and surren-
der themselves to the first woman they find . . . for their delivery."[24]

Nor did pregnant women confine themselves to simple household
chores. "You often see women just a few days before their delivery
sweating in the fields or stumbling homeward under some heavy load of
fodder," wrote Dr. Christian Pfeufer in 1810 of the Bamberg area.[25] And
fifty years later, another rural doctor in the same region said, "Pregnant
women here do not take it easy at all and perform even their heaviest
duties until the end of the pregnancy, often until the arrival of labor
pains."[26]*

The justification for this custom, doubtless in reality the result of eco-

---

* Studies done by the Children's Bureau of the U.S. Department of Labor around the
First World War found that rural women routinely did field work right up to the onset
of labor.[27]

nomic constraints and husbandly indifference to the wife's health, was that it made for an easier labor. In Finland peasants believed that hard work throughout pregnancy, "but especially in the final months . . . eased the birth by separating the [pubic] bones from each other and by opening up the genital canal."[28] Women in Württemberg were taking it easier during pregnancy by 1909, when Pastor H. Höhn made his survey. And where they weren't, the reason was, he said, because "heavy work makes for a light labor."[29] Again, around Metz, women rested up during the beginning of pregnancy and then exerted themselves toward the end in the hope of "ensuring that the infant descends and gets out easily."[30]*

So at the level of folklore, communities were able to elaborate justifications for keeping hugely pregnant women in the fields. What the women themselves thought about this custom, however, is another matter. And the only evidence I know came from the pens of those working-class English mothers who in 1914 answered a Women's Co-operative Guild questionnaire. "I did fairly well for a working man's wife," wrote one mother of six, "but the recollection is anything but pleasant. Fancy bending over a washing-tub, doing the family washing perhaps an hour or two before the baby is born." Another woman, typical of many who responded, said that, because of her husband's unemployment, she had to work while carrying her last-born, "standing all day washing and ironing. This caused me much suffering from varicose veins, also caused the child to wedge in some way, which nearly cost both our lives."[33] It is therefore unlikely that earlier generations of peasant women relished the "antenatal care" they were receiving.

Setting the Scene

WHO WAS ON HAND?

When Samuel Sewall's daughter gave birth on the last day of January 1701, in Boston, present were her mother and mother-in-law, plus the midwife Mrs. Wakefield, and Mesdames Usher, Pemberton, Hubbard, and Welsteed, and "Nurse Johnson." Thus, at least eight other women found themselves in the lying-in room.[34] Around the same time Guillaume de la Motte was called to deliver the wife of a butcher in the little Norman town of Montebourg. There had been a complication, de la Motte tells us, for he had to perform some obstetrical maneuver "in the presence

---

* For evidence that heavy work late in pregnancy is genuinely harmful, see Heinz Küstner's data.[31] Bonnie S. Worthington cites evidence from Texas that "mothers who engage in very heavy physical activity during the last weeks of pregnancy tend to deliver more than the expected number of small-for-gestational-age babies."[32]

of more than thirty people."[35] It is fair to say, then, that traditional births were community events.

And they brought together whatever collective lore the community possessed. "Women of the people are like queens," said a French doctor who knew the countryside well, "in that everyone is able to attend their deliveries. When a peasant woman feels her first pains, the neighbors come running, filling up her narrow hut. Some of them walk her around, others rub her, massage her. Some blow into her mouth to prevent the uterus from climbing up."[36]

Thus labor had begun. The crowds were gathering. First came the older women; then after the delivery had been successfully completed, the younger wives.[37] The women insisted on heating the room full blast, on the peasant theory that exposure to drafts could be fatal. "How marvelous it is," wrote man-midwife Bernard Faust in 1784, "when mothers leave the windows of their bedrooms open. Then the stand-offish old women, who otherwise crowd round the mother in a room they have heated to the boiling point, will now stay home, for they dread these cool rooms, cleansed with fresh, clean air, more fearfully than if one were burning asafetida."[38]

These women were there, of course, to help support the mother in labor and generally to offer encouragement. Which sounds fine. But our positive notions about "encouragement" differ considerably from the chronic fatalism and fear of supernatural forces that one finds among traditional peasants. All were preoccupied with what could go wrong. "Do not whisper in front of the mother," to avoid alarming her, commanded article 8 of Kaufbeuren's 1737 midwife ordinance.[39] "As labor continues," wrote a Frankfurt doctor in 1844, "the mother is diverted with tales of heroic deeds from the practice of her midwife, with horror stories of obstetric content which in no way contribute to assuaging her, and with accounts of the malpractice and negligence of various doctors in the neighborhood."[40] If no midwife lived in the village, said Dr. Schleis von Löwenfeld, "the oldest women there take the responsibility on themselves. The whole room fills up with women. This one advises one thing, that one advises another."[41] We hear in these quotes two kinds of culture clashing over the question of who would be with the mother and what would they tell her. And Dr. Jean-Marie Munaret's advice to physicians was to foreshadow an epochal change in the birth experience of the average woman: "Tell the crones who customarily occupy the bedchamber to leave. They befoul the air, make your client uneasy, torment her, and will get in your way during your maneuvers, only to criticize you afterward if you are unsuccessful."[42]

But for the time being, they would stay.

Sometimes men were present, sometimes not. For example, in eastern Languedoc in the nineteenth century, only women were present at births—to wit, "relatives, friends and maybe an inexperienced daughter." But in central Languedoc, "the delivery brings together in the main room of the house the whole family, including men and children. It is, especially in winter, the occasion of a big party [*veillée*], where the men play cards, the children play and check from time to time to see how labor is progressing. A big cauldron is on the fire to clean the mother and infant afterward and to wash the bed linen."[43]

In other places the husband was absent, as in the Sologne: "If the intimidated husband wants, as is customary, to withdraw discreetly to some tavern to await the outcome, his wife says to him ironically, 'Because you were there for the planting, you should be there for the harvest as well.' "[44] My impression is that, while men did participate occasionally in births, the scene as a whole was set by women. And the ensuing postdelivery celebration, about which we shall later read, was exclusively a "women's festival."

BIRTH POSITION

In what position did women actually give birth? Today in hospitals the "lithotomy position" is standard (so called because patients once lay flat with their legs up in order to have bladder stones removed). Yet that position for birth is a recent innovation. Before hospital birth triumphed, a wide range of birthing positions prevailed at home.

Following the Hippocratic view, people believed in the Middle Ages that the infant helped in its own delivery. Toward the ninth month of pregnancy, the fetus started to run out of food in the uterus and so would decide to make its way to the outside, turning itself from the head-upright position, where it was thought to have passed most of its gestation, to a head-down position, which would permit it to crawl out of the uterus. Birthing pains, therefore, consisted of the fetus's efforts to break the bag of waters and to crawl through the birth canal to the outside. To better facilitate the child's passage, the mother would give birth standing or squatting, both positions favoring gravity.[45]

Then, in the fifteenth century, midwives in German cities began to adopt the birthing stool, taking the idea from Italy where such stools had been used since ancient times.[46*] Why they decided upon this innovation is unclear. Possibly their new professional organizations, whose formation I described in the previous chapter, thought stools more appropriate for sophisticated urban mothers. In any event, by the sixteenth century

---

* According to Heinrich Fasbender, the first mention of a birthing stool in history occurs in the works of Soranus of Ephesus in the 2nd century A.D.[47]

birthing stools were generally used in the cities of Central Europe.[48] Else-luise Haberling explains how the stools worked. After a mother's pains had reached the point of expelling the infant, the midwife would ask her to climb upon the stool. "The midwife placed one assistant so that the mother could lean back against her. This assistant was always experienced, either an apprentice of the midwife or a neighborhood handy-woman. . . . She would hold the mother from behind with her arms, and supplement the birth pains by pressing lightly or heavily against the fundus [top] of the uterus, according to the midwife's instructions." Two other women stood at each side of the stool to encourage the mother and help the midwife.[49]

Outside the cities, mothers in Central Europe seemed to prefer giving birth in the classic modes of standing or squatting. In the 1890s, Dr. Max Höfler wrote of the Tölz area of Bavaria that "until a few decades ago local women delivered in the traditional squatting position. Their excellent pelvic conformities and their good constitutions may have contributed to this easy form of delivery."[50] Accounts of standing are even more numerous. When, for example, peasant women around Memel went into labor, they would grab onto a cloth knotted between the roof beams, and sway back and forth as "those present encourage them to press down."[51] At roughly the same time, peasant women around Bamberg birthed either standing, or while sitting on their husbands' laps.[52] Even in the 1920s peasant women in the isolated Swiss Lötschenthal delivered while standing, supporting themselves from a sling.[53] Thus, there persisted until late in time a "Central European" pattern of birthing stools for city women and of standing, with support, for rural women.

A similar mélange of tales, contrasting city and country, trained and untrained midwives, could be produced for other countries of Europe as well. The reader, however, has by now a sense of the basic variations—standing, kneeling, sitting, and so forth; and I shall simply mention that sometimes peasant women gave birth recumbent, lying on a pile of straw beside the bed, but only to spare the sheets! Hence in the village of Gy in the Sologne, "most of the women give birth on sacks at the foot of the bed or in front of the big fireplace."[54] In "numerous hamlets and mountain villages" of the Valais, mothers lay upon a pile of fresh straw or, in some places, "covered the straw with old newspapers or a sheet. People would never use clean sheets, either for the delivery or for the lying-in period."[55]

In Hungary, too, it is striking how mothers wanted to spare the bed linen. Women would spend the first "period" of labor in bed, while their pains were merely opening the cervix. And then just as soon as the child began to be expelled, they would spring from bed and deliver on the ground. Or they would deliver on top of the straw after the linen had been removed. Even when doctors and midwives persuaded younger women to give birth in regular beds, "the older [midwives] still cling to the notion that the child will come out quicker and easier in standing, kneeling, sitting, or lying on the ground. A number of midwives, moreover, promote delivering on the earth floor in order to have as little clean-up afterward as possible."[56] The reader thus sees how complex is this question of birthing "horizontally." Some women avoided it for reasons we know now to be valid: the infant does come more easily when the mother squats or sits up.* Others shunned it for reasons of economy: not to soil the valuable linen. Others still birthed recumbent, but outside the bed. In other words, many factors played a role: a doctor did not simply ride up and knock the mother flat with his forceps.

Finally, a word about England. Customary birth positions there have not been studied systematically. On the evidence I have seen, city women usually delivered on proper birthing stools, while women in smaller communities knelt, or sat on a couple of plain stools pushed together. Willughby wrote that, "Several midwives, chiefly about London, use midwives stools," which he opposed, preferring mothers to lie in bed for normal deliveries: "Let me persuade and intreat the midwife not to torment the poor woman, at the first coming of her pains, by putting her to kneel, or to sit on a woman's lap, or on the midwife's stool, but suffer her to walk gently, or to lie down on a truckle bed." Elsewhere he wrote that kneeling was "the country mode of delivery."[58] Another writer, who knew mainly London, also cites birthing stools.[59]

As on the Continent, in England some traditional postures survived long after birthing in bed had become *à la mode* in the cities. Mary Wrigley of Collyhurst, for example, gave birth in 1772 upon the knee of the midwife's assistant.[60] A surgeon in a Welsh mining community said in the 1860s that "the most pernicious practice among midwives here is that of delivering the women on their knees on the floor of the bedroom; much unnecessary hemorrhage takes place, and consequently the recoveries are very tardy."[61] And in 1875 the *Lancet,* the British medical weekly founded in 1823, reported that women in the "northern counties" continued to give birth on a kind of stool, formed by tying together the "two inner front legs of two chairs." The chairs were then pushed apart from behind, and the mother sat at the angle. "Two of her female friends or attendants then sit on the chairs on either side of

---

* One author found that letting mothers assume the position of choice, as opposed to the horizontal position, shortened labor by 25 percent.[57]

her, she placing her arms on the shoulders of the two supporting." The birth attendant was to sit on a low stool facing her. "Now, I have known of instances where surgeons have been told 'they were not required,' because they would not attend in such a position."[62] This was 1875, mind you!

The larger point to be retained from these tales of kneeling, squatting, and bizarre arrangements of chairs is that women traditionally gave birth in positions that they deemed comfortable, up to a point. (In those days the welfare of the fetus was simply not at issue.) Beyond that point the woman's personal preferences ceded to the midwife's insistence upon a birthing stool or to the state's insistence that she use a stool. Which poses us with a problem for later in the book: when finally the bed vanquished these traditional postures, was it because women were driven to lie horizontal by male physicians avid to "intervene in the natural process of childbirth"? Or was it because all along women probably found the bed more comfortable but avoided using it for fearing of soiling it?[63] As the next section shows, the midwives were themselves not exactly reluctant to intervene.

The Midwives Intervene

Now we have the mother upon the birthing stool or lying on the straw next to the bed. Her labor pains have begun. What happens next?

The midwife might first of all "break the waters," which means puncturing with a fingernail or pointed thimble the sac of amniotic fluid that surrounds the infant in the uterus. This puncturing is not quite the same as "inducing" labor today, because labor had already started. The midwives did it to speed up the birth. Willughby related that, "One Mrs. K. F., a London midwife, being to go to another woman, in hopes to deliver her woman quickly (as, upon my inquiry she confessed privately to me) did tear the membranes. All the waters issued suddenly forth. The child, being deprived of moisture, perished in the womb."[64] Willughby believed this to be a common practice: "There be some midwives that, through ignorance or impatience, or being hastened to go to some other woman's labour, do tear the membranes with their nails, or cut them with scissors."[65]

The skeptic may claim that Willughby, as a man midwife, did his best to slander his female competitors. Yet comments on midwives puncturing the sac abound. In 1769, Gerhard Thilenius explained, in his manual for midwives, how the contractions will naturally break the waters. "I cannot sufficiently rebuke the unfortunate custom of the midwives puncturing the sac arbitrarily and without reason."[66] The city of Kaufbeuren forbade, in 1737, its midwives from keeping one fingernail long for the purpose of rupturing the waters.[67] And even in the 1920s an elderly Swiss midwife proudly showed a visiting doctor a thimble with a jagged top which she used to puncture the sac.

"Where did you get this idea, Marjosa?" he asked. "Is it your own invention"?

"Oh no," she said. "Even my grandmother used it."[68]

Many midwives did not just content themselves with breaking the waters, but went "exploring." In the words of Hamburg's Doctor J. H. Wigand, they "push the head back up in the uterus; they make too much room between it and the pelvis, and permit not only the waters but the other contents of the uterus to run out [such as the umbilical cord]."[69] Why so much meddling? Wigand said, "Most mothers are not in a position to evaluate the competence of a midwife, the less so because the midwives so outrageously slander one another and deny that their colleagues possess even the simplest of skills. Thus women judge a midwife on the basis of her industriousness in doing a delivery." A top midwife, in the eyes of Hamburg's mothers, was "none other than one who works herself into a sweat from head to toe. The midwives know how to exploit this preconception. They stick their hands continuously into the vagina. They stretch it, pull it, and manipulate it as though it had a strong, stubborn will of its own. They sigh and groan so expressively that one would despair of ever seeing the infant actually born."[70]

In contrast to recent "golden age" interpretations, the actual midwives of traditional Europe and England intervened furiously in the natural process of birth.* Constantly tugging and hauling at the mother's birth canal, at the infant's head, and at the placenta, they were captives of a folkloric view that the best midwife is the one who interferes most. Lest the reader be in doubt, massaging the area between the thighs, dilating the vagina, or attempting with one's hands to "steer" the infant's head, are all pernicious, useless practices. They confer benefits to neither mother nor fetus and risk tearing the mother's soft parts or infecting her. Even though one occasionally encounters today older practitioners who believe in "massaging the perineum," the consensus in medicine is against these usages. In fact any meddling with the birth canal is now seen as risky, and such practices as applying forceps are justified only by the need to

---

* For example, Jane B. Donegan writes, "The midwife's role was confined primarily to offering comfort and reassurance to her patient, encouraging and supporting her without interfering in the normal process of parturition."[71]

get the infant out as quickly as possible so as not to risk reducing the blood supply to its brain.*

Neither midwives nor doctors in traditional times knew anything of "infection." But rather than sitting with hands folded, the midwives had a reputation for terrible impatience. Ideally, mothers shouldn't bestride the stool until labor is well advanced, but in practice many midwives clapped their clients onto stools when the pains first began, exhorting them to bear down for hour after useless hour. Remember that only after labor has been underway for ten hours or so will the cervix have opened enough to let the baby be pushed out. C. F. Senff, who was not unsympathetic to midwives, wrote in 1812, "It is known how impatiently midwives usually await the completion of a birth, how they customarily drive [the mother] to bear down more strongly, how they place her prematurely upon the birthing stool . . . above all when they have been called to another delivery."[74] "Mothers are so exhausted by being forced to bear down prematurely," wrote a Sulzbach doctor, "that by the time they reach the end, where they need to press down, they are completely worn out."[75] And, of course, given the contempt with which unwed mothers were held, it was they who felt most the kiss of the midwife's lash. Dr. Wigand described them bearing down "with all their might, legs and arms held rigid," because the midwives would "waste little time or patience" on them.[76]

The authorities in Central Europe struggled constantly against the midwives' impatience. The former were interested more in seeing live infants at the end of the delivery than in the mother's happiness as such; yet they were on her side. In 1669 the city of Darmstadt ordered that midwives not "drive the mother on prematurely but coax her when it is time, in the event she refuses to press down for fear of pain. The midwife must also not reach in tyrannically or clumsily."[77] In 1703 the city of Frankfurt similarly instructed its midwives that even if things went slowly, "you should not become impatient nor . . . urge the mother to bear down until she feels recurrent pains. Nor should you bore into her cervix with your fingers or pull at the mother's body with your hands in order to pull the child out forcibly."[78]

These German towns struggled throughout the eighteenth century with their interventionist midwives, as doctors began to realize that a natural

---

* For a simple guide to what maneuvers *are* appropriate in delivering a baby, see a midwives' manual, such as that by Leo Eloesser et al.[72] Straightforward instructions for "keeping flexion," "helping extension," and such are available in obstetrics textbooks.[73] No current authority makes any mention of "massaging" the perineum or manually dilating the birth canal.

birth required no intervention save catching the child and cutting the cord:

- As of 1782 it was ordered on the Oettingen-Wallerstein estates that, "because the dangerous practice has established itself among midwives of forcibly tearing apart the cervix and the external genitalia . . . they are emphatically prohibited from any action except supporting the perineum."[79] (The perineum is the skin between the thighs, and pushing against it with one's hand during a contraction was thought to prevent the infant from coming out so rapidly as to tear the mother.)
- The city of Regensburg forbade midwives in 1779 to place mothers on a birthing stool before the waters had burst; nor were the midwives to "bore into the cervix" with their fingers "for the sake of widening it or even of tearing it or of opening the waters with their fingernails."[80]
- In 1797 the city of Lippstadt noted that "many midwives . . . widen the mother's birth canal with their fingers in the intention of thereby easing the passage of the head, or they tear the waters, or they press back the coccyx [the "tailbone"], or they press down on the abdomen."[81] All these practices were forbidden, as indeed they risked rupturing the mother's uterus, tearing her cervix, or giving her a horrible infection.

We cannot merely dismiss these criticisms as mean-spirited bad-mouthing on the part of jealous doctors, for everyone agreed that midwives were to do home deliveries. The only question was how.

It would be tedious to iterate similar examples from other parts of continental Europe, though the literature abounds with horror stories of the midwives' fumbling and fiddling at the mothers' private parts. Let me, however, note the alarm with which qualified midwives themselves viewed their colleagues' officiousness. Louise Bourgeois, the chief midwife in the Hôtel-Dieu in Paris, said in 1626; "I do not doubt that there are some very skilled midwives, but not in such numbers as the others. One can tell them apart by knowing that any woman who fears the Lord will more cherish honor than lucre, and will never attempt to hurry up a mother in order to rush on to others. [A good midwife] will not act as those who always have their houses full of young women and mothers without husbands and who are always pressing them to hurry."[82]

Later authors spelled out in detail the French midwives' practice of "working the mother" to have her deliver as fast as possible.[83] What are the causes of urinary incontinence? asked Jacques Mesnard, a surgeon in Rouen. "Most often the bad maxims of the midwives, who shove their finger too forcibly against the mother's pubic bone, thinking thus to dilate the birth canal, and who push against the tailbone from the posterior wall of the vagina . . . which causes the organs to become inflamed and ulcerated."[84]

When, in the years after the Second World War, Rose-Claire Schüle surveyed midwife practices in the Valais, she was appalled at how much of this meddlesomeness had survived: "First they grease up their hands, and then grease up the vagina and the cervix of the mother"—all this in order to "soften" the passages. If labor is slow, they "carefully undertake the dilatation of the cervix with their bare hands, not disinfected but lubricated. . . . Needless to say, the trained midwives call the doctor."[85]

The most dramatic testimony of the traditional midwives' spirit of intervention comes from Percivall Willughby, who in the seventeenth century was writing for an audience of midwives and in no way trying to justify their abolition. Don't intervene in normal labor, he urged. You don't need to thrust your hands into the vagina at every birth pain. "Neither must [the midwife] go about to hasten the birth by using any force to the woman's body, to dilate the passages by her hands and fingers." Let "Dame Nature" do the work, summed up his advice. "The midwife's office, or duty, in a natural birth is no more but to receive the child, and afterward to fetch the after-birth, if needed."[86]

Because Willughby attended mainly obstetric emergencies, his observations need generally not detain us here. But Mrs. Wolaston's delivery in Threadneedle Street in London, which he attended in 1657, gives us some insight into the midwives' world: "When the midwife perceived that I was sent for, she resolved to hasten her work. She caused several women perforce to hold the mother by the middle, whilst that she, with others, pulled the child by the limbs one way, and the women, her body, the other way. Thus, at the last the child, by violence, was drawn from her and made at the separation (as she told me) a report, as though a pistol had been discharged."[87]

It is clear, I think, that Europe's traditional midwives actually did interfere throughout the course of a normal labor. The medical evidence to this effect may not merely be dismissed as self-interested and biased. The matter is important because the quality of attendance at childbed affected immediately the lives of all mothers in the past, who are the subjects of this part of my story.

One final point remains about the midwives' officiousness in managing normal labor. It was, in the beginning, the *doctors* who had told them to meddle. The Roman obstetrician Soranus believed that the midwife should keep stretching the vagina with her fingers and pull open the labia. Once the mother's cervix had completely dilated, the midwife should tug away at the child's head in every pause between contractions. In the meantime her assistants should keep pressing down on the mother's abdomen, in order to push the infant out.[88] Whether Soranus was merely repeating what was accepted custom in his day, or whether this wretched advice passed into folk obstetrics on his initiative, is unclear.

But by the sixteenth century, when medical writing on midwifery recommenced, doctors firmly believed in these meddlesome views. Zurich's Jakob Rueff, for example, urged midwives to rub their hands (and the mother's abdomen) with oil of roses before doing internal examinations, and, if the mother's pelvic muscles seemed rigid, to dilate manually both the vagina and the cervix.[89] The sixteenth-century French medical writer Jean L. Liébaut urged midwives to help squeeze the infant from the uterus by pressing high up on the abdomen, and to "open up the mother and relax her parts with a finger." He placidly advocated puncturing the amniotic sac with a finger as well.[90]

The tragedy is that, once the doctors changed their minds and advocated no interference with "Dame Nature," they were unable to wrench the midwives from this thousand-year tradition which the doctors themselves had begun. The obstetrics manual of the skilled Berlin midwife Justine Siegemundin, published in 1690, counseled no manual dilatation of the vagina. But her advice fell on deaf ears.[91] Percivall Willughby was first in England to instruct "these great tuggers of women's bodies" not to intervene in normal labor.[92] Yet they continued to do so until our own century. By the end of the eighteenth century, medical opinion had repudiated the "haling and hauling" of the midwives. But interventionist lore had filtered ineradicably into village culture and was not to be removed.

Retrieving the Placenta

After the infant is born, a third stage of labor remains: the birth of the placenta, that large, purplish organ that connects the fetus to the mother's bloodstream. Normally the placenta will come away from the wall of the uterus a few minutes after the child is out, and even if it stays behind as long as half an hour, there's no cause for alarm. In traditional midwifery, however, people believed they should detach it immediately by hand. This is the final source of "intervention" in normal labor.

When the placenta seems stuck to the uterine wall, the usual reason is that the uterus has not fully contracted. Occasionally, however, one of the placenta's big bumpy surfaces (called "cotyledons") is bound to the underlying tissue of the uterus.* In such cases, pulling on the umbilical cord, or tugging at an edge of the placenta, may cause a hemorrhage or turn the uterus inside out. The mother could die of shock. At a minimum, reaching in one's hand can convey infection. So there is no doubt these practices are pernicious.

But routinely done in the past. Nicolas Saucerotte said in 1777 that "it is without doubt attributable to the mother's desire to be quickly delivered as soon as her child has entered the world, and to the joy which her attendants experience, that most midwives extract the placenta immediately after the child's birth."[94] One long-practiced London midwife told a doctor "that she endeavoured never to let her patient suffer long . . . for the moment the child was born, she took care to pull at the after-birth until it came away."[95] Regensburg's 1779 midwife ordinance warned that "after the successful birth of the child, you should quietly await the afterbirth and not, as earlier was the custom, immediately reach into the uterus with your hand, tear it apart with your fingernails, and forcibly haul it out."[96] Early in the twentieth century the rural Swiss midwife Marjosa was still routinely fetching the afterbirth, telling her clients, "It's high time we go after it; otherwise it would have started to climb up." The mothers were thereupon content that Marjosa's quick intervention had prevented this major complication—the placenta wandering up toward the heart![97]

Because of such interference, inverted uteri following normal deliveries were familiar. "I was, in the greatest haste, sent for to a woman six miles distant from me," wrote Edmund Chapman in 1735. On arriving, he found she had been dead an hour. "The midwife told me that the afterbirth stuck so fast in one part, that she was not able with all her strength to take it from her, though she had gained most of it." Chapman thereupon asked to see the body. "I found, to my great surprise, that the uterus was inverted, and entirely out of the body, hanging down between the thighs, with the placenta adhering to its fundus." And so he learned the whole story. After an easy delivery, the midwife "had pulled hard at the string, and so brought down the uterus, which as soon as she could take any hold of, she did. And then pulling with fresh violence, and not being deterred by the loudest cries, the poor miserable woman in a few minutes fell into strong convulsions and deliriums, and so expired."[98]

The uterus had been hauled out together with the placenta, said Louise

---

* F. Ahlfeld reported, in 1890, that manual detachment of the placenta was truly necessary in only four of every thousand deliveries.[93]

Bourgeois in 1626, at least three times in Paris "in the last four or five years." Midwives would run their hand into the uterus "and pull out whatever they encounter, which is frequently a part of the uterus to which the afterbirth is clinging." The consequences were awful. "I am terribly sorry for these poor women," said Bourgeois, "whom I see working away. They have no possibility of resting up, because they know that if they do not work, they cannot eat, and so they shall languish for the rest of their days."[99]

Training might have forestalled such grabbiness, which the local authorities in the village of Vallstadt near Wolfenbüttel well knew, as they demanded again a trained midwife after one of the two untrained granny midwives had, in 1805, "incautiously removed the afterbirth, inverting the uterus and killing the mother."[100] But the resentful traditional midwives refused this kind of guidance. In December 1782, a doctor in Saxony was called by a mother's family to help out a midwife. The midwife evidently felt insulted by his arrival and paid no attention to his warning to leave the dangling cord alone. "Suddenly she seized it and pulled so powerfully that the placenta came after, but torn. Now she crowed to me that she possessed enough skill as to be able to dispense entirely with outside assistance." But as the doctor bent to examine the placenta, the midwife called to him, "Look, the rest is coming now." And as he turned, he saw, to his astonishment, "that she had pulled down the uterus as well, so that the cervix was now hanging out of the birth canal." The mother died later of an infection.[101]

These stories make the midwives, who were merely following traditional lore to pull on whatever one could, appear monstrous. Again, I wish to emphasize that these malignant practices were originally taught in academic medicine and probably later diffused into the folkloric practice of the midwives. For a thousand years official medicine had instructed that the placenta must immediately be removed, else the uterus would contract and make impossible its delivery.[102]

Thus it does not surprise us that in 1771 the town of Runkel-Wied determined that "the afterbirth is never to be left to nature, but instead must immediately be retrieved by hand." Moreover, the midwife was to dive in there once again to see that no "congealed blood and the like have been left behind."[103] In other words, these midwives fiddled and meddled with the cord, in part, because they thought their medical supervisors wanted them to do so. Unfortunately, however, when medical views changed, the midwives refused to change with them and, for another hundred years, obstinately turned normal deliveries into dangerous encounters.

Resting Up

The upper middle class women whose experiences have monopolized our views of women in the past, would spend one to two weeks in bed after giving birth. Women from the popular classes were generally up in one or two days. That is the gist of this section.

First, I must clear away some underbrush. If a mother's uterus has properly contracted, or "involuted," after delivery, there is no reason why she cannot get up and walk around within a few hours. She may resume a normal schedule as soon as she feels like it thereafter: no physiological reasons confine her to bed.

Only recently has medical opinion become so liberal. Most people in the past *believed* in the nine-day bed rest, even though few were able to follow it.* The doctors said a woman should lie flat out for at least a week, not even moving to let the bed be made. After two weeks, wrote Francis Ramsbotham, "she may begin to put her feet on the ground."[104] The midwives also cherished nine days for lying-in, and they would call daily, or twice daily, for that time.[106] Midwife Josefine Biedermann, for example, was outraged when, on the sixth day, a mother hoisted herself from bed to run a small errand.[107] Looking back on earlier confinements, one English mother wrote in 1914 that "it was thought certain death to change the underclothes under a week. For a whole week we were obliged to lie on clothes stiff and stained, and the stench under the clothes was abominable, and added to this we were commanded to keep the babies under the clothes."[108] This was English midwives' traditional lore, said Dr. Lapthorn Smith: "The prehistoric nurse will not allow [the mother] to lift her head from the pillow, and as a result large clots and decomposing debris from the uterus remain for ten days in the vagina."[109] Thus, the birth attendants were insistent.

We know now that these long horizontal sojourns could harm the mother by letting the blood pool in her leg veins, possibly coagulating into clots which could damage her lungs—or kill her—with a "pulmonary embolism." Yet even though no good medical reason existed for keeping women flat out, people thought there was one, which is what matters. When Ramsbotham wrote that mothers regarded the ninth day of their convalescence as "critical," he was probably alluding to infection, or "puerperal fever."[110] As you shall see, the risk of post-delivery infection loomed terrifyingly; and because the onset of symptoms could be delayed, only after about nine days could women really relax.

In these prolonged convalescences, the practice was to make the mother

---

* Maternity patients were discharged from hospitals in Lyons only after ten days.[105]

sweat. Her attendants would stoke the oven up high and then wrap her in a feather bolster, so that the sweat poured off for days. "Sometimes the first three weeks of lying-in are viewed with great anxiety," wrote Cadolzburg's Dr. Rieger, "for the new mother is brought to bed, and the 'nine-day sweat' which she is supposed to go through is sweated out with all care and attentiveness."[111] When, however, women like this remained abed for considerable periods, we may suspect it was because something had gone wrong in the delivery. The priest of the village of Tromarey makes precisely this point: "It takes most of our women quite a while to get back to normal after giving birth because they were delivered so roughly."[112] An infected mother would have chills. What could be more natural than "sweating the poisons out of her." But the justifications offered for these prolonged convalescences are beside the point. If you could afford it, you stayed in bed for a week or two after birth.

And if you couldn't afford it, which was true of most women from the popular classes, you were up on the second or third day. Your presence was indispensable. In the town of Sulz-on-the-Neckar there lived "common women who pay so little mind to childbirth," said Dr. Wunderlich, "that I once saw someone who had delivered that morning up in the afternoon carrying a bucket of water from the well."[113] You would be astonished, wrote Moritz Thilenius in 1769, "to see peasant women going about their household tasks that same evening after delivery. I once saw a mother, who had delivered late the night before, caring for the livestock the next day, without paying it any mind."[114] If these women were at work again quickly, it was because they had to be. "They're back at it after two or three days," wrote one observer of a Swiss village in the 1930s, "because very few husbands know how to milk a cow. They understand less about running a household than the average city dweller."[115]

In truth two to four days seems to have been the average lying-in period for traditional farm and artisanal women. A number of comments, which I shall not quote at length, converge on that figure. Said Dr. Caradec of one area of Brittany, "Happily local women give birth easily, because it is not unusual to see them resuming their household tasks after three or four days."[116] In the Steiermark province of Austria, not only did women "continue to do the heaviest kind of tasks, even after labor pains have begun," they were also up again "the second day after in order to do housework."[117]

One final note. Later you will read about "women's fêtes" celebrating the newborn's baptism or the mother's happy delivery. Naturally, somebody had to do all that cooking for the fête. While the neighbors may have brought dishes, it was often the mother herself who stumbled from bed shortly after delivery to get things ready. Thus, in the Bamberg countryside, "One often sees the mother quite casually rise from bed to prepare the so-called 'baptismal blowout' [*Gevatterschmause*], while the other people in the house and her friends accompany the infant to baptism."[118] A horrified doctor who reported the same thing happening in the countryside of Baden, warned, "Such behavior cannot fail to damage the health of the mother and her child."[119] Perhaps it hurt them, or perhaps not. The point is that peasant and small-town women had little time to recover from a typical birth.*

It has become fashionable today to argue that in past times women somehow had "control" over their own deliveries, and that today they have none. Hence, these traditional procedures are thought to have been better for women.† The message of this chapter, however, is that women have never really controlled their own births, that birth has always been subject to a web of custom and community regulations which reduces the scope of choice open to an individual mother. Today hospitals have rigid protocols about what procedures to use under what circumstances. The implicit protocols of these traditional midwives were no less rigid: place the mother on the birthing stool as soon as labor begins, fiddle and manipulate throughout, and finally tug the placenta out of her. The surrounding community expected the mother to work right until the onset of labor pains, and to resume her daily routines shortly after the child had been expelled. When custom counts so heavily in how people organize their lives, it is ridiculous to think that traditional mothers were "in control."

---

* Catherine M. Scholten says that in Colonial America women were confined to their beds "ideally for three to four weeks."[120] Both this estimate, and her suspicion that doctors were involved in some sinister conspiracy against parturient women, strike me as unlikely.

† For example, Ann Oakley, in a 1979 article, wrote, "The female control of reproduction is cross-culturally and historically by far the most dominant arrangement. It has, in the industrial world, been transformed into a system of male control."[121]

CHAPTER 5

Pain and Death in Childbirth

EVEN THOUGH pregnancy is a natural, physiological process and not a pathological one, it can be nonetheless *highly dangerous*. In this chapter I shall discuss the dangers, with the understanding that they touched only a minority of births. Yet word gets around. If a woman knew ten or fifteen other women, she probably knew someone who had died giving birth, or who would later die. Risks of this magnitude create a collective sense of fearfulness. There is no doubt that the typical woman in the years before 1900 faced her approaching delivery with foreboding.

Women's Fears

When a Massachusetts woman, Sarah Stearns, faced birth for the first time, she wrote in her diary after taking communion with relatives, "Perhaps this is the last time I shall be permitted to join with my earthly friends."[1] Mrs. A., a New Yorker, accompanied her husband in the 1840s to England, where she found herself pregnant for the first time. She would not divulge her age to Dr. W. B. Kesteven, who examined her, but she certainly communicated her uneasiness. He wrote, "I felt unusual confidence in endeavoring to dispel the *ordinary despondency* of pregnant women approaching the time of delivery, which in the present instance had obtained an unusual hold upon the patient" (my italics).[2] Looking back around 1914 upon earlier pregnancies, a working-class Englishwoman said, "I always prepared myself to die, and I think this awful depression is common to most at this time."[3] Granted that these are merely isolated quotes, a scattering of evidence that might belie a more fundamental optimism about childbearing. Yet in the literature this sense of ominousness turns up again and again, while I have seen little optimism or enthusiasm, especially among first mothers.

When "childbed fever" started to spread, expectant mothers became wild with apprehension. A Dunkirk doctor described an epidemic that broke out in 1855: "The fate of the new mothers preoccupied many of the women who had not yet delivered. They sought to know the number of stricken, passing it on and exaggerating it, and ended up knowing how many despite our efforts to keep it secret." Marie David, a poor Dunkirk woman, was so obsessed by the death of several women of her acquaintance that, at the first sign of her own infection, she cried out "I know I'm going to die," and in fact died a week later.[4]

These appropriate apprehensions became woven into the fabric of women's culture, so that the collective wisdom about how a normal pregnancy should be approached inevitably contained rules for cheating death. One forestalled death, first of all, through prayers and rites. When in 1702, Magdalena Geisenhöfin, in the village of Pfarrstetten, learned of a new pregnancy, she was "not a little disturbed, because this time, like the last, things could turn bad and unpleasant. So after her pains began, a ring was put on her finger which had been placed in the miraculous goblet of our St. Magnus."[5] Alsatian women would wrap about themselves during labor long scrolls of paper, supposedly cut to the "True Length of Christ," on which prayers had been inscribed.[6] And in Styria, as labor approached, women stuck consecrated objects under their pillows, prayed to Saint Margaret, the patron saint of childbirth, or drank "holy water" that had been blessed on 27 December. Labor once begun, they fastened on themselves portraits of saints and prayed from a special book on which was written, "Whosoever carries this prayer about will not die suddenly . . . and every pregnant woman will give birth easily."[7] In this manner did English village women also pray to St. Margaret or the Virgin Mary "to reduce pangs of labor."[8]

The skies were searched for prognostications. "If Ash Wednesday's completely cloudy, all new mothers will die in the same year," said the Württembergers.[9] This collective lore about childbirth amounts to what Mireille Laget has called "a collective awareness of the brutality that the mother experiences."[10] Repeated from generation to generation, this folklore alerted women to the risks that their womanhood entailed.

I have already described the scenes of village women clustering about a mother in her delivery. When a woman actually lay dying, terrible scenes would make their mark on the collective consciousness! Mrs. M. gave birth on a bed of straw in a cold farmhouse near Steinau sometime in the 1860s. The midwife had manually removed the afterbirth and ruptured her uterus in the process. Immediately after the midwife had withdrawn her hand, the woman said to her husband, "My dearest, I think I'm going to die. She's torn everything out of my belly." And then she said, "My hands are dying, my feet are dying." Ten minutes later she died.[11] The sources tell of another, terribly difficult delivery which I shall not describe in detail. The midwife had called a barber-surgeon, who ruptured the mother's uterus with his instruments. All of a sudden the woman cried out, "Oh, my God. I think I'm going to die. You've torn out my insides. I beg you in Christ's name, just let me get my breath a bit," and then she died.[12]

But how justified was this fear? How many deliveries in fact ran into trouble? Plenty.

Complications

A preliminary word about how many deliveries encountered complications. What constitutes a "normal" delivery is partly subjective. As we shall see, an infection after delivery might seem normal to the mother, yet abnormal to her doctor. What seems to the mother an abnormally long labor, fourteen hours perhaps, might appear—in the light of statistics—routine.

How often did the midwives themselves think that a complication was present? The statistics on how often they called in doctors to help range widely: from 7 percent of all deliveries (a German village around 1900) to 23 percent of all deliveries (trained English midwives in the 1920s). The less trained the midwife, and the longer the doctor would have to travel on horseback, the fewer the calls for help. The doctors, for their part, thought that about one birth in ten involved complications.[13]

The mother's own judgment of the frequency of complications accords fairly closely with these estimates of "one in ten." Of the mothers who went to Margaret Sanger's birth control clinic in New York, 21 percent said that at least one of their previous labors had been difficult (table 5.1). Each of these women had given birth an average of three times.

TABLE 5.1

Complications of Pregnancy in 28,000 Births (New York City, in the 1920s, as Reported by the Mothers)

Complication	Percentage of All Pregnancies in Which the Following Complication Appeared:
Eclampsia, nephritis, vomiting	1.7
Mental-nervous disorders	.2
Gastrointestinal, cardiac disorder	.2
Bleeding, placental disorders	1.6
Sepsis (genital and breast)	.2
Difficult labor	20.8
Total complications	24.7

SOURCE: See notes to tables, page 376.
NOTE: The rates for eclampsia and mental disorders have as their denominator the 39,000 total pregnancies, as opposed to the 28,000 pregnancies carried to term.

Thus, from the mother's viewpoint, the typical birth had a 7-percent risk of complications (if one had only three children).

How frequent were other complications aside from difficult labor? Not very. For the New York women they added about another 5 percent to the 20-percent chance of difficult labor, putting at 25 percent the total risk from complications over one's fertile years (table 5.1 gives an overview). Remember, this is the overall risk of obstetric trouble, rather than the risk for each pregnancy.

In other words we must not conclude that if today "95 percent" of births are without complication,[14] the same was true of the past. The granny midwives of small-town Europe may have called the doctor no more than 5 percent of the time, which we may take as the minimum of genuinely terrible complications. But trained midwives saw problems much more often. And the mothers themselves believed they had at least a one-in-four lifetime chance of some unpleasant "abnormality," usually a painful "difficult" labor.

SLOW LABOR

What is a difficult labor, and what causes it?

Of the various causes of slow labor, least significant is the baby's position in the mother's body. The first part of the infant to appear in the birth canal determines the "presentation." Of the many aspects of our story, this one has probably changed least over the centuries. Most children are born head first. But perhaps 2 percent to 4 percent of the presentations can get the mother into serious trouble.

Here's how. In a normal delivery, as the ninth month approaches, the infant's head slides down into the mother's pelvis. The child will be lying on its left side, its chin resting on its chest (so that the neck is "flexed"). Then as labor begins, the mother's contractions force the baby's head down through the pelvis and into the birth canal. The chin remains pressed against the chest, but the head turns so that it is straight up and down. Thus, the first part of the child to emerge is the base of its skull, the occiput. Then as the rest of the head emerges into the outside world, the chin slowly rises from the chest and pops out, too.

Sometimes, however, not the head at all but the infant's buttocks are the first part to engage in the pelvis, so that the buttocks themselves, or the feet or knees, are the first part to be born. Although this kind of "breech" presentation sounds ominous, it actually has little impact on the speed of labor; but the infant's head becomes the last part to be born and is especially at risk of injury.[15] Breech presentation occurred then, as it does now, in about 3.5 percent of all labors.

In two kinds of presentation the infant has great difficulty being born, and unless the mother has skilled help, or unless her natural contractions are able spontaneously to correct the presentation, she will die undelivered. In perhaps one half of 1 percent of births, the child's *face* presents at the vagina, its head severely extended backward rather than flexed forward. As long as it stays in that position, it cannot be born. In fact some four fifths of the face presentations did in the past correct themselves sooner or later, permitting a spontaneous delivery. In Marie Lachapelle's midwifery service at a Paris maternity hospital, 88 out of the 101 face presentations, in the years between 1812 and 1820, were ultimately delivered spontaneously.[16] But this delivery often entailed agonizing delays for the mother and lacerations of the muscles of her "pelvic floor."

Another kind of presentation was far less likely to correct itself spontaneously—a "transverse lie." It happened in perhaps 1 percent of deliveries that the infant lay crosswise inside the mother's pelvis rather than lengthwise, so that its shoulder was first to appear in the birth canal. Thus, the arm would be the first part to be born, and in that position an infant is undeliverable. Sometimes the mother's contractions can correct the problem spontaneously, but usually she needs an operation, or she will die undelivered. Marie Lachapelle's midwives were able to deliver spontaneously only 12 of the 118 Parisian mothers with this condition.[17] The others required operations.

The following little tabulation, based on thirty-one thousand deliveries in the rural Swiss county of Sursee from 1891 to 1929, shows approximately the frequency of each of these various presentations:

Head, nose down (occiput anterior)	92.9 percent
Head, nose up (occiput posterior)	1.4
Face	.6
Breech (feet, knees, hips)	3.1
Transverse	2.0
Total	100.0 percent[18]

Thus 93 percent of all births would be perfectly straightforward head presentations, where the child's nose is pointing downward as it emerges from the mother. Nor should there have been any grave problem with the "breeches," which composed an additional 3 percent. Only when the child is born with its nose pointing upward (occiput posterior), or when the face blocks the vaginal outlet, or when the infant lies crosswise, would the mother risk being unable to deliver or experience a terribly slow delivery. Such situations add up to only 4 percent of the total.

In absolute terms, 4 percent doesn't sound like much, but considerable variability existed from place to place. Of thirteen studies, each of more than ten thousand deliveries, face and brow presentations could amount to as much as 1 percent of the total, as in London in the 1840s and 1850s. While only .2 percent of the mothers who gave birth in Dublin's Rotunda Hospital in the 1820s had transverse lies, *over 2 percent* of the Austrian mothers birthing toward the end of the nineteenth century had them.[19] Thus, for unexplained reasons some groups of women could find themselves at risk of malpresentations.

Keep in mind as well that, even though these percentages appear low, a large number of women could find their lives dramatically affected by malpresentations. In Vienna, for example, from 1898 to 1902, 1,500 women underwent the horrors of a transverse lie (excluding births at the General Hospital). Thus, even though only .7 percent of the 225,000 women who delivered in those years were affected, they add up to a considerable sum.[20] Among the 108 mothers who recorded their pregnancy histories in a Württemberg village toward the turn of the century, 8 transverse lies occurred among some 475 deliveries. Assuming each happened to a different woman, almost one out of ten women in the village was struck by this major kind of emergency![21] So rather than being remote risks that would never descend into an ordinary woman's life, these malpresentations—of the face and shoulder in particular—could easily occur in the community.

"Difficult labor" means that the birth went on for a long time rather than ending in twelve hours or so—the average today. Normal labors can vary greatly in length, some taking place in just an hour or two, others needing much longer. First mothers, for example, typically labor about six hours longer than do women who have already born children (fourteen hours versus eight).[22]* We have no reason to think that women in the past had weaker uterine muscles than women today, or that they produced larger children (in fact, the average infant was smaller at birth). So if the average birth dragged on sixteen hours or so, the reason is that in those days birth attendants were less likely to intervene.[24] Augustus Granville, for example, supervisor of a home midwife service in early nineteenth-century London, said he did not believe in interfering before fifty hours![25] Such "watchful waiting" meant, of course that births would last longer. Perhaps one third of the nineteenth-century births on which we have information lasted more than twenty hours. Today only one labor in ten lasts that long.[26] (It is at around twenty hours that doctors today intervene, because thereafter the infant's chances of dying increase significantly).[27] Or, as one writer says, "It is unwise ever to allow the sun to set twice during any one labor."[28]

The practical implication of these statistics is that the average woman before 1900 was likely to spend about five hours longer in labor than she would today. She had perhaps a one-in-three chance of laboring more than twenty hours, and the books are full of confinements that lasted longer than forty-eight hours.

These protracted labors, or "dystocias," might have been caused by the rigidity of the cervix—that is, its unwillingness to let the uterus's contractions push through the bag of waters. Or the dystocia could have come from the weakness of the uterus's own contractions, or from an overly small maternal pelvis—so that the child's head had literally to be pounded through. Or dystocia might come from an overly large infant head, as "hydrocephalus," for example—an excess of cerebrospinal fluid—balloons out the skull. There are, in other words, many potential causes of slow labor, which it is unnecessary to discuss in detail. Moreover, with the exception of pelvises contracted by rickets, we often don't know the cause in historic times.

Slowness did not necessarily mean disaster. In April of 1711, Guillaume de la Motte, the man midwife who lived in a small town in Normandy, was called to the home of a gentlewoman. Her contractions were infrequent, and he spent the night there. At 6:00 A.M. she had a few violent pains; he could feel the child's head; but the waters broke only twenty-four hours later; and only two full days after that, was the infant finally

* Labor for white primiparas at the Johns Hopkins Hospital between 1937 and 1945 lasted an average of thirteen hours; for multiparas, eight hours.[23]

born. It was a boy, who was "doing fine, although his head was terribly elongated." The mother, "as exhausted as I was," also did well.[29] One granny midwife in the American South said that "anyone can stand a day of being in labor; it's on the second and third and fourth days when you're 'plum wore out' and 'feel like you can't do nothing else' that you wish you could die and don't see how you can stand it."[30] But for these women, and many like them whose only problem was slowness to dilate the cervix, things ultimately went well.

When the cause of the delay, however, was some mechanical obstruction, such as an overly small pelvis or a malpresentation, the birth scenario would unfold more ominously. In August of 1697, de la Motte was called to the home of a poor woman in Gréneville parish. He found her with a "continual cough, her abdomen hard, tense, and swollen up to her throat; her eyes were deeply sunken, her lips purple, her breath stank, and her extremities were cold and showed almost no pulse"—all signs of a raging infection and shock. She had apparently been long in labor, unable to give birth because the infant's arm was "sticking out [of the vagina] almost to the shoulder, large, black, squishy, and cold." De la Motte delivered her; and, surprisingly, she recovered.[31]

Such long labor was not a death sentence. But the longer it went on, the less became one's chance of emerging from it successfully. The mother would become "distressed," her heart pounding, her breath rapid; she would be dehydrated and feverish as "acidosis" (an accumulation of acid in the bloodstream) commenced, making her feel exhausted. As successive contractions cut off the oxygen exchange in the placenta, the child, too, would become distressed. Something would have to be done.

What Could Be Done?

What could midwives and doctors do, before the advent of the caesarean delivery, to shorten difficult labor?

FIRST POSSIBILITY: DO NOTHING

In many traditional societies women unable to deliver spontaneously were once simply abandoned, left to die undelivered.[32]* Europe before 1800 was not necessarily a traditional society, in the sense of nineteenth-century Morocco, Algeria, or the South Sea islands, for it possessed an

---

* John Robertson cited testimony of two South Seas missionaries;[33] and Edward Ford, writing of the D'Entrecasteaux Islands in 1940, said, "No treatment is known for the complications of labour and in obstructed labour the case is regarded as hopeless and death is awaited."[34]

impulse to activism in the face of obstetric disaster that can be traced right back to the Greeks and Romans. Yet many granny midwives and helping neighbors simply did not know what to do if a mother ran into trouble, and so she would be left to die. Louise Bourgeois, a skilled midwife, deplored other midwives who were "so presumptuous as to think that if after a few efforts they could not deliver a woman then, for better or worse, all is lost." Such midwives would even send a surgeon away, if friends had summoned him, "and thus let die mother and child."[35] Percivall Willughby often found "the mother undelivered, and she and the child dead before I could come unto them, through the ignorance of such midwives." Willughby and his daughter traveled all night through the rain to Congerton on one occasion, coming by daybreak to the place: "But this lady was dead, undelivered, before our coming. I much desired to see her corps, but the midwife would not permit it. I knew this midwife not to be very judicious in her profession, and I believe that she was ashamed that her work should be seen Anno 1655. This midwife was gentle in habit of cloths, but ignorant in the ways of practice of midwifery."[36]

When confronted with an unfamiliar situation, many midwives just gave up. Administrative officials in out-of-the-way places like Agde, Mende, and Barre in Old Regime France said that "the ineptitude of these [midwives] is so great that if the delivery is not natural, the mother and child die."[37] Moritz Thilenius noted that "in cities, or in a place where there is a skilled midwife, it happens very seldom that a woman dies during the birth." In the countryside, however, "the midwives do not know what to do in a malpresentation, and usually they leave things to nature too long. . . . Their ignorance is the reason that many mothers die with their infants during the birth."[38] Once when François Mauriceau arrived at the home of a forty-three-year-old woman, in labor for nine days with her first child, he found the situation of the infant normal. The thing to do, he explained to the relatives, is deliver her by turning. But they protested, "thinking it better to let her die than to torture her unnecessarily. This request was unreasonable, but in view of the mother's deplorable state I was obliged to abandon her to her fate." (The mother did deliver spontaneously a day later, but died of "gangrene.")[39] Thus, there is no doubt that if mothers in traditional Europe got into difficulty, they might be just written off.

SECOND POSSIBILITY: "FOLKLORIC REMEDIES"

Folkloric remedies mean any traditional solution for dystocia that did not involve vaginal intervention. Simplest of these folkloric solutions were the magical ones. One of the most common "charms" of the Irish country people involved "loosening every place, person, or thing in or about the house, unlocking all the locks, unbarring doors and windows, untieing all knots and even setting free the cows in the byre"—according to the logic that setting free things externally might induce the uterus as well as to set free its contents.[40] For difficult labor in Hungary's Heveser County, the husband would step three times over the wife, then fumigate her vulvar area by burning the band from his underpants or by burning hairs from his own and his wife's armpits. If these remedies did not help, he might have intercourse with her.[41] Among the Slovaks of Nograder County, the husband would let the wife drink from his own mouth, put the band from his underdrawers around her abdomen, and then urinate in his boot and have his wife drink from it.[42] And so on. Magical solutions for dystocia were found everywhere among the people, and interest us not necessarily because they worked, but because they represent a determination to help a mother in straits.

The next line of folkloric defense would be drugs. Several times in this book I refer to a peasant preoccupation with "polypharmacy," dosing oneself with a variety of "infusions" and "potions" for every complaint imaginable. Confronted by medical problems, traditional Europeans felt most comfortable in taking drugs compounded from local plants. Some plants do contain chemicals that seem to have an elective effect upon the uterus. I shall consider these in the chapter on drugs for abortion, but here I wish merely to point out that some of these "potions" could have reinforced the contractions of the uterus. It is clear, for example, that ergot, a black fungus found growing on stalks of grain, strengthens the uterine muscle; and indeed, alkaloids derived from it are much used today in delivery rooms. Europe's peasants took ergot long before it was rediscovered in 1808 by the medical profession.[43] They took as well a long list of other chemicals for difficult labor, some of which might have worked, others being almost certainly useless or toxic. "In Mittelfranken people prefer for difficult labor the ankle bone of a rabbit which has been shot on one of the first three Fridays in March. You shave off three knife-tips of bone and give it to the mother." Or, "Give the suffering mother two slices of the roots of a white lily." Or, "Give the mother a couple of spoonfuls of the water in which two eggs have cooked."[44] In another part of Bavaria, country people would reach in difficult labor for their bottles of *essentia dulcis* and *spiritus apoplecticus* and for their vermifuges and cinnamon sticks and so on.[45] The list is endless. The point is that when things did not go as planned, after prayers and magical amulets, the mother would usually get some disagreeable concoction to drink.

If drugs failed, the last line of folkloric defense would be to try and shake out the fetus by rattling the mother around or turning her upside down. Dr. W. R. Wilde on the "lower orders" of Ireland: "In some localities it was not in former times uncommon, when the labour was very tedious, to get two or three stout men to shake the unhappy patient backwards and forwards in her bed with great violence. . . . A ploughman was more frequently chosen for such purposes than any other person; but, to prove efficacious, he should be taken direct from the plough."[46] Willughby tells of "a poor creature, not far from Ashburn, that was willing to suffer any affliction to be delivered. . . . Her conceited midwife's last refuge was . . . to toss her in a blanket, as some have served dogs, hoping that this violent motion would force the child out of her body."[47] In the Karasjok district of Lappland, if the child refused to come out, people would grab the mother's feet and knees, turn her upside down and shake her up and down three times, thus presumably correcting a complicated presentation.[48] The French equivalent of this practice was to tie the mother upside down on a ladder.[49] In the Tana district of Lappland, the mother would lie atop a blanket, and two men, then grabbing the edges, would jerk her back and forth in it.[50] When in Finland the child's head refused to come out, the mother was encouraged to shake it out by jumping down from the oven bench or from the plank bed in the bathhouse.[51] One can imagine the ruptures of the uterus, tears of the birth canal, and hemorrhages that attended this kind of folkloric intervention.

THIRD POSSIBILITY: PULLING ON WHATEVER PRESENTS ITSELF

If folkloric devices failed, the next step would be for the birth attendants to try to pull out the child by any part they could get hold of. There is a rich peasant tradition of tugging on whatever presents itself. "If the midwife finds any unusual presentation," wrote one observer in 1752, "she becomes confused and . . . begins to pull, even if it is a polyp growing to the uterus, whereby often the mother pays with her life."[52] It happened in one place that the mother gave birth successfully but that, after the placenta was out, another mass, a polyp, presented itself in the vagina. The midwife tore it away. Then a second, smaller polyp appeared, which the midwife pulled away as well. Although the mother fainted at this point, her bleeding had stopped. Everyone was reassured, so she was put to bed, and the family sat down to a celebratory dinner. "Scarcely were they at table when I rode in on my horse," recounted the doctor. "They received me joyously, told of the preceding events, and invited me to sit down to eat. I, however, wished to see the mother first. They took me to her room where she gave me her hand but was unable to speak for weakness. She appeared deathly pale and was ice-cold. Nor could a pulse be felt. I ordered the covers to be pulled back, and we found her swimming in blood."[53] This story illustrates how much in the natural course of things it was for obstructions to be pulled away.

If, in fact, all the preceding shaking and hanging and drugging failed, the midwife would just try to pull out with brute force whatever part she could grasp.[54] An inviting target for pulling was the infant's head, just having popped out of the birth canal, the shoulders stuck behind. There are straightforward ways of handling this kind of "shoulder dystocia," but one of them is not to pull on the head with all one's might and main, lest one detach it. De la Motte found himself often called in such cases: "On 21 July 1704 I was summoned to deliver a woman in Saint-Colombe parish. . . . I found on arrival that the midwife had pulled off the child's head, without having tugged greatly. She was so contrite and afflicted that I tried to console her and omitted giving a reprimand."[55] (Given such traction as actually to separate the head from the body, just think how frequent were birth injuries to the spinal and neck nerves!)

If the child's arm was born first (a transverse lie), tugging would be ruinous. Imagine the scene. The midwife would go to examine the mother, bend down, and find a little hand sticking out of the vagina. What was the midwife to do in such a situation? The best academic knowledge of the time said to push the arm back in the uterus and wait for this malpresentation to correct itself naturally. If the mother's natural contractions did not turn the child to a better position, the birth attendant should "turn" it, about which more in a minute.[56] The standard village solution to this problem, however, was to pull mightily on the arm, hoping thus to pull out the child—anatomically impossible. Or, to cut off the arm and then see what happened.[57] Around Soissons, said Dr. Augier du Fot, if an arm or a leg appears first, the midwives simply cut it off.[58]

Here is a typical, in fact fairly experienced, German midwife in 1822, delivering a mother with a transverse lie. The neighbors and family agreed, after the local granny had proven unable to cope, to send for midwife Veronika Paul, who lived in a nearby village and was reputed "often to have acted skillfully in difficult labors." She arrived about twelve hours later, examined the mother, and stated that she "had successfully conducted perhaps ten or eleven deliveries of this kind." After a few manipulations, Frau Paul successfully brought one of the child's hands out of the vagina and then proceeded to pull on it "with such force that the arm tore off and the child's torso remained behind in the mother." Now followed a series of fruitless attempts, at the end of which the mother died.[59] The point is that even the renowned Frau Paul's solution to difficulties was to pull as hard as she could on anything she could reach.

The three midwives in England who delivered Mary Hector, wife of a barber-surgeon, in July of 1670 were unable to resist pulling at a prolapsed

arm, finally cutting it off at the shoulder. When Willughby arrived on
the scene, they attempted to dissimulate and brought the baby to him
"very handsomely put into a shirt, and the arm was put up into the
sleeve unto the shoulder, and the hand tied at the wrist, and decently
laid by the child's side.

"It was so well done and shrouded that to one that knew nothing
and had only looked on the child's body, thus shrouded, this ill work
at a distance, could not have been perceived that the arm was cut off
at the shoulder."[60]

Thus deeply rooted in traditional midwifery was the impulse to pull
at whatever one could. I belabor this matter only because, in recent times,
we have heard so much about the "wise women" of yore and their special
kind of knowledge that represented centuries of practical experience, etcetera.* In fact, traditional lore existed for normal deliveries and was useless
when anything went wrong.

FOURTH POSSIBILITY: AN OBSTETRIC OPERATION

If this traditional wisdom failed, the next recourse for the villagers
would be to perform an obstetric operation. Although there is only one
"traditional" operation as such—embryotomy—some important "modern" operations had been known in village culture since the sixteenth
century. What operations might have helped a laboring mother in dire
straits?

Version. Version, or "turning," was the first procedure to which doctors
and midwives would have recourse, if the mother had an unnatural presentation, the child's head was too big, or her own contractions too ineffec-
tual. I am speaking here of "internal" version, which means actually
reaching the hand into the uterus to turn the child about. Some of the
ancient Greek doctors, for example, preferred to turn the child onto its
head ("cephalic version"), so that it could better "aid in its own delivery."
Others preferred to turn it feet down, and then simply to extract it by
the feet ("podalic version" with "extraction"). But during the Middle
Ages, academic medicine lost sight of version, and only in 1550 did Ambroise Paré describe turning the infant feet down as the best way to deal
with malpresentations.[62] It is likely that skilled urban midwives had not
lost sight of version, for sometime before 1550, Dr. Ortolff of Bavaria
alluded to turning as though it were perfectly familiar to his midwife
audience and required no further explanation. In 1513, Eucharius Rösslin
cursorily mentioned in his textbook both podalic and cephalic version,

* One example among many: "If she [the typical housewife of some premodern golden
age] was exceptionally skilled, she became a midwife, herbal healer or 'wise woman,' whose
fame might spread from house to house and village to village. . . . So there could be no
Woman Question in the Old Order."[61]

confident that his readers already knew the procedure.[63] So it is academic medicine, recovering from its long uninterest in matters obstetrical, that in the sixteenth century rediscovered version. Paré's textbook was widely read; and in the period I am calling traditional—roughly 1500–1850— internal podalic version was the procedure of choice in obstructed labor.

What did version mean to the women of a village? In 1771 the town of Runkel-Wied instructed its midwives on version as follows: "In case of malpresentation, lack of pains, hemorrhage and the like, the midwife will have to perform version. She should abstain from such phrases as "The child has stuck to the uterus and so cannot get out," and instead just quickly stick her hand into the uterus and turn the child, that is, hunt for first one foot, then the other. She then pulls on both feet together and, as the mother presses down, pulls the child downward and out of the mother's body, taking care to make sure the infant's heels are directed toward the midwife, the toes toward the mother."[64] This last precaution was to ensure that the infant would be pulled out with its face directed downward, so that its chin would not risk getting caught on the mother's pubic bone.

The Runkel-Wied code makes it sound simple. In reality, version was horribly painful, in the absence of any anesthesia (not until 1847 were ether and chloroform used obstetrically). Here is a story from the Herisau district of Switzerland around 1800. A forty-two-year-old woman, pregnant for the tenth time, had already been five days in labor. The granny midwife finally summoned Dr. I. G. Oberteufer, who tried for three hours to turn the child from its transverse lie. No luck. He called his father, who was also a doctor; and the two of them pulled away at the mother again for another several hours. Still no luck. Finally they told her, "We are unable to deliver you, but let us send for a couple of birth attendants from St. Gallen." "No thanks," she replied, saying that she preferred to die instead.[65]

One doctor, who did a lot of rural deliveries, wrote in 1901: "I still think back with horror to a difficult version I was obliged to do in a transverse lie without anesthesia. The awful cries of the woman, who called out for death, the terrible agitation of the relatives, which can easily infect the doctor himself and move him to ill-considered actions, the demanding nature of the operation, will always remain in my mind."[66]

So word got around of how painful version was. Sometimes women had to be tricked into it, if there were no other way to deliver them. De la Motte was called in 1704 to a farmer's wife whose infant lay crosswise, an arm protruding. As soon as he began his explanations at her bedside, she interrupted him, knowing full well why he was there, and said in her agony that she wanted only to be delivered "by the ribs" (a reference to caesarean section). If he wouldn't do it, he should leave. De la Motte shrugged and turned to four men, "who were there among innumerable women," asking them if they would help to save their good friend. So he took all his knives and hooks from his bag, and acted as though he were about to perform the section, asking the woman to cooper-ate by lying on the straw. She did; but, instead of operating, he reached his hand into her birth canal. The four men were scarcely able to hold her, for she was "one of the largest and strongest women I have ever seen," and struggled fiercely. But de la Motte successfully turned the infant, which had been dead for some time, and the mother survived.[67] Among village women version had such a reputation for being painful that they preferred to undergo a caesarean section.

In those pre-caesarean days, versions had to be done perhaps twice in every hundred deliveries. Of the figures I have seen, the lowest is .4 per 100 home deliveries in London in the 1840s, the highest, 3.6 percent in the town of Memmingen toward 1800. Several large series of statistics, such as Sursee County's 32,000 births, cluster around 2 percent.* Thus, a mother who bore five children would have perhaps a one-in-ten lifetime chance of experiencing version.

Keep in mind that most traditional midwives felt perfectly competent to do version, that it was not a procedure reserved for doctors. The New England midwife Jane Hawkins, involved in a later witchcraft trial because one infant had been a monster, testified that the baby "which was of ordinary bigness, came hiplings [breech] till she turned it."[73] "I deny not," Edmund Chapman, a London man midwife, said in 1735, "that many women midwives may know how to turn a child, nor that they may, in some subjects, perform it with success. But then considering the many unforeseen difficulties that may happen, especially the head's sticking against the bones of the pelvis . . . ," Chapman thought it better that doctors be called when version was necessary.[74] A German midwife, accused of having through inexperience torn the uterus while doing ver-sion, replied proudly that she had already done twenty-four versions.[75] A final piece of evidence: In Prussia around 1890, doctors were debating whether to recommend that version by midwives be made illegal. The licensed midwives responded in their own defense that all the granny

---

* The risk, however, would fall more heavily on mothers who had had infantile rickets. For series on version, see Höfling, who includes the births from a maternity hospital—613 versions in 76,000 deliveries;[68] C. F. Danz and C. F. Fuchs, who—evidently in the 1840s—recorded 18 versions in 4,700 deliveries;[69] Rudolph Beck, whose study was based on 32,000 deliveries, 1891–1929; and half of the versions were for transverse lies;[70] Otto Büttner, on the basis of 18,000;[71] and John Hall Davis, for the western district of the Royal Maternity Charity in London.[72]

midwives did them, and that the legal midwives would lose the respect of the patients if they could not do them, too![76]* So it is clear that both trained and granny midwives alike regularly performed version.

Forceps. But what if version was impossible? Let us say, for example, that the mother had been in labor so long that the infant's head was wedged tightly in her pelvis, so that the birth attendant would be unable to slip a hand past to grab the feet. Or say that the birth attendant did not wish to risk rupturing the mother's uterus—as would be easily possible with version—or to subject the mother to great pain. What could be done?

Before the invention of forceps, the only recourse would be to destroy the infant by perforating its head, evacuating the contents of the skull, and then letting the mother deliver the rest of the body naturally—a horrible procedure, and one to which I will come in a few pages. After the middle of the eighteenth century, however, the birth attendant had an option that might spare the infant and would reduce the mother's risk of being lacerated either by the sharp knives of infant-destruction operations or by the bony fragments of the infant's skull. This option was the obstetric forceps, invented by members of the Chamberlen family, a London dynasty of male midwives which commenced late in the sixteenth century. The Chamberlens had been greedy and, for many years, kept their invention secret, operating under the cover of a sheet. But by the 1730s news of the forceps got out; and shortly thereafter, two man midwives, William Smellie and André Levret, invented improved models which were far better than the Chamberlens' originals.[77]

A forceps is simply a big set of tongs with two curved blades. Each blade is fitted separately about the infant's head. Then the blades are locked together, and the doctor pulls. All this sounds simple, but the doctor can get into trouble if the child's head has not yet descended into the pelvis, or if the mother's cervix is not yet entirely dilated. Doctor Jean-Marie Munaret knew of many rustic occasions in France where "a number of persons" would pull together on the forceps, "tearing off part of the infant." "The women of the countryside fear this instrument more than do city women. What is certain is that one can do a lot of damage with it."[78] Precisely. With its tremendous grip, the forceps offered the advantage of terminating long labors quickly. But exactly for that reason it could be deadly.

Forceps deliveries at home, without anesthesia, could be fearsome. Midwife Lisbeth Burger told how she and the father had to hold the wife down while the doctor delivered her with forceps: "The groaning and whimpering of the mother dominated everything in the room, the jerking

* The reported midwife version rate in Ostpreussen was .3 percent.

and shaking of her tortured body. . . . After all that pulling and levering, holding and bleeding, the child finally emerged from the mother's lap. Torn and hemorrhaging, exhausted to death, the poor mother lay back against the cushions."[79] The London man midwife William Hunter used to show his students a pair of forceps, rusty from disuse, and say that "it was a thousand pities they were ever invented," because "where they save one they murder twenty."[80]

Initially, forceps were used only slightly more often than version—an interesting comment on the doctors' aversion to them, in view of the greater risks of version for the mother. By the end of the nineteenth century, however, forceps were applied in Central Europe in perhaps 2 percent of all deliveries, while version had begun to disappear.*

Because the forceps appeared so late in time, it never became—unlike version—part of the tradition of skilled midwives. Although reports crop up from time to time of midwives with forceps in their kits,[83] most midwives left forceps to the doctors, indeed hated them. "In the use of instruments," wrote Friedrich B. Osiander in 1787, "I found few [of the local midwives] of assistance. Some clasped their hands together and ran away when I talked about applying forceps. In scarcely a quarter of the nineteen forceps deliveries which I have done around here in the last four years— all of which ending happily for the mother—did the midwife on the scene give me any help." He complained especially that none of them was up to holding the first forceps blade in place while he applied the second.[84]

There were many reasons for the traditional midwives' uneasiness about forceps, not least of which was their resentment about being diminished, in the eyes of their clients, by the doctors. Nonetheless, long before the midwives were legally forbidden to use instruments, they voluntarily shied away from forceps. On 28 May 1768, London man midwife John Knyveton wrote in his diary, "I have ushered into the world eleven children [in the last two weeks], two or three of them not quite normal in presentation—in one the midwife wished me to use the forceps, but this I feared to do, the perineum being very tight."[85]† She might have applied them herself, but didn't, giving us some understanding of why the midwives ultimately lost out as the doctors' equals. It is well known that some of these British midwives, such as Elizabeth Nihell, bitterly fought the male doctors and their forceps. Yet my impression is that most midwives were more concerned for the health of their patients, and for the infants,

---

* In one area of London in the 1840s and 1850s there were more perforations of the fetal skull than forceps deliveries![81] In several million births in Bavaria from 1878 to 1890, forceps were used in 1.6 percent.[82]

† According to Jean Donnison, it was in England at this time "custom" that forbade forceps to midwives.[86]

than for their own economic position. And they saw that, despite what William Hunter said, the forceps could bring deliverance from suffering. Margaret Stephen, a London midwife, wrote in 1795 that "the forceps are of the greatest utility. . . . There is none of all the instruments I ever saw so well calculated to save the lives of children."[87]

Did forceps inspire fear or confidence in women? One of the early French obstetricians, Jean-Louis Baudelocque, would give a woman one of the blades of the forceps to hold, and not start the operation until she had handed it back. But his successors discontinued this practice. "We have found that no demonstration is able to instill confidence, and that only actions themselves—that means the skillful and painless application of the forceps, plus a happy result—are able to remove their fear."[88] A century later Berlin's Max Hirsch thought the attitude of women had changed completely: "I do not deceive myself in saying that the fear of forceps is not especially great among the common people, that, to the contrary, the application of the instrument is often requested for the quick termination of the delivery."[89]

Mothers swallowed their fears, or at least some of them, with good cause. The mortality from forceps deliveries at home declined steadily. In the 1830s in the province of Fulda, one's chance of dying in a forceps-assisted delivery was one in twenty-five; in Oberhessen, one in thirty-three.[90] By the 1890s elsewhere in Germany, the chance had sunk to one in one hundred; thereafter one in two hundred, one in five hundred, until by the 1920s the risk of dying through the application of forceps had become negligible.[91]

Embryotomy. If the mother could be delivered neither by version nor by forceps, one possibility alone remained: to destroy the infant with a mutilating operation, or "embryotomy." If the baby's head was pierced with scissors and then pulled down with a sharp hook, the procedure was called "craniotomy." "The conditions almost always met are these," wrote Joseph DeLee. "The woman has been in labor many hours or even days, unclean hands have frequently examined her, attempts at delivery with the forceps have failed, the vulva is torn and bruised, the cervix hangs in shreds, the urine is bloody, the child is injured or perhaps dying. Here there is only one course—craniotomy."[92] When Adrian Wegelin, a St. Gallen doctor, was called to a twenty-eight-year-old woman, pregnant for the first time, she had been in labor for ten hours. The child's head, "unnaturally swollen," was in the pelvis, refusing to advance. Consider Wegelin's options: "version was impossible" because the head was jammed in the middle of the pelvis, leaving no room for his hand. He and another colleague, summoned to the scene, tried forceps but were able to apply only one blade, which kept slipping off and was finally bent out of shape!

The only thing left was to perforate the skull, which he did by boring a hole in the frontal bone and then pulling the child down with a hook. It took the mother six weeks to recover.[93]

One can see why such odium has attached to embryotomy across the centuries. It meant often killing a live child, although Catholic doctors were supposed to attempt it only after the fetus had died.[94] It meant terrible gashes in the mother's soft parts, for the hooks and scissors for opening and crushing the skull could always slip, tearing her birth canal. And it enormously augmented the risk of infection. As a result, doctors avoided embryotomy almost at all costs, and rarely did it. In the Sursee district of Switzerland, for example, it was done only twenty-two times over a period of forty years in thirty-two thousand deliveries—once every two years, in other words.[95]* Fleetwood Churchill calculated that embryotomy was performed, on the whole, once in every nine hundred deliveries, although the British certainly did it more often than the Germans (one in every two hundred, as opposed to one in every two thousand—because the British were loathe to use forceps!).[97] Why, therefore, am I dwelling at such length upon an operation that doctors did so little? Because the midwives performed embryotomy quite often.

The skilled urban midwives of earlier centuries always carried iron hooks in their bags to extract *dead* infants. If the mother had not delivered spontaneously, and various potions had availed nothing, the midwife was supposed to call other midwives and her female supervisor to the scene. If all agreed that the infant was dead in utero, hooks would be thrust into the child's head, through the eye or the mouth, in order to haul it out. If the child presented buttocks first, the hooks would go into its back or its ribcage. The midwives were to pay careful attention not to "wound the uterus or to pull it out."[98]

But, in fact, many traditional midwives, not just these skilled urban professionals, seemed to have been conversant with the knives, sharp hooks (crotchets), and blunt hooks needed to decapitate the infant or evacuate its cranium. These procedures were done in the uterus on both live and dead infants. Dr. W. R. Wilde of St. Mark's Hospital, Dublin, wrote in 1849 that, "I have heard my father, who was in extensive practice in [County Connaught] say that he had known midwives constantly attempt forcible extraction of the fetus, with the hook of an ouncel or steel bar."[99] Willughby had several stories, such as: "A good woman dwelling at Brincliffe, nigh Sheffield, through a difficult labor, fell into the hands of an ignorant woman. She cut the child into several pieces in her body. By this midwife's knife, and the child's bones, the woman's

---

* One rural Swiss doctor who was often called to obstetric emergencies never had to do an embryotomy in ten years' practice.[96]

body was hurt in the extraction of several parts of the child's body. And, through the raising of the neck of the womb, it became ulcerated."[100]

According to de la Motte, it was because of the laziness and incompetence of the French rural surgeons that the midwives had gradually taken over the sharp hook. These midwives "push their temerity to the point of using hooks just as boldly as the surgeons themselves, and much less appropriately. In every parish and village where these midwives hold sway, there are women suffering from involuntary losses of urine, uterine prolapse, and lacerations."[101]

If the midwife did not routinely carry a hook, one would be found somewhere in the village. "In almost all difficult deliveries . . . [the midwives] use a sharp hook which they usually borrow from a weighing scale," said Dr. Augier du Fot of Soissons.[102] The French surgeon Jean-Louis Baudelocque complained that in difficult labors "the midwives and surgeons of the countryside, who generally own few instruments, resort for the sake of getting the head out to the iron hooks which the peasants use to suspend their lamps."[103]

In citing this testimony about midwives' use of embryotomy tools, I don't wish to suggest they were more incompetent than the surgeons, barbers, and shepherds, who were in there slashing away as well. The evidence of some surgeons' unsuitability for obstetric operations is astounding. When summoned to a mother in trouble in Sarstedt, near Hanover, the surgeon ordered merely hot fomentations the first time; impatient at the second call, he proceeded to cut away a portion of the infant's occipital bone (at the back of the head), and then left, prescribing warm drinks.[104] So midwives did not have a monopoly on brutality or meddlesome incompetence, but they stood far closer to the women of the villages and small towns than did these surgeons, and were prepared to use any instruments except forceps to deliver them.

This section has opened an obstetric chamber of horrors. For if traditional women encountered complications in birth, they would be in real trouble. Of all the procedures mentioned here, only version offered much hope of relief, unless a fairly up-to-date doctor lived nearby who knew how to use forceps. When, therefore, we repeat the truism that "most births were normal," let us remind ourselves that the substantial minority that were not could entail death or mutilation for the mother.

Further Complications

Two special circumstances deserve attention: women whose pelvic bones were contracted, and older women giving birth for the first time.

The reader will recall from chapter 2 the estimate that in some areas

TABLE 5.2

Contracted Pelvises among Women in Mid-nineteenth-century Parisian Maternity Hospitals: Obstetric Outcomes

Size of Pelvis	Number of Mothers with Contracted Pelvises	Percentage of Spontaneous Deliveries	Percentage of Mothers Dying
More than 10 centimeters	301	72	19
9–10 centimeters	215	42	22
8–9 centimeters	94	12	22
Less than 8 centimeters	55	4	49

NOTE: Measurements were made across the *diametre sacro-sous-pubien*, which I take to denote the diagonal conjugate.
SOURCE: See notes to tables, page 376.

perhaps one in every four women suffered from a pelvic contraction, and some of these contractions were doubtless caused by rickets. Such a narrow pelvis would reduce a mother's chances of being delivered spontaneously. "Some women have a pelvis so small," wrote a Cassel doctor, "that the opening through which the child must pass is too narrow. . . . The child is in a normal position, the sac of waters appears, the waters burst, but the head remains immovably fixed and the strongest labor pains avail nothing."[105]

Perhaps half the women with contracted pelvises ultimately delivered themselves spontaneously, as table 5.2 shows. The other half required some kind of operation, or they would die undelivered. The normal distance between one's sacral promontory (in back) and the bottom of the pubic arch (in front) is about 12.5 centimeters, or 5 inches. This is the "diagonal conjugate" of the pelvis—the front-back diameter that a doctor or a midwife can measure most easily. As table 5.2 further reveals, of 665 mothers with contracted pelvises in nineteenth-century Parisian maternity hospitals, half had only modest contractions (diameters of 10 centimeters or greater). They delivered themselves spontaneously about three quarters of the time; they died, however, much more often than normal mothers, presumably because their labors lasted longer, putting them more at risk of infection. (Their 19-percent maternal mortality contrasts with the overall 6-percent maternal mortality prevailing in Parisian maternity hospitals around that time.[106]) But the smaller the pelvis, the graver the outcome. Thus, of mothers whose pelvises were less than 8 centimeters in diameter, only 4 percent were able to give birth naturally, and half of the severely contracted mothers died.

Women with severe contractions posed nightmarish problems to their doctors and midwives. Margery Barker of Derby, for example, had a small pelvis and spent several days in labor. Willughby was summoned. He found "a narrow passage and the child had not at all descended, being hindered by the broad end of the [sacrum] inverted, and not flexible, and the child too large for so straight a passage." So he delivered her by version. Amazingly, however, she went on to become pregnant again, but this time Willughby was out of town. After six days in labor, she died undelivered. When Willughby got home, "the midwife told me that the child never descended or came within the bones [of the pelvis] and that her body being narrow, she knew not how to deliver her."[107] Many such stories dwell in the old volumes of this now-forgotten medical literature. They are of interest only because they hint at the suffering of these thousands of anonymous women. At the beginning of this section I talked about the large number of women who experienced "delayed," "obstructed," or "difficult" labor, despite their child's presenting normally by its head. These bone-deformity diseases offer much of the explanation: the pelvis had simply grown too small.

A second circumstance contributing to all these lacerations and delays in labor was the mother's relatively advanced age. Obstetricians like to talk of the early twenties as the "optimum" age for childbearing, when a woman's cervix dilates most rapidly in labor, the muscles of the uterus and abdomen press down most powerfully, and the womb most quickly regains its normal shape afterward. Having a first child becomes progressively more difficult as one gets older; so that by thirty-five, a mother giving birth the first time is considered an "elderly primipara" and watched carefully for complications.[108]

It therefore illumines the carnage of childbirth in the past to know that in European villages, perhaps 40 percent of all births occurred to women over thirty-five, and 37 percent of all first births did so![109]

Consider the risks. Whereas only 4 percent of mothers in general have labors lasting more than twenty-four hours, almost one quarter of first mothers over thirty-five have such labors.[110] Whereas only 9 percent of the mothers in general in the Innsbruck Maternity Hospital had a forceps-assisted delivery in the 1880s, 28 percent of the older first mothers had such a delivery. The "perineum" of older first mothers in that hospital was torn three times as often as was that of mothers in general.[111]*

That so many women did not give birth until late in life was owing to the fact that they married so late. Given the primitive obstetrics of village society, the cost they paid for this delay was considerable. Between 1795 and 1802, St. Gallen's Dr. Adrian Wegelin was called to a hundred obstetric emergencies—a third of them to first mothers, most of whom were over thirty-five (twelve were over forty). "In February 1801, I was

* "Older" in this source means "over thirty."

ORIGINAL INVOICE

REMIT TO:

ACTION BOOKS
RS UNIVERSITY
RUNSWICK, N.J. 08903

INVOICE DATE	INVOICE NO.		
8/31/91	378318		
ACCOUNT NO.	SHIP NO.	PAGE	
43246		1	

PURCHASE ORDER NO. EXAM COPY

SHIP TO:

GREEN, DR LINDA
NORMANDALE COLLEGE
9700 FRANCE AVE S

BLOOMINGTON   MN
                   55431

SHIP DATE	TERMS	CLASS	TYPE	FEDERAL I.D.
8/31/91	NET 30	8	8	43-090-8220

LE DESCRIPTION	PRICE	DISCOUNT	AMOUNT
S - PPR	18.95	10.00	17.05
**************			
ON BOOKS			
4 RARITAN CENTER			
.J. 08837			

POST/HANDLING	TAX	MISC.	PLEASE PAY THIS AMOUNT
3.23			$20.28 TOTAL

transaction publishers

RUTGERS UNIVERSITY
NEW BRUNSWICK, NEW JERSEY 08903

Telephone: (908) 932-2280
Fax: (908) 932-3138

TRAN
RUTG
NEW

BILL TO: GREEN, DR LINDA
NORMANDALE COLLEGE
9700 FRANCE AVE S

BLOOMINGTON   MN
55431

01-TRN-03 5/84

36773677

PURCHASE ORDER NO.			SHIP VIA	SMAN.	TERR.
EXAM COPY			U.P.S.	9999	999
ORDERED	SHIPPED	BACK ORDERED	STOCK NO.	TI	
1	1		848-5	WOMEN'S BODI	
				*****:	
				RETURNS TO:	
				TRANSACTI	
				BLDG. #42	
				EDISON,	

B/O =	BACK ORDERED ON ORIGINAL
NYP =	NOT YET PUBLISHED
OP =	OUT OF PRINT
O/S =	TEMPORARILY OUT OF STOCK

RETURNS TO
BUILDING 424
RARITAN CENTER
EDISON, N.J. 08818

TOTAL MERCHANDISE

17.05

AAAAAAAAAAAAAAA   ZONES :

summoned to a forty-year-old first mother who had already been in labor about fifteen hours." The child's head had not advanced, the pelvis was somewhat contracted, and the cervix still stiff. The midwife had tried steambaths, enemas, and opium with no luck. Wegelin delivered the child with forceps, "but because of the rigidity of the birth canal, the perineum suffered. However the tear did not extend to the anus."[112] Thus, if so many women were once afflicted with torn cervixes, discomfort in sitting because of improperly healed perineal tears and chronic pelvic inflammations, the reason was partly that so many women were older when they started to bear children.

Convulsions and Bleeding

Even if the child slides smoothly down the birth canal, the traditional mother would still have three other perils to fear: infection, hemorrhaging, and convulsions. Infection is sufficiently interesting to warrant having the next chapter to itself. But the average woman in a typical village would know as well of the "fits of pregnancy" and of the risk of bleeding to death.

HEMORRHAGES

Keep in mind that the placenta is connected directly to the mother's veins and arteries; and that when it comes away, the mother's blood vessels gush freely for a moment, until the uterus contracts and closes them off. So normally the mother loses no more than a pint of blood. But if the uterus does not contract in time, blood will pour endlessly forth and risk sending the mother into shock.

Losing a couple of pints of blood (around one liter) is not highly unusual and occurs in perhaps 5 percent of vaginal deliveries today.[113] But today women can get transfusions; doctors know how to stop bleeding with drugs or by performing, if necessary, an emergency hysterectomy. None of these possibilities existed before 1900, except perhaps for the slow-acting drug ergot. In those days excessive hemorrhage was a major calamity.

Thus Lisbeth Burger, the German small-town midwife whose memories date from around the turn of the century, tells us with what alarm she approached the bakery where Frau Schulz had just given birth. "In front of the door a couple of neighbor women are standing, muttering and whispering. The ten children have just come back from school and are standing around bewildered. Inside, the house has a terrible look. There's a huge pool of blood in the kitchen, and tracks go into the shop and through the living room. And the bedroom! It looks like someone has been murdered. The bedding is all awry, a wash basin, the floor . . . everything covered with blood. Frau Schulz is lying in bed, pale as wax and sunken as warmed-over death. So I send all the children and neighbors away."[114]

How common were these hemorrhages? De la Motte said that "it is only too common to see women perish from blood loss. . . . The number is not small who pay for this accident with their lives after giving birth. During a time when everyone thinks only of rejoicing in the happy delivery of a cherished infant, their strength is running out with their blood, and death arrives gently before one would even have thought it possible"— a reference to how little blood needs to be lost to send a mother into shock.[115] François Mauriceau mentioned hemorrhage ninety-four times in his obstetrical cases—the largest number of references he makes to any single complication.[116]

The presence of village folklore on hemorrhage suggests that it must have been fairly frequent. For example, the townspeople of Fulda said to themselves that when the mother's "heart blood" (Herzgeblut, referring probably to bright red arterial blood) starts seeping away, "she is no longer to be saved."[117] In one part of Finland villagers coped with hemorrhage by putting a woman's clean shirt onto a hunting dog that had just come back from the forest, and then drawing this wet garment onto the mother herself.[118] Midwives around Tübingen pressed "blood stones" [Blutsteine] into the hands of hemorrhaging mothers. So implicitly did they trust the bloodstone that the relatives around the bed of one bleeding mother refused to let Friedrich Osiander intervene. He was forced to watch the woman bleed to death.[119]

Today some bleeding occurs in the last half of pregnancy in about 3 percent of all births,[120] usually owing to the premature separation of a normally implanted placenta (placental abruption or "accidental hemorrhage," as it is called in England). Some antenatal bleeding, however, is the result of the pathological implantation of the placenta, not on the upper walls of the uterus where it belongs, but directly over the exit from the uterus. When the placenta thus completely or partially blocks the opening of the uterus, it is said to be a "placenta previa," which means a placenta that "comes first." And even though, among the main varieties of prenatal and postnatal hemorrhage, it is least common, it is the most fearsome to deal with: the child cannot be born without dislodging the placenta. But when the placenta is dislodged, it touches off a big hemorrhage, one which, moreover, especially disconcerts the birth attendants because the child has not yet even been born. Thus did de la Motte, called in February of 1696 to a neighboring parish, find in the barnyard when he arrived "a number of women, who rushed out with a terrible cry that told me better than anything they might have said of the extreme danger in which the poor mother found herself. I quickly dismounted and went to her room. I found the placenta, which had just been pushed from the vagina by a contraction, and a flow of blood which continued abundantly." He immediately delivered the child by turning it, and the mother survived.[121]

The management of placenta previa thus required a cool head and plenty of experience. We have no reason to think that the skilled urban midwives lacked either. Many premodern midwife ordinances give them full responsibility for treating antepartum hemorrhage. Thus Bremen's 1738 ordinance said that "if a woman is stricken with heavy hemorrhages in the last months of pregnancy, and these are not successfully stilled with bloodletting, lying quietly and other means, the midwife is to deliver her in the appropriate manner."[122]*

But the mother with placenta previa who came into the hands of an unskilled granny midwife was probably done for. Popular culture was marked by a profound unwillingness to act in the presence of hemorrhage. Louise Bourgeois, a skilled Parisian midwife, was called to treat a woman whom a granny midwife had been looking after for hemorrhage for four or five days: "I found her in a cold sweat, with the pulse of a dying person. . . . The midwife had said to her it was necessary to let nature take its course and that the midwife had already had many cases like this." The woman died a quarter-hour after the arrival of the surgeon whom Louise Bourgeois had summoned.[123] A rustic English gentlewoman was seized by a violent hemorrhage. The midwife's first idea was further to drain from her "ten to twelve ounces more at the arm." When that failed, one of the mother's friends "was of the opinion that she ought to be delivered; but the midwife resisted, and said that she never yet had forced a labour, and that she would not begin then, terrifying the unhappy sufferer by telling her, that if she was delivered, she would certainly die." She died anyway, before Edmund Chapman, whom a desperate family had summoned, could arrive.[124]

I have dwelt upon placenta previa because these stories show how inadequate was traditional obstetric folklore in coping with grave emergencies. By the nineteenth century, a number of solutions existed for managing placenta previa; but before then, delivery of the mother as rapidly as possible by turning the infant was the only way.[125]

Other occasions for blood loss loomed as well, for placenta previa represented only about a sixth of all obstetric hemorrhages (table 5-3). To-

* The reference concerns any antenatal hemorrhage, not just placenta previa.

TABLE 5.3

*Hemorrhage in Pregnancy and Delivery (in
the Nineteenth and Twentieth Centuries)*

	Cases per 1,000 Deliveries	
	Placenta Previa	All Hemorrhages
Before 1850	.9	6
1850–1900	2.3	18
1900–1940	2.8	22
Current	5.0	—

NOTE: These are averages of statistics in separate studies.
SOURCES: See notes to tables, pages 376–77

gether, all these kinds of major bleeding occurred maybe six times in
every one thousand labors.

One final point. Most of the trends I describe in this book are "happy"
ones in that they represent steady improvements for women over the
years. The frequency of hemorrhage in pregnancy, however, seems to
have increased in the nineteenth and the twentieth centuries. The numbers in table 5.3 should not be taken too literally, because part of the
apparent increase from "before 1850" to the 1930s was doubtless the
result of better clinical observation. So maybe the rate of blood loss between 1900 and 1940 was not fully three times higher than before 1850.
Perhaps placenta previa is not five times more frequent today than in
the Rotunda Hospital of Dublin around 1800. But is it likely that the
doctors of the Rotunda, scientific leaders of their day, missed *four fifths*
of the placenta previas among their mothers? Not very.

My impression of a real increase over the years in hemorrhagic complications is reinforced, moreover, by results from the German state of Baden,
which from year to year are comparable. Placenta previa rose in Baden
from 2.7 per 1,000 deliveries between 1871 and 1900 to 3.8 between
1901 and 1925.[126] Other doctors, too, thought that the incidence of hemorrhage in delivery was on the upswing.[127] In this small but important
area of my story, therefore, I shall not be able to argue that the years
around 1900 saw a lifting of women's traditional burdens.

ECLAMPSIA

I know that by now the reader is weary of complications. Yet a few
words need to be said about the one that looms today as the most frightening of all because its causes are still not understood, and its consequences
are still awful: the "fits of pregnancy," or eclampsia. A pregnant woman
will start to exhibit the warning signs—the appearance of protein in her

urine, the swelling of body tissues, especially at the wrists and ankles, rising blood pressure. And then, suddenly, without warning, she can break into convulsions and die. Dorothy Bayly of Boylston was a victim. On 29 January 1671 she went into labor with her first child. At eight o'clock that evening she "fell into convulsion fits, and without any intermission continued in them until past one the next day, and senselessly died in them."[128] A poor woman in London's Ship Street who in 1833 got them during labor kept crying out, "Oh my head." Her doctor said, "The convulsions recurred every three-quarters of an hour: during the paroxysm, the body and limbs were strongly convulsed; she frothed at the mouth; her features were distorted, and her hands forcibly clasped."[129] Eclampsia strikes women most often in their first pregnancy.[130] "On 23 March 1669," said François Mauriceau, "I was called to deliver a woman of twenty-five, in labor with her first child. She had been taken with furious convulsions for a day and a half, losing all consciousness and had almost bitten off her tongue with her teeth."[131] Thus even the prospect of a mother going into fits would alarm everyone around. A convulsing mother was a major obstetric disaster.

How common was eclampsia in the past? What was the likelihood that it would impinge on the life of the average woman who lived in the typical village?

Statistically, it occurred perhaps once in every six hundred deliveries; thus, one would have to follow quite a few labors before encountering it.[132] In small communities lifetimes could pass without mothers hearing of the "convulsions of pregnancy." Marjosa, for example, had never seen one in her decades-long practice as a midwife in the Swiss Lötschental.[133] An eighteenth-century London doctor said that it was "seldom seen by a country practitioner, but in cities it is sometimes met with among ladies of a delicate and emotional character." (There is no relationship between "character" and eclampsia.) He himself had encountered only four cases.[134] Yet Mauriceau in Paris describes thirty-one cases of eclampsia and presumably had heard of many more.[135]

Awareness of convulsions was apparently part of women's culture because folkloric remedies existed for it. Give the mother "melissa tea" or let her hold the "bloodstone" in her hand, said the peasants around Bamberg.[136] At a meeting of black midwives in small-town Mississippi, a doctor asked how many had ever "seen a pregnant woman with fits?" About half raised their hands.[137] Midwife Alma Thomas had encountered eclampsia only once. She was alone with the mother: "Now came some terrible minutes. Any midwife who has experienced convulsions will know what it means to be quite alone. I can still see it so vividly even today. What did one of my colleagues say to me recently? That she had a mother go blind on her? My God, if only that doesn't happen."[138] So small-town midwives certainly knew about eclampsia, even if they didn't see it very often.

How about mothers themselves? A working-class housewife in prewar England told the Women's Co-operative Guild about her own bout with the premonitory symptoms of eclampsia—swelling so that she "could not get a pair of gloves or boots on," sediment in the urine and such— and then went on to describe a young friend's experience with convulsions: "She took ill at the eight months, and had a very bad time, falling out of one fit into another, and at last, after her baby was born, she lay two days quite unconscious." I quote this at length because the writer went on to say that not having sought medical advice was "sheer ignorance" on the part of her and her friend, plus "the idea that we must put up with it till the nine months were over." This statement suggests that both the warning signals themselves (now called "pre-eclampsia") and eclampsia were known to average women.[139]*

Eclampsia may have increased over the years, or at least until the 1940s, when effective treatment began to forestall "pre-eclampsia" from turning into full-blown convulsions. According to table 5.4, both first mothers (who are more at risk) and mothers of established families had convulsions more often in the twentieth century than in the nineteenth. These composite data are not terribly precise, because the circumstances of one study can differ greatly from another. But the state of Baden kept statistics on eclampsia quite carefully from 1886 to 1925, and over that time its frequency doubled.[140] So there is little doubt that the direction of change was up.

In view of intense medical efforts during those years to reduce the risk factors in eclampsia, *any* increase should startle us. Why did it occur? What might have changed in women's lives to put them more at risk? One North Carolina doctor ascribed, for example, the rise in eclampsia among blacks in that state to the advent of good times economically: rather than eating from their gardens, as people did during bad times, they would stuff themselves on "salt pork, molasses and corn meal," and thus became eclamptic more often.[141] There is no scientific basis for this particular "fat back" theory. Yet changing diet is an obvious candidate.

What is truly astonishing in women's encounter with eclampsia is that not until the 1940s and 1950s did medical treatment begin to make much difference in survival. In the middle of the nineteenth century, the major therapies for eclampsia were purging and bleeding, and the mortality was

---

* Once called "toxemias of pregnancy," eclampsia and pre-eclampsia are now classed among "hypertensive disorders," because no toxin has ever been found.

TABLE 5.4

Incidence of Eclampsia, or Convulsions (in the Nineteenth and Twentieth Centuries)

	Number of Cases per 1,000 Deliveries	
	Mainly First Mothers (Primiparas)	Mainly Mothers of Established Families (Multiparas)
Before 1850	4.1	1.8
1850–1900	4.4	2.0
1900–1940	8.4	3.3

NOTE: These are averages of statistics in separate studies.
SOURCES: See notes to tables, pages 377–78.

around 20 to 25 percent. In the 1930s, the major therapies were barbiturates plus early delivery, and mortality still hovered at 20 percent.* Contributing most to saving convulsing mothers from death has been magnesium sulfate therapy, first introduced around 1916 but not widely used until after the Second World War. Second, morphine sulfate is now given in shots to calm the mother, and no effort is made to deliver her until the convulsions are over. The result is that today the mortality from eclampsia is about 5 percent.†

Most important, however, has been the prevention of eclampsia from happening at all—the main point of antenatal care. But look how recently this prevention has been accomplished. Not until 1948 did doctors decide in one hospital in Sydney, Australia, to make a determined effort to cut down eclampsia, and so they had in the next five years only one case in 15,000 deliveries. But before 1948 the rate among booked patients in that hospital had been 2.5 per 1,000, which was the level prevailing in early nineteenth-century Europe.[145]

Death in Childbirth

I rely heavily on the doctors in this account. How do we know we can trust them? Or that they are not viciously distorting the historical record in order to libel their enemies, the midwives? We know that in

---

* Of 198 cases from the late eighteenth and the early nineteenth centuries cited by Churchill, 50 died.[142] Joseph DeLee wrote in 1933, "Over 20 percent of women afflicted with eclampsia die, and this has been hardly affected by changes in treatment in the last one hundred years."[143]

† In thirteen contemporary series it ranges from 0 percent to 10 percent; they average out to 5 percent.[144]

the past midwives attended most births. And we know from statistics that many mothers died in those deliveries. These statistics are the most stunning of any indictment of the traditional midwives.

Before 1800 perhaps 1 percent to 1.5 percent of all births ended in the mother's death. The exact average of the studies I have consulted is 1.3 percent. It would be unusual, over a long period of time, for more than 2 percent of all births to end in the mother's death, although that apparently happened in London's Aldgate district in the sixteenth century, and in colonial New England.* It would similarly be unusual for maternal mortality to be lower than one half of 1 percent, though villages existed in Germany where that sometimes occurred. If we assume that the typical woman who lived to the end of her fertile years gave birth to an average of six children, her lifetime chances of dying in childbirth would be 6 times 1.3, or 8 percent.†

What does an 8-percent risk mean in terms of the other risks to which women were subject in their fertile years? Although I shall cover this question in detail in chapter 9, I note here that in the Brabant countryside, for example, one quarter of the female deaths at age fifteen to fifty were due to obstetric causes.[155] Among the ruling families of Europe in the seventeenth and the eighteenth centuries, one death in four among fertile women came in childbirth.[156] Thus, childbirth was a leading cause of death, usually second to tuberculosis, among women of childbearing age.[157] A 1.3-percent risk of dying in any given delivery may not

---

* London's maternal mortality rate of 12 per 1,000 deliveries was not much out of line with other parts of England in the eighteenth century. Northampton in 1737–72 had 13 per 1,000; Manchester in 1760–72 had 8 per 1,000.[146] David Levine and Keith Wrightson found 18 maternal deaths per 1,000 deliveries in the village of Terling, 1550–1724;[147] they consider this rate "surprisingly low." John Demos writes of the early Massachusetts settlers that "something like 1 birth in 30 resulted in the death of the mother."[148] This extraordinarily high figure seems, however, to be confirmed by John Jewett, who placed maternal mortality in Massachusetts in 1641 at 25 per 1,000 births, and in 1741 at 14 per 1,000.[149] Philadelphia's rate in 1808–15 of 4 per 1,000 was much lower.[150]

†Arno Trübenbach calculates the percentage of mothers in two Thuringian villages ever to die in childbirth as follows:

Urleben		Wiegleben	
1601–1700	4.9	1701–1800	4.0
1701–1800	7.8	1801–1900	6.0
1801–1900	4.0[151]		

This table is based on deliveries of *bodenständigen Mütter*, maternal deaths within six months of a confinement. Sigismund Peller calculated that before 1800 11 percent of all fertile women among Europe's ruling families died in childbirth.[152] For a group of German villages from 1780 to 1899, Arthur Imhof puts the risk at 5.5 percent.[153] A number of studies converge on the figure of 6 children per completed family.[154]

TABLE 5.5

*Urban versus Rural Maternal Mortality
Rates (to 1850)*

Maternal Deaths per 1000 Deliveries			
Villages		Cities	
German villages		London	
1650–1699	10	1583–1599	24
1700–1749	4	1629–1636	16
1750–1799	12	1670–1699	19
1800–1849	8	1701–1746	14
		1747–1795	12
Brabant villages		1828–1850	4
1624–1640	19		
1641–1700	N.A.*	Edinburgh	
1701–1756	17	1750s	14
1750–1791	18	1770s	8
		1790s	6
		Königsberg	
		1769–1783	13
		1784–1793	10
		1794–1803	8
		1804–1814	7
		Berlin	
		1720–1724	11
		1746–1757	12
		1758–1774	12
		1784–1794	7
		1819–1822	7
		1835–1841	4

* Not available.
SOURCE: See notes to tables, pages 378–79.

sound like much; but, in terms of a woman's lifetime, it matters a lot.

Note in table 5.5 that maternal death rates declined sooner and much more rapidly in the cities than in small towns and the countryside. London's dropped from twenty-four per one thousand births in the late sixteenth century to twelve by the late eighteenth, and to four by the 1830s! There were similar substantial declines in eighteenth-century Edinburgh, Berlin, and Königsberg. In the countryside, by way of contrast, no decrease at all occurred during the eighteenth century. Maternal mortality remained steady at almost 2 percent in a sample of Brabant villages. It seems to jump around—evidencing no down trend—in a sample of German villages and small towns. And in Sweden no decline took place until after 1800.[158] The contrast between cities and countryside shows

clearly, I think, the positive effect of various improvements in midwifery—
such as medical training for midwives, forceps and the like—which were
diffused first in the cities. This relationship between lesser mortality in
cities and progress in obstetrics remains to be proved in detail. Yet it
strikes me as likely that if women in London were dying less in childbirth
in 1790 than in 1590, it was because by the late eighteenth century a
number of skilled doctors were on hand, the midwives were probably
far more competent, and a whole host of maneuvers, such as version,
were available to spare the mother the horrors I have reviewed in this
chapter.*

After the 1870s maternal mortality began to decline everywhere, a result
of the wave of medical progress that started with Joseph Lister's discovery
in 1867 of antisepsis. Unfortunately, around the same time, the number
of women dying from infected abortions also began to increase dramatically. And because most of those abortion deaths were included in "maternal mortality," the overall statistics give the false impression that the
death rate of mothers in full-term deliveries was not going down at all.
To the contrary, it decreased steadily after about 1880. The evidence
for all this will be presented in the following chapter, but here I want
merely to remind the reader how greatly women's chances of dying in
childbed did decrease.

Switzerland was one of the few countries to exclude, from its maternal
mortality statistics, deaths from infected abortions. The Swiss data began
in 1901, when the maternal death rate was only one half of 1 percent.†
Contrast that with 1 to 1.5 per 100 death rates around 1800. By the
1930s it had declined to 3.7 per 1,000; by the 1970s, to .2 per 1,000,
or 2 per 10,000.[162] The Swiss maternal mortality rate will soon be measured
in "N deaths per 100,000 deliveries," which means that 100,000 mothers
have to give birth before even one death occurs. In other words, a negligible
rate. The Swiss experience holds true widely: slow decline in the years
after antisepsis was introduced; rapid decline after the invention of the
sulfa drugs in 1936; fall to almost zero with the ultramodern obstetrics
of the post-1960s.‡

---

* There were by the end of the eighteenth century "some hundreds of male midwives
in London alone," according to Thomas R. Forbes.[159] Friedrich Colland thought that maternal
mortality had declined in late eighteenth-century Vienna's Allgemeines Krankenhaus, because version and forceps had replaced embryotomy in the management of obstructed
labor.[160]

† In Edmond Weber's data, which include abortion deaths, Swiss maternal mortality
from 1876 to 1888 was 5 per 1,000 births.[161]

‡ The statistical evidence for a post–1880 decline in maternal mortality will be presented
in the next chapter. One might note, however, that in some national series of statistics
including abortion deaths the down trend is so powerful that it shows up despite the
countervailing rise in abortion. See, for example, Brennecke's Prussian data, showing a

So that you may form a picture in your mind's eye of exactly how deaths in childbed have changed over the years, imagine the major diseases that women would face in the 1860s, just before the assault on infection began; in the 1930s, as doctors had learned to prevent and treat some of the most common maladies; and today, when women fail to survive childbirth only in the most anomalous circumstances. Table 5.6 compares the causes of maternal deaths over the years:

· Infection slaughtered over half of the mothers who died in home deliveries in the 1860s in one part of Baden. Then, as now, hemorrhage figured importantly, and third on the list came other "medical" diseases like tuberculosis to which the mother succumbed doubtless as a result of her weakened state.

· The 1930s statistics come from New York City. Infection was still something of a worry, mainly in deliveries involving instruments, and especially in caesareans. Many women also died of "heart failure," a result of their having contracted rheumatic fever earlier.* Finally,

---

decline from 8.2 maternal deaths per 1,000 births in 1855–59 to 4.2 in 1890–94.[163] Similarly, in Mecklenburg-Schwerin, maternal mortality (uncorrected for abortion deaths) declines from 10.0 in 1870–74 to 4.7 in 1905–09.[164] National series, on the other hand, for Belgium, Iceland, Sweden, and England show no decline before the 1920s and the 1930s. In England at least, this is because the rise in abortion mortality was so overwhelming.[165]

The supposed failure of maternal mortality to decline before 1935 produced speculation about how much the increasing percentage of primiparous women in the childbearing population might have "prevented" death rates from falling, since primiparas do have higher mortality rates than two-, three- and four-paras, due to the slowness of their labors and their increased risk of birth-canal injuries. Mary Dublin, however, accepting official mortality statistics at their face value, concluded nonetheless that changing age and parity structures had little impact on maternal mortality.[166] Recent work by Linda Berry concluded that compositional changes in the population of childbearing women explain only 1 percent to 15 percent of the variation in changing maternal mortality.[167] See also Edward Jow-Ching Tu's 1979 study.[168] If these studies had attempted to remove septic abortion deaths from the data, they would probably have found compositional effects playing even less of a role. Janet Campbell observed quite correctly that the potential increases in overall maternal mortality that are due to a higher percentage of first births are compensated for "by the decline in the risks associated with 8th and later confinement."[169] A special investigation concluded in 1937 that "the falling birth rate has resulted during the last 10 years in an increase in the proportion of first confinements, and at the same time in a fall in the proportion of confinements of women who have previously had many children. The opposing effect of these changes on the total mortality risk directly attributable to pregnancy and childbearing have been almost complementary."[170] This report did find a slight tendency for areas with a higher percentage of primiparas to have a higher maternal mortality.[171] Some authors see in these minor geographical variations the effect of social class—thus, J. M. Winter's argument that maternal mortality was higher in London's West, than in its East End because more births in the West End were first births.[172] In my view, however, these differences were probably owing to middle-class women's lesser previous exposure to infection, and consequent greater risk of dying of a postpartum infection to which they had no acquired immunity. See chapter 6.

* The White House Conference on Child Health and Protection concluded that "in the age period 18 to 43, rheumatic fever accounts for about 90 percent of all heart disease."[173] To what extent septic maternal deaths were concealed by a diagnosis of "heart disease" is another question, considered in the appendix, pages 302–3.

TABLE 5.6

Causes of Death in Childbirth: Change over Time*

	Baden (1864–66)	New York City (1930–32)	United States (1976)
		(In percentages)	
Infection	57	33	4
Phlebitis–embolism	?	6	17
Hemorrhage	17	12	15
Eclampsia–"toxemia"	6	15	21
Shock-traumatic delivery	8	11	6
Other obstetrical causes	—	1	24
Related "medical" diseases	11	22	13
	100%	100%	100%
Number of maternal deaths per 1,000 deliveries	5.4	4.5	.1

* Abortion and ectopic pregnancy (a pregnancy outside the uterus) excluded.
SOURCES: See notes to tables, page 380.

the New York working-class mothers whom these statistics cover probably suffered the consequences of the puzzling increase in eclampsia I have discussed.

· By the 1970s, American mothers, in giving birth, would be able to put death from their minds. When, very rarely, their doctors encountered maternal mortality, the fits of pregnancy would be the most common single cause. Diseases that seem to come out of the blue—like stroke or "amniotic fluid embolism"—compose the other culprits. These are tragedies that an average obstetrician almost never sees. The banal, predictable deaths—infection and shock—have been banished from the delivery room.

It is impossible that these momentous changes have been without impact on the way women view sexuality, the pleasures of raising children, and the nature of their relations with men. Today the bearing of children is largely a joyful, privileged experience, one valued the more because men do not have access to it. The point of this chapter has been to show that, as recently as a hundred years ago, things were very different.

CHAPTER 6

Infection after Delivery

AFTER her father had beaten her and thrown her down the stairs, the young woman, now late in pregnancy, traveled on foot "in the bitterest cold and with little clothing" from Torgau to Berlin. There in the late winter of 1825 she was admitted to the Royal Maternity Hospital. She gave birth and died of an infection.

Her doctor ascribed this death to "fear, shame, worry and grief, after her father had mishandled her, plus being abandoned to danger, want and desperation."[1] In retrospect, however, it is likely that she died of "childbed fever," which was then epidemic in the hospital. Since the dawn of time, women have risked these bacterial infections in giving birth. In fifth-century B.C. Athens, for example, the wife of Dromeades came down on the second day after delivery with an acute fever and chills. On the third day she complained of pain around her abdomen and of nausea; she became delirious; her breathing was irregular; her urine was "thick, white, and muddy." By the fifth day her fever was even higher. The chills continued until the next day when, "her extremities cold," her breathing "rare and large," her body in spasms, she died.[2] The underlying cause of death was almost certainly a post-delivery sepsis, the modern term for what was once called "puerperal fever" or "childbed fever." These infections have plagued women through the ages.

If we want to understand how the physical experience of women has been historically different from that of men, we must deal with the technical subject of these bacterial infections. Sepsis was a source of universal anxiety to women giving birth. Statistically, it loomed larger than cancer and struck with the same apparent whimsy. Post-delivery infections would set in around the third day after birth, when the mother had relaxed, thinking she had passed through the delivery without incident. "There is nothing more sudden than the changes in the condition of these women," said Dr. J. S. Parry of Philadelphia's Blockley Hospital in 1874. "In the morning they are cheerful and smiling, and seem to be well, yet they are consumed by fever; pulse rapid, features pale and shrunken, and death is written upon their foreheads. They sink and die without a struggle."[3] These deaths, wrote a French doctor around the same time, "are the saddest spectacle that one can see because the women retain a great articulateness" right up to the very end.[4]

To the extent that our limited sources speak on the feelings of the women themselves, mothers seem to have been greatly apprehensive about childbed fever. An Alsatian proverb, alluding to the long incubation period of some of the infecting bacteria, said that "heaven stays open nine days for the woman in childbed," meaning that if she did not develop symptoms within that time, she would be all right.[5] Styrian villagers believed that "if one woman dies in childbed, so must two others also die soon afterwards"—a reference to the communicability of "puerperal fever."[6] It vexed the English obstetrician J. Matthews Duncan that "the death of a woman in childbed, as every one here well knows, always attracts a great deal of attention . . . but if the cause of death is known to be puerperal fever—or anything pertaining thereto—then, indeed, quite a panic is created in the neighbourhood, and both doctor and nurse come in for more than their full share of blame."[7] This, of course, was what upset women from Styria to Mayfair: that childbed fever seemed to spread epidemically like plague. "I don't want to die like the others," screamed Catherine Dancard, a new mother of thirty-two years, in Dunkirk as an epidemic broke out there in September of 1854.[8]

The Frequency of Infection

All very dramatic, you might say, yet how common *was* post-delivery infection? What was the likelihood that the typical housewife, as opposed to some half-starved, fugitive maid in a septic maternity hospital, would contract an infection after giving birth? I shall argue in this section that few women could expect to pass through childbearing without having had one infection—or at least without helping out a neighbor who had been struck with one.

Most such infections were called not "puerperal fever" but "weed" or "milk fever." These were the milder sort. A traditional medical theory held in common by both populace and doctors said that fever after delivery was caused by the milk rising in the mother's breasts. Hence the term "milk fever," which meant not a breast infection but a fever produced by the milk leaving the blood (where it was thought to reside) and entering the breasts or other parts of the body. Hungarian peasants, for example, explained that the fever arose when the milk "climbed into the head."[9] Moritz Thilenius, a German doctor who wrote in the middle of the eighteenth century, said that fever after delivery was normal: "During birth one's condition is febrile, and it remains so afterward. Usually around the third day the fever really breaks out and is called milk fever or milk chills. It customarily is very mild, and as soon as the milk is flowing and being sucked out, vanishes without a trace."[10] The French man midwife de la Motte seemed to think milk fever (*la fièvre du lait*) normal, as he explained that an official's wife whom he delivered in January 1706, got over hers after the fifth day. But she did not really, for she thereupon "was surprised by a chill, which was followed by an extraordinary fever, and a diarrhea which added itself to the fever." It is clear that "milk fever" for this mother meant the beginning of an infection that was to spread from her uterus, the local source of infection in most "milk fevers," and turn into peritonitis ("her belly hard, swollen and painful").[11]

Doctors dismissed these infections as unimportant. Said London's Robert Bland, "Many of the women" delivered by midwives through the offices of the Westminster General Dispensary in the 1770s "were afflicted with severe afterpains, or had what is called the milk fever; but as these complaints were generally relieved in three or four days, and did not seem to have any influence in retarding their recovery . . . no notice is taken of them."[12] And almost a century later in London, these less dramatic forms of sepsis were still so common as to be considered normal. "In all the cases here investigated," wrote William Squire in 1867, urging the introduction of the clinical thermometer in obstetrical practice, "the most constant and most obvious disturbance of temperature is that which ushers in, and accompanies, the formation of milk."[13] In the United States some kind of infection after delivery remained terribly widespread right up until the 1870s and 1880s, when doctors finally understood that fever was caused by bacterial invasion. Looking back on his experiences in those earlier times, a doctor from Portland, Maine, wrote in 1905 that "Every lying-in woman was expected to have 'milk-fever' on the third day of the puerperium."[14]

Of course, there is no such thing as milk fever. These were mild infections. Today these small rises in temperature occur in only a small percentage of all births (outside of the first twenty-four hours) and usually accompany "endometritis," which is an infection of the lining of the uterus.[15]* Thus, most "milk fever" was probably endometritis, though a quarter of all such fevers come from somewhere outside the genital tract, such as the bladder or the breasts.[16] But it was not localized endometritis that was so feared. It was the possibility that the infection would spread from the uterus to the bloodstream, to the abdominal cavity, or to the veins of the pelvis and the legs. Historically, "puerperal fever" denotes these serious complications of endometritis, and it is they that made childbearing such a potential menace for so many women. How common were they?

One problem is that the doctors and midwives of the time failed to recognize many infections as obstetric in nature and called them instead "enteritis" or "pneumonia," reserving the term "puerperal fever" for peritonitis, which they associated with a distended, agonizingly tender abdomen. Thus, German doctors in the Hadamar Maternity Hospital recorded, between 1822 and 1844, only five cases of "puerperal fever" among their newly delivered mothers. In addition, they saw after delivery:

10 cases of "gastric fever"
 6 cases of "purely rheumatic fever"
 6 cases of "purely catarrhal fever"
 1 pneumonia case
 3 cases of "pleuritis vera"
 4 cases of facial erysipelas
 2 cases of "rash" (*Friesel*)
17 other cases of gastrointestinal upset "without fever"
11 "rheumatic afflictions of various kinds"[17]

These were not just coincidences. It will be apparent to even the casual observer that most of these "non-obstetrical" illnesses in new mothers were in fact post-delivery sepsis. In some cases a pelvic infection had seized the muscle of the colon, causing constipation or diarrhea—hence, "gastric fever." In other cases a bloodstream infection had reached the lungs or heart—hence, "pleuritis" or "purely rheumatic fever." In still

* A mild elevation of temperature within twenty-four hours of birth often occurs in the absence of infection; that kind of "physiological" pyrexia is *not* being considered here.

other cases a streptococcal infection had caused a skin rash called "erysipelas" (*Friesel*). But all these infections lacked the classic signs of peritonitis and so were thought unrelated to the delivery.

To avoid a dramatic undercount of infection cases, the historian should assume that virtually all infections occurring within a month after delivery were obstetric in nature. Thus, deaths assigned to pneumonia and such should really have been included in "puerperal infection." As one New England doctor said of the death certificates of new mothers, "We find that the puerperal state is complicated in a surprisingly large number of fatal cases with malaria, pneumonia, typhoid fever, etc. It is strange to notice that the diagnosis is made after labor, never before it."[18] Thus, if we fail to expand our definition of "puerperal fever," we will be helpless in the hands of such "fudgers" as Glasgow's Dr. Alexander Miller, who reported his six maternal deaths in one thousand deliveries as follows:

1 death from hemorrhage and shock, a placenta previa
1 death from TB
1 death from enteric fever
1 death after three weeks from "cardiac syncope,"
   i.e. heart failure
1 death from "cerebral congestion"
1 death, a forceps delivery, from puerperal septicemia

Dr. Miller congratulated himself that "my maternal mortality may safely be reduced to two, viz. those of puerperal septicemia and placenta previa, and I trust you will agree with me when I say that I could hardly be blamed with that death. As regards the other, I have regrets that I did not insist more on a proper nurse at the time."[19] In retrospect it is likely that he was associated not with one but with *four* infection deaths: the septicemia case he tried to assign to the nurse, the "cerebral congestion," the "heart failure" three weeks after delivery, and the "enteric fever." All four mothers had probably been infected by bacteria introduced into the bloodstream at delivery. The technicalities of this mother-by-mother "retrospective diagnosis" quickly benumb the general reader, but the point I wish to make is that, in assessing numerically how many mothers had grave puerperal infections, we cannot limit ourselves to what the medical people of the time called "puerperal fever."

It is likely that about 4 percent of all home deliveries during the era of traditional midwifery involved a *serious* infection for the mother. The logic is as follows: The average maternal mortality from sepsis before 1860 seems to have been around eight per one thousand deliveries (see Supplementary Table 6.A, pages 311–12). Estimates of the percentage of serious fatal infections range from 9 percent to 40 percent, depending on the time, the place, and the definition of what a "serious" infection entails. I have from the literature the impression that overall about one fifth of the infected mothers died.* Hence 8 times 5 equals 40, or 4 percent.

If we further assume that the average mother who survived to age forty-five was likely to give birth around six times, we must make her *lifetime* risk of contracting a grave puerperal infection 6 times 4 percent, or around 25 percent. This is not a negligible risk: a one in four chance of, at some point in one's childbearing years, coming down with one of the very nasty infections I shall describe in a moment.

Kinds of Infection

A simple uterine infection can mushroom into a life-threatening illness in four different ways:

1. By *peritonitis*, in which the bacteria spread from the infected uterus, tubes, and ovaries to the glistening white lining of the abdominal cavity called the "peritoneum."
2. By *bacteremia*, in which the bacteria spread from the infected veins of the uterus into the general bloodstream, disseminating poisons called "toxins."
3. By *septic thrombophlebitis*, which is the infection of a blood clot in an inflamed vein. As pieces of this infected clot break off, they are carried in the bloodstream to distant parts of the body, causing further infections in such sites as the lungs. When pus-forming bacteria are at work in the bloodstream, this is called "pyemia." Pyemia and bacteremia are sometimes lumped together in the general term "septicemia."
4. By *cellulitis*, which is an infection of pelvic connective tissue. This may be accompanied by large pockets of pus ("abscesses"), which are painful and enervating under the best of circumstances and, under the worst, can rupture into the abdominal cavity, causing a grave illness.

I must emphasize that in real life, as opposed to textbooks, these forms of infection all overlap. A mother seriously ill with some post-delivery bacterial onslaught was likely to find an infection between the leaves of her "broad ligaments" (cellulitis), the bacteria having at the same time pushed through the lymphatic vessels of the uterus to her abdominal cavity (peritonitis), while simultaneously infiltrating her pelvic veins and causing long, painful clots to form (thrombophlebitis); from all of these

---

* Of the 172 cases of "well-marked puerperal fever" that Robert Lee saw from 1827 to 1832 in private practice and at various hospitals in London, one third ended fatally.[20] Of the mothers who were infected in the Frankfurter Frauenklinik from 1913 to 1922, 9 percent died. Walter Sigwart, who reported this study, said he thought that infections ended fatally perhaps 10 percent of the time.[21] Of the 110 puerperal fever cases in Amt Sursee from 1891 to 1929, 39 percent ended fatally; yet presumably only the grave cases were reported.[22]

sources her general circulation was being overwhelmed (bacteremia or pyemia). If she died, it would be from a bacterial invasion of her lungs, from the poisonous effects that bacterial toxins produced on all vital organs, from septic shock, or from all of these. The terminal mechanisms of these overwhelming bacterial invasions are still poorly understood, even today. In 222 autopsies on patients at the Paris Maternity Hospital in 1829, for example, the vast majority had some form of peritonitis. About half the women had long blood clots in their veins (thrombophlebitis).[23] In 163 post-delivery autopsies in a Viennese maternity hospital around the time of the First World War, about half the mothers had some venous thrombosis; about half had peritonitis; many had both.[24] The point is that the various kinds of infections ran together.

While the mother was still alive, however, one of these four general types of infection would appear most saliently. On the basis of her symptoms, the doctor would normally settle upon a diagnosis of "peritonitis" or "septicemia" or whatever. These observations interest us because autopsies were rarely done before the middle of the nineteenth century, and then only on women who had died in maternity hospitals. Lest my preoccupation with determining the exact nature of the infection strike the reader as unnecessary and boringly technical, let me point out that the kind of infection a mother had mattered considerably to her subsequent health, assuming she survived. As a gynecology text of the 1880s said, "It is the rare exception to examine a multiparous female pelvis without finding some traces of a previous cellulitis or peritonitis."[25] These "traces" were either abscesses, adhesions, or chronic tubal infections. And, to the mother, they would be an enduring, painful souvenir of her infection. A bloodstream infection that does not produce great buckets of pus may, on the other hand, leave a different kind of souvenir: a permanently damaged heart or kidney disease. So even though the details of these infections may seem gruesome to readers of today, they were of great moment in the lives of women in the past.

For a long time the view held sway that "childbed fever" meant some kind of pain or swelling in the abdomen. Even in the 1930s a group of English doctors studying maternal deaths refused to consider several post-delivery "scarlet-fever" deaths as resulting from childbirth because "signs of abdominal or uterine sepsis were not observed."[26] This overattentiveness to the belly means that historical descriptions of "puerperal fever" focus almost entirely upon peritonitis. Hence we consider it first.

PERITONITIS

In the spring of 1774, Jean Reid delivered her third child in the Edinburgh Infirmary and fell ill two days later, starting with "pains in the lower part of the abdomen." She felt "coldness and shivering" and had a headache.

By the third day she suffered nausea and vomiting; diarrhea appeared. She complained of "pain in the region of the uterus and of swelling and fullness of the belly." Her lochia stopped.

By the fourth day the uterus was sore to touch; she was terribly thirsty and had a "deep crimson colour on her cheeks."

By the fifth day her pulse was beating 160 to the minute. The doctor noted a "dry burning heat of her skin." Also "Reid had on many parts of her body small red tumours under the skin, moveable and painful."

By the sixth day "the back of her right hand was swelled and red." No pulse was to be felt. She was "breathing very quick," yet was in no pain and remained coherent until she died later that day.

At autopsy "the cavity of the abdomen contained about two pounds of a fetid milky fluid."

The doctor finally noted that Reid's "small tumors on the skin . . . seemed to have some resemblance to the erysipelas then endemic in the Infirmary," and that "the surgeons of the hospital found that an erysipelas supervened on every incision."[27]

Several points may be made about Jean Reid's death of peritonitis and associated bacteremia and shock. The infection probably radiated out from the lymph channels of her uterus to the abdomen. The pain of peritonitis probably had a reflex action on her colon, stopping its muscular activity and causing unabsorbed fluids and fecal gases to build up. That's what produced the "swelling and fullness of the belly." Judging from the erysipeloid infection on her skin and the "erysipelas" that all the surgeons in the hospitals were complaining of, it is likely that she was infected with a highly virulent hemolytic streptococcus. As it seized the huge, vascular surface of her peritoneum, it poured bacterial toxins into her circulation. Meanwhile the natural defenses of the peritoneum were putting up a fierce local fight against the bacteria, which explains the large amount of pus in her abdomen, but the bloodstream infection was too much. Shock from the toxins had begun. Her pulse was racing as the heart attempted to compensate for the diminishing amounts of blood that her veins were returning. And as the peripheral tissues got less and less oxygen from the heart, they started sending back carbon dioxide, which she was clearly trying to blow off through her panting. The exact cause of her death was unclear, and still is today for patients in this kind of shock.

Untypical of peritonitis is the little amount of pain she seemed to have. Although one study found that about one tenth of all peritonitis patients have no abdominal pain at all, and that, like Jean Reid, about one third of them have pain for only one or two days, the majority experience protracted, severe pain.[28] One French doctor, on the basis of patients in the maternity wards of the Hôtel Dieu in Paris, said that the "sharp cry" that the pain of peritonitis produced was so distinctive as to "establish of itself the diagnosis."[29] Among the small-town and peasant women whom de la Motte helped deliver in early eighteenth century Normandy, severe pain accompanied the "tension of the abdomen" in cases of "inflammation of the uterus" after childbirth. "The new mother suffers . . . a great pain in the hypogastric region [just above the pubic bone] so that she has trouble resting in any position save on her back, and when she wants even to turn herself on her side, she feels a mass, about as heavy as it is painful; it falls about like a weight. But this pain is mild compared to what she feels in the lower back and kidneys when she moves . . . all of which makes it insupportable for her to lie in any position save recumbent."[30]

Case studies are full of peritonitis victims like Mary Lord of Manchester, whose abdomen was "so exceedingly tender that she could not bear it to be touched."[31] Mary Tanner of London was attended by Augustus Granville for puerperal fever in mid-January 1818. "She dreaded the approach of my hand, and even the bedclothes seemed too great a weight."[32]

Nor need peritonitis signal its onset with "shaking chills," in which the mother's teeth literally chatter for minutes on end as her body copes with the soaring fever.* Jean Reid had several bouts with chills, but the Chicago obstetrician Joseph B. DeLee felt that "the severest forms of infection have the fewest number of chills."[34]

Keep in mind, finally, that even though Jean Reid's abdomen was filled with pus and fibrin at the time of her death, some of these bacteria can invade so rapidly that the body's defenses have no time to throw off any pus. So swift can the invasion be that the intestines never become ballooned, nor the abdominal muscles sore and defensive, and the swollen, boardlike abdomen, which doctors like de la Motte thought distinctive of peritonitis, will never appear.† Yet the mother's death will nonetheless be due to abdominal infection, and not to "apoplexy," which is what the eighteenth-century diagnosis in those cases would have been.

---

* David Charles and Maxwell Finland, for example, say that, "except in cases of diffuse peritonitis, chills are infrequent."[33]

† According to G. F. Gibberd, "The more invasive the organism the less the inflammatory reaction, and for this reason haemolytic streptococcal infections are characterized by relatively unobstrusive localizing signs: in the most fulminating infections there may not be any."[35]

SEPTIC THROMBOPHLEBITIS AND PYEMIA

A woman does not have to be a new mother to get the formation in her veins of clots ("thrombophlebitis"); she can have cancer, or be on the Pill, or be immobilized in bed for a long time. In fact, an infection is only one of the causes of this disease; but in the women who interest us, the peasants and small-towners of traditional society, it was likely to have been the main cause of the thrombophlebitis.

Even without an infection, thrombophlebitis can be a dangerous business. A large clot forms along a vein—a mixture of fibrin, platelets, red cells, and white cells. Clots tend to break off from it, to coast along the major veins that lead back to the heart, and to be pumped by the heart into a pulmonary artery (the arteries leading to the lungs). These clots are called "emboli." Blocking the blood flow to the lungs, they tend to cause shock. The victim of pulmonary embolism experiences agonizing chest pain and dies. Even today, aspects of embolism are not fully understood. I dwell on this because "embolism" became a favorite medical diagnosis of maternal deaths: it implicated no one and suggested that the mother had been struck down by an inscrutable fate over which her birth attendants had no control.*

What concerns us now, however, is when this big clot in one of the pelvic or leg veins is septic. Mrs. A., a London woman of thirty who gave birth in June 1828, probably had one in her right leg. Her labor had been "tedious"; she began bleeding afterward, and her birth attendant had to remove the placenta by hand. Thus, the conditions for infection were created, but for a little over a week she was well.

On the ninth day she experienced "a violent febrile attack," was delirious, and displayed a "painful diffused swelling soon after around the right knee joint."

I shall not take the reader into all the details of her case. Let me just say that she displayed the typical signs of a violent bloodstream infection, with "a peculiar expression of wildness in the countenance," racing pulse, "hurried and anxious" respiration and so forth, until the thirteenth day, when "a painful circumscribed swelling had taken place in the middle of the calf of the right leg, where the integuments were hot, and of a dark red color."

Four days later, however, she appeared to recover and was much improved over the next week. But the first of July brought an unpleasant return of all the symptoms of fever and the swelling right leg. Now her right wrist was swollen as well with septic arthritis, "and for a week

* J. M. Munro Kerr wrote, "It is a simple explanation, and salves the conscience of the person in attendance."[36]

she suffered excruciating pain in the left ankle and right shoulder joint, and then died on 24 July, "completely worn down with diarrhea, fever," and the various swellings on her body.[37]

It is probable that a septic clot had been slowly accumulating in Mrs. A.'s right leg. Now and then pieces would break off and drift in the bloodstream up to the lungs. There the germs would proliferate further and spread to other parts of the body, such as the wrists, the shoulder, the ankle and knee joints. Unlike peritonitis, thrombophlebitis usually develops only a week or two after delivery and takes a leisurely pace to run its course.* The mother is ground down by repeated attacks of septicemia, which announce themselves in a spiking fever, repeated chills, and a suddenly accelerated pulse.

Sometimes phlebitis in a leg vein will cause the arteries that supply blood to that leg to shut down, giving it a pale color. The English called this "marble leg" or "white leg." The medical term is *phlegmasia alba dolens.* "The next day her left leg began to swell," wrote Percivall Willughby, who in December 1670 had been called to the childbed of Jane Spencer, a weaver's wife. "It became very painful, and cold. It was like a blown bladder, and glistened."[38] Another working-class English woman described in 1914 her sufferings with her second baby: "I had what is known as 'white leg' during the lying-in period. . . . A chill will produce this state, and this was the cause in my case, owing to getting out of bed on the second day rather than call mother upstairs when I needed her."[39] Even though, as I have observed, white leg need not be caused by sepsis, in the past it usually was.†

BACTEREMIA

The reader will now be sufficiently acquainted with the signs of bloodstream infection that I need not dwell long here. As you shall see in a moment, some of the bacteria involved in childbed infection are horribly virulent. When the blood circulates through a patch of infected tissue, it picks up the toxins the bacteria generate, and carries them all over the body. Or the bacteria themselves ride along in the general circulation, breaking down red blood cells, accumulating on the valves of the heart, and invading the lungs. "Endocarditis," "pleuritis," swollen spleen, and the like all develop—complications that today are seen mainly in terminal

---

* In my own "200-year sample" of obstetric infections (see supplementary tables, pages 297–300), for example, deaths whose salient characteristic was the peritonitis took an average of twelve days to run their course; thrombophlebitis and pyemia took seventeen days.

† Joseph DeLee believed that "extreme asepsis in the conduct of all obstetric cases will effectually prevent the vast majority of all the forms of phlegmasia alba dolens."[40] See also the discussion in the supplementary tables, page 303.

infections accompanying such underlying wasting diseases as cancer. These complications would be too depressing to discuss, had they not been so common in the past, especially in the lying-in chamber.

The details attending the death in childbed of Mary Wollstonecraft, an early feminist, are sparse, yet highlight the ubiquity of these infections. A midwife delivered her on Wednesday, 30 August 1797, of her second child in her comfortable London home. Unfortunately, the placenta was retained. Her husband, William Godwin, sent for a doctor from the West-minster Lying-In Hospital, who extracted it "in pieces, till he was satisfied that the whole was removed. In that point however it afterwards appeared that he was mistaken," wrote Godwin in his journal. It was not until the following Sunday that Wollstonecraft began to have shaking chills, "symptoms of a decided mortification, occasioned by the part of the pla-centa that remained in the womb," Godwin wrote. But, in fact, they were most likely occasioned by a bacterial invasion of her bloodstream, introduced by the hand of either the midwife or the doctor. We have no further details about the course of the illness and know only that Mary Wollstonecraft died a week later on 10 September, among the better-known of victims of puerperal septicemia.[41]

CELLULITIS

Although infection of the connective tissue of the pelvis was common, we know little about it historically because a physical exam is required to differentiate it from low-grade peritonitis or endometritis. In the era of traditional midwifery, doctors did not physically examine their patients. (They examined their faces, their stools, and their pulses and then pre-scribed enormous doses of mercury and aloes.) I mention cellulitis here because it had particularly disagreeable long-range consequences.

When this tissue is infected great pockets of pus may accumulate. They slide up the back of the abdomen or mass on both sides of the uterus—locking it firmly into place—or travel along the tissue planes in the front of the abdomen to "point" right about the hipbone. If they fail to drain there, these abscesses may drain via the vagina or the rectum, or they may not drain at all but, instead, wall themselves off as painful lumps of pus for the long duration. Or if they do none of those things, they may simply rupture into the peritoneal cavity at some inopportune mo-ment, such as in a subsequent delivery, endangering the woman's life.

As the body wrestles with the cellulitis, there will be afternoon fever, sweats at night; the abscesses will be palpable as big lumps beneath the skin that seem to migrate about. After about five or six weeks, "the exudation becomes sensitive, the spontaneous pains recur, sleep is lost, and locomotion, defecation, and urination occasion acute suffering. The fever becomes violent, chills announce the presence of pus, and finally, about the seventieth or eightieth day, perforation of the abscess takes place."[42]

It was these abscesses that partly occasioned the long-term debility from childbearing of which so many women complained in the past. "What is called the after-birth had grown to my side," wrote one member of the Women's Co-operative Guild in 1914 about an earlier delivery. And the doctor, who had arrived "nearly drunk," failed to get it all away. "I had milk fever first, and then childbed fever. I lost all reason, never knew a soul for just three months. Then I had to go under an operation to have the substance got away [presumably the abscesses drained], which left me in a very bad way, the child being eight months old when I was able to get up."[43] James Young, an Edinburgh gynecologist, speculated, long after the scientific era of obstetrics had begun, that "about 60 percent of hospital gynecology is a legacy from vitiated childbearing, and of this a very large part falls into the category of infection."[44]

Such a victim was Hannah Philips of Birkenhead, England, whom a midwife had delivered of her sixth child late in April 1850. The afterbirth had stuck, and the midwife had done something "which gave her great pain, to remove it; believes she passed her hand into her." Five weeks later Mrs. Phillips showed up at the local hospital with a "great pain in the lower part of the belly, particularly on the right side; can only lie on her back, with her legs drawn up; she is worn and emaciated, with hardly any milk; has a constant desire to sit on the commode, with a feeling as if there is something to come away." She had a low fever and night sweats. A rectal exam turned up a "fluctuating phlegmon"; "on the 8th of June, while sitting in the nightchair, a large quantity of pus came away through the rectum, after which she experienced great relief."[45]

The point in reciting these horrid details is to give a sense of the afflictions in childbearing with which average women had to cope in their daily lives. Because the uterus in childbirth is like an open surgical wound, women were far more prey than men to bacterial infections.

Does the Kind of Bacteria Matter?

Let me descend into the technical world of bacteriology for a moment and note that the kind of bug that infected a mother can tell something about how violently she was delivered, or how much blood she lost, or how torn up was her birth canal. These questions are of interest as I attempt to assess the "typical birth."

Some bacteria are generally benevolent to humans and perform important tasks in our bodies as "commensals"—defending the vagina, for example, against pathogenic invaders, or swarming in the colon to help break food down into waste products. But, if I may presume briefly to lecture the reader, once these bacteria find themselves in a sheltered body cavity which has no experience with them, they can multiply and do terrible damage with the toxins they generate. Technically, these helpful organisms are "opportunistic": they will grab any opportunity to establish themselves in a blood clot, a fragment of dead tissue, or a foreign body, and multiply furiously, safe from the oxygen of the bloodstream. Some of these bacteria are called "anaerobes": they do best away from healthy cells that the blood is still nourishing with oxygen. Others, called "aerobes," thrive in the presence of oxygen. So the way in which germs respond to oxygen in the cells is a crucial distinction.

I need to make one more distinction. Other bacteria are not normally found in the body at all. Whenever they succeed in invading tissue cells, they touch off infection, whether oxygen is present or not. One family of these "pathogenic" bacteria has had an enormous importance in the history of childbirth: the "group A beta hemolytic streptococcus." Doctors once thought that this streptococcus caused almost all the grave cases of childbed fever. And the point of this section is to say that that view is false.

But before I launch into the evidence, I want to explain why this particular micro-organism has such a long name and why it was so dwelt upon before the 1940s.

The streptococcus was one of the first bacteria to be identified. Louis Pasteur saw it under a microscope in the lochia of an infected mother in 1860 without realizing its significance (because healthy mothers, too, have all kinds of microbes in their lochia). A couple of other doctors identified it in the blood of an infected mother in 1869, but were unable to cultivate it in their laboratory. Then ten years later Pasteur did succeed in culturing streptococci from the blood of a dying mother—and made it possible to link systematically the microbe to the infection.[46] But what he did not realize at the time—and what nobody picked up until much later—is that there are many different kinds of streptococcus.

One kind, when grown in a culture of blood cells in a laboratory dish, will cause a clear open circle to form: it has dissolved, or hemolyzed, the red blood cells—hence, the term "hemolytic streptococcus." Some bacteriologist added "beta" to the hemolytic part, because another kind of streptococcus, the "alpha" sort, only partially dissolved the red blood cells. Until the 1930s this beta hemolytic streptococcus was terribly feared because it was so often recovered from the blood of sick mothers. Then a bacteriologist named Rebecca Lancefield discovered that a number of groups of beta hemolytic streptococci existed, and that the most virulent by far was "group A." This group produces most cases of "strep throat" and rheumatic fever, though other groups can be quite dangerous, too. And this is the group that produced many cases of puerperal fever.

One further point: all hemolytic streptococci flourish in the presence of oxygen; and unlike many other microbes, they can live freely for long periods of time in the open air, losing only some of their virulence. Because of this hardiness, the hemolytic streptococci would inevitably be among the first bacteria to be discovered: they are easy to grow "aerobically" (that is, no special precautions need be taken to isolate them from air).

The hemolytic streptococcus was reputed to be a terrible killer of women in childbed for two reasons:

1. It is highly "contagious," in the sense of being capable of passing directly from mother to mother, because it can survive in particles of dust, or under the rim of the bedpan, or wherever. It can thus make entire rooms, or entire buildings, septic: if you enter them, and expose a protected body cavity, you'll get the bug. Hence, the frightening mortality of wounded soldiers in nineteenth-century field hospitals where the hemolytic streptococcus abounded. And the mortality of women confined in nineteenth-century lying-in hospitals, where strep equally abounded, was also ghastly. I return to that subject in a moment.

2. Before the end of the 1920s, nobody gave much thought to the special techniques required for culturing those bacteria that flourish *away* from oxygen. These anaerobes, the reader will recall, die off quickly when exposed to the atmosphere. Unless, therefore, one takes special precautions to preserve them from air immediately after one takes the patient's blood or lochial sample, they will vanish, and the lab report will come back "sterile." It was actually in the late 1890s that two German bacteriologists first reported anaerobes in a new mother. In 1910, Hugo Schottmüller published a major paper in which he demonstrated without doubt that these anaerobes were the main pathogens in fatal postabortal infections and in some postpartum infections as well.[47] But then twenty years passed before the medical community really latched onto this discovery.

Meanwhile, doctors continued to culture patients' samples *aerobically*—an easy technique. And, of course, they discovered such aerobes as the hemolytic streptococcus in hospitals, whither the infected multitudes bring them, and where conditions for doing such laboratory tests existed in the first place. But most patients who became infected gave birth before the 1930s at home, and not in hospital. And nobody took their blood samples, especially not anaerobically. So nobody knew to what extent other organisms aside from hemolytic strep figured in the kinds of infection that most women acquired. Then in the 1930s blood and lochial cultures started regularly to be cultured both aerobically and anaerobically, and the picture of the causative organisms in childbed fever changed dramatically.

All this is familiar to students of bacteriology. How may one ascertain what organisms women died of before the invention of all these laboratory tests I have just described?

There are several tactics. First, one looks for other kinds of infections one knows to be caused by streptococci turning up at the same time as puerperal fever. If they both appear together in a lying-in ward or a village, one might reasonably assume that the childbed fever was caused by the same organism that caused the other infection. Erysipelas, for example— a reddish skin infection associated with some swelling—is caused by strep. Scarlet fever is a classic streptococcal infection of the bloodstream by one of the strains of group A strep that possess a specific enzyme causing a skin rash (hence, "scarlet" fever). To what extent did these other streptococcal infections occur in the past at the same time and place as puerperal fever?

From the seventeenth-century on, puerperal fever was spotted at the same time as scarlet fever and erysipelas all over Europe. Sometimes doctors and midwives themselves infected with scarlet fever would pass it into the birth canal of the new mother; sometimes people coming into contact with sick new mothers would later develop erysipelas or "ulcerated sore throats"; sometimes the puerperal fever itself seemed to be a form of erysipelas.[48]

Erysipelas and scarlet fever turned up especially in the maternity wards of big general hospitals. For example, of the six women who died of puerperal fever in Vienna's General Hospital in 1806, "four had simultaneously scarlet fever."[49] Until the 1870s the Paris Maternity Hospital was plagued with scarlet fever and erysipelas; for example, in 1843 "there seemed to reign among the student midwives an erysipelatous constitution . . . one [student] succumbing after evidencing symptoms of meningitis." (From January 1843 to April 1844, 267 mothers died there as well.) Another visitation of "puerperal scarlatina" occurred in the hospital in 1860–61.[50] And so forth. We may conclude that the puerperal fever was caused by the same organisms responsible for the erysipelas and the "scarlatina"— namely, the streptococcus.

In home deliveries, too, the coincidence of erysipelas, scarlet fever, and "puerperal fever" was observed. Robert Storrs of Doncaster reported that "a medical friend" of his "had a number of cases of fever, and amongst them one had a very large abscess of the neck, which required his daily attendance. One evening, when engaged in this duty, he was fetched from thence to attend a lady in her accouchement, and contrary to his own wish, was prevented from changing his clothes before visiting her. Four-and-twenty hours after delivery this patient was seized with symptoms of regular puerperal peritonitis, of the lowest character." But there is more. "This lady's maid, who attended her most affectionately throughout this dreadful state, happened to cut her finger, which she brought into use in sponging her mistress." And, of course, the infection that the maid had contracted led, as the author tells us, to her own death five days later "from the first shivering fit."[51]

Statistically, an "epidemic" of puerperal fever would more likely be accompanied by erysipelas than would an isolated case—an indication that the streptococcus was probably more involved in epidemics. My own 200-year sample included isolated infections and epidemics in both home and hospital. In hospital, 22 percent of the epidemics saw some mention of erysipelas, but only 3 percent of the isolated hospital cases did so. In home infections, erysipelas occurred in 31 percent of the epidemics, in only 14 percent of the isolated cases.* (Doubtless in reality, erysipelas occurred even more often but remained unmentioned by observers.) Hence, in both home and hospital, the streptococcus probably lay behind maternal sepsis when it erupted "epidemically."

Yet even though epidemics were more likely to be written up in medical journals than were isolated cases, epidemics were not the norm. Most sepsis deaths were "isolated," in the sense of not being part of a larger pattern of contagion. In Saxony between 1887 and 1901, for example, 88 percent of the midwives responsible for a puerperal fever death *did not cause a second death* that same year. And in only eight of the thirty-six hundred reports on sepsis deaths in that period, did the midwife responsible have four or more deaths on her slate for that year.[52] (Doctors did so little general-practice obstetrics in that part of Germany that no counterpart information is available for them.) How may one establish what germ caused all these thousands of "isolated" sepsis deaths in either home or hospital?

One tactic is odor. Some germs, such as group A hemolytic streptococcus, produce virtually no noxious odors when they infect people.† Another less virulent group of hemolytic strep (group B) creates a fetid smell.‡ Other organisms, however, throw off an overpowering fecal stench which the doctors often commented on. And when one encounters these comments, one is entitled to infer that the infection was caused not by

---

* For the sources, see supplementary notes.
 † "The lochia are not offensive in infections due to Streptococcus haemolyticus group A alone."[53]
 ‡ Charles H. Rammelkamp calls "a foul-smelling discharge" characteristic of group B infections, along with other symptoms.[54]

the familiar streptococcus but by the much less familiar anaerobic bacteria which flourish in the bowel.*

Mrs. Harpur, whom a midwife delivered in November 1669, was probably stricken by such an infection. Because the placenta would not come away, friends of the mother sent for Percivall Willughby, who found "the issuing humours so stinking, having a cadaverous, suffocating scent, that the room was not well endured by the incommers, for that it caused in some of them a heaving at the stomach."[57]

After a thirty-four-year-old widow named Bridget gave birth at New York's Bellevue Hospital in the early 1870s, she developed an infection. Dr. Fordyce Barker examined her. The cervix was "not painful on pressure, even when compressed between the fingers on the cervix and the fingers of the other hand over the fundus uteri. The odor on the fingers withdrawn from the vagina was so unexpectedly offensive, that Dr. Barker instantly vomited most freely."[58] (What a bedside manner the man had!)

Such odors were not uncommon. "One normally locates the [purulent] deposit with the first incision in the abdomen," wrote Lukas Boër about post-mortems on puerperal fever victims in Vienna's General Hospital: "It is yellow, or brownish-yellow, . . . stings the fingers somewhat and smells foul."[59] Boër was repeating a common medical fantasy about how things like cancer and pus were thought to "sting" the examiner's fingers; yet the essential finding here is that he thought fetid pus normal in the abdominal cavity at autopsy, so it may well have been a non-group A organism. In Odessa toward the end of the nineteenth century, such odors were deemed customary in infected new mothers. "The usual course is as follows: on the third or fourth day the puerpera starts to be feverish. At the same time the lochia change color and are soon odiferous; the uterus becomes soft."[60]

Because about two thirds of all obstetric infections tend to be "mixed," involving several different organisms simultaneously, malodor from the vagina does not necessarily mean that the same organism is producing the bloodstream infection.[61] But it does mean that something more complex than a simple hemolytic streptococcus infection is in progress.

A third tactic is to look for gas. Some members of especially the clostridia family—a family responsible for tetanus and botulism among other things—give off large amounts of gas once they establish themselves in

---

* These organisms are the strictly anaerobic inhabitants of the colon. The coliform group, which includes *Escherichia coli,* does equally well in the presence or the absence of oxygen and does not produce an odor. Thus, past medical opinion, which traced noxious smells to "a typical *E. coli* infection," was incorrect. This mistaken view crops up occasionally even today. Gilles R. G. Monif, for example, talks about *E. coli* as producing "a characteristic fetid odor."[55] But a recent review of the literature is explicit on the subject: "E. coli pus has no odor."[56]

tissue layers. *Clostridium perfringens* (known to British readers as *Clostridium welchii*) in particular causes "gas gangrene," and mothers infected by gas gangrene offer one of the most horrifying spectacles the researcher is likely to encounter.* A young German doctor visiting the newly constructed Maternity Hospital in Paris saw A. Leclerc, a young woman of twenty-two, carried away by such an infection. I shall spare the reader the details, but it is significant that when the doctor told Madame Lachapelle, who was the chief of the service, that such an infection was "quite new" for him, she replied that when she used to be in the Hôtel Dieu, "gangrene of the pelvis was often observed." And indeed in the new Maternity Hospital, this doctor said, "it seemed to arouse no particular excitement."[63]

But these grim anaerobic infections could establish themselves easily at home, too. So that a "poor woman, living in miserable quarters" who gave birth in Ravensberg County around 1750, contracted about the eighth day after delivery great pain in her body and all her limbs. By the following day her body and her legs had swelled up, and the day after that she died. "Immediately after death the body ballooned up to the point of exploding, and a stinking pus flowed from the nose and mouth."[64]

Thus, odor and gas characterize anaerobic bacteria. But so much has the streptococcus dominated the attention of both clinicians and scholars that not until the 1930s was it recognized how often these anaerobes cause serious infections. Unlike the group A streptococcus, which normally does not inhabit the body, the anaerobes abound in the colon and the vagina. For them to touch off a fulminating uterine infection, some rather special circumstances are required. It is really these circumstances that I expect to interest the general reader—rather than all the arcane ways in which one germ is different from another germ.

For an anaerobic infection to take hold, one of the following conditions usually exists:

1. The blood supply to tissues in the mother's birth canal is interrupted. Let us say that the birth has been protracted; pressure from the infant's head has prevented tissues in the cervix and vagina from getting enough oxygen; they start to die, thus offering a perfect nest for these germs. Remember that they thrive in the absence of oxygen.

2. Foreign bodies may be present, such as stitches repairing a perineal tear.

3. Following an operation or following the bruising and tearing of a violent delivery, tissues are "traumatized"—which is to say, destroyed.

4. An already established infection from *aerobic* organisms, such as

---

* In most fatal infections of the blood, death ensues from the action of the toxins that the bacteria produce before enough gas appears to become clinically visible.[62]

group A strep, devitalizes genital tissues and enables these normally benign anaerobes to gain a footing.[65]

These qualities explain the special role of anaerobes in septic thrombophlebitis: for example, they nestle snugly into the clot, safe from the oxygen of the surrounding bloodstream, and are thus carried inside small emboli from the clot to distant sites. These qualities explain why retained placental fragments often resulted in infection. Dead placental tissue offered a perfect growth site to organisms that otherwise would have been swept out of the uterus as the lochia drained. And the association between obstetric operations and subsequent infection is also illumined: it was not just that the man midwife's hand or instruments were contaminated. The damage to body tissues done by the operation created a growth site for germs that otherwise would probably have remained innocuous.

The reader will recall how frequent trauma was in those days. We have seen the midwives madly dilating away at the vagina. We have learned about the numerous labors that stretched on for days as a result of contracted pelvises and of many physicians' policy of "watchful waiting." You are familiar with the horrible high-forceps deliveries and the traumatic infant-destruction operations that prevailed before the advent of caesarean birth. In all these situations sites for the growth of anaerobes were created. It would not have mattered if some anaerobes got into the uterus in quick, straightforward labor. But such labors were far less common in traditional midwifery than is normally assumed.

Nor was there in traditional midwifery any shortage of fecal contamination. One eighteenth-century authority advocated facilitating delivery by reaching into the rectum and pushing against the child's chin.[66] Of fifty-nine handywoman midwives who were polled in Glasgow around 1907 and who carried a Higginson's syringe, "22 admitted using it impartially for douching or for administering enemata, frequently for the same patient and always without any effort to disinfect the nozzle save by external rubbing."[67]

All this rather unedifying information on feces and smells makes it not unreasonable to assume that the high percentage of anaerobic infections that began appearing after the late 1920s, once blood and cervical samples started being cultured *both* aerobically and anaerobically, was not somehow the result of circumstances peculiar to the late 1920s but was a reflection of a state of affairs *that had always existed.* The bacteriological data are presented in the supplementary table 6.B (pages 313–14). By highlighting various anaerobic organisms, as well as some other germs that normally live peacefully on the skin or in the vagina, these data make the point that "the kingdom of the streptococcus" was a myth.

The great majority of serious maternal infections were caused by the normally utilitarian micro-organisms that constantly surround us.*

Yet even today group A strep remains a fearsome potential source of *epidemics*. Even though antibiotics have greatly reduced its presence since the Second World War, it is still found in the throats and noses of about one in every five people.[69] It continues to cause a lot of "septic sore throats" and, from time to time, to touch off epidemics of puerperal fever. In April 1965, for example, twenty new mothers were stricken in the Boston Hospital for Women, the first epidemic in thirty-three years. All survived.[70] In January and February of 1968, nine new mothers fell ill with group A streptococcus infections at New York Hospital-Cornell Medical Center. All survived.[71] This specter from the past can reach into the delivery room even today.

Who Infected the Mothers?

Did the doctors or the midwives infect the mother? For some historians the answer is simple: "The meddling male doctors infected them as they intervened in the natural process of childbirth with their forceps."† Although this answer is not wrong, it seizes one of the less likely probabilities. There were four possible sources of infection.

SELF-INFECTION

The least likely agent was the mother herself. Around the turn of the century the diagnosis of "self-infection" flourished: by this was meant *not* that the mother had explored her vagina with her own two fingers, giving herself an infection (which could easily happen); but, rather, that a pre-existing lesion in her genital tract had flared up, or that germs from elsewhere in her body had reached the uterus or peritoneum via her bloodstream. Before the various kinds of streptococci had been fully differentiated, people thought that some of the strep that naturally reside in the vagina had penetrated the uterus, touching off a serious bloodstream

---

* Samples taken from the genital tract reinforce the view that strictly anaerobic and coliform bacteria predominate in puerperal infections. The first investigators to take reliably both aerobic and anaerobic uterine cultures were Joan Taylor and H. D. Wright, who found forty-one positive samples (taken from forty-eight septic mothers) in London's University College Hospital, 1928–29, and the hemolytic streptococcus in only one third.[68]

† Jean Donnison states this thesis most cogently, and it runs through much of the recent social history of medicine.[72] Richard W. and Dorothy C. Wertz claim that "puerperal fever is probably the classic example of iatrogenic disease."[73]

infection.* In fact, the streptococci found in the blood almost certainly belonged to different groups than those in the natural vaginal flora.† When group A organisms in particular were responsible, they had come from outside.

If a mother had gonorrhea, she might end up after birth with some of it in her bloodstream, as the relatively uninvasive gonococcus drifted upward into the uterus. But this happened rarely, considering how common gonorrhea was before the Second World War. As one New York doctor said, "It is a wonder to me why we do not have more infections from gonorrhea."[77]

If a woman already had another infection elsewhere in her body, the microbes might conceivably touch off a peritonitis via the bloodstream; although in many instances—for obscure reasons—this does not seem to happen (impetigo won't produce rheumatic fever, for example). In any event, doctors liked to snatch at this possibility—a tempting exculpation for flaws in one's own technique.‡

The major argument against self-infection as an important mode of infection is that too many long series of cases are on record where no mother died of sepsis or even got "puerperal fever." One traditional Swiss midwife in the Lötschental area had never even seen a maternal death. Childbed fever was unknown there. Nor could the skeptical German doctor who interviewed her find in the church's burial register any mention of a maternal death ever having occurred there in the past![79] To whatever the good luck of these Lötschental mothers may have been owing, they had never been victims of self-infection.

More cold water is splashed on the theory of self-infection when we learn that no sepsis deaths had occurred in the outdoor service of the Edinburgh Maternity Hospital in its thirty-three hundred deliveries between 1839 and 1847.[80] A German midwife claims to have gone thirty years without a single case of serious infection—and since I do not implicitly doubt the doctors' accounts, I see no reason to doubt hers.[81] Inger Solheim, a midwife in Lappland who died in 1880 at the age of one

---

* As late as 1933, J. M. Munro Kerr felt that the debate over "extrinsic" versus "intrinsic" infection was "not settled"; he even considered the view that "all streptococci are interchangeable."[74] Rarely did a month pass around 1900 without the *Zentralblatt für Gynäkologie*, the main German gynecological journal, printing some inflamed contribution to the debate over self-infection.

† Charles A. White and Franklin P. Koontz said that beta hemolytic streptococci are normally found in only 1 percent to 3 percent of symptomless obstetric patients.[75] B. P. Watson stated explicitly, "Infection with the Group A beta hemolytic streptococcus is practically always exogenous in contrast to infection with the anaerobic streptococcus which is practically always endogenous."[76]

‡ Doctors in Berlin's Virchow Hospital noted that a mother with a septic sore throat ended up three days postpartum with a hemolytic streptococcal infection of her bloodstream as well.[78]

hundred, was said to have practiced for sixty years without a maternal death.[82] Thus self-infection was probably unusual.

Several other villains, however, played major roles in infecting the mother. The sources are too scanty to let us weight them in any order. I wish rather to emphasize that, from our present state of knowledge, all these villains seem equally important, and that only one of them involves that classic scenario, the meddlesome doctor unnecessarily applying his contaminated forceps.

THE TRAUMA OF AN OBSTETRICAL OPERATION

As we have seen, operations before a caesarean delivery were brutal affairs, leaving birth canals torn by forceps, lacerated by jagged bones as fetal skulls were crushed, and bruised and necrotic from version. All that devitalized tissue offered a ready site for infection. And a hundred sets of statistics demonstrate that the higher the percentage of instrumental deliveries, the higher the infection rate. Among the home-delivery deaths in my own 200-year sample, one third had involved operations. Of the sepsis deaths from 1929 to 1933 in Scotland, 40 percent entailed instrumental or manipulative deliveries.[83] Of the twenty-seven mothers who died of infection in the Giessen Maternity Hospital between 1814 and 1818, ten had been delivered with instruments or by an intervening hand in the uterus.[84] Of the mothers delivered instrumentally in Paris's Lariboisière Hospital between 1884 and 1886, 33 percent later ran high fevers; only 2 percent of the mothers who delivered spontaneously were later febrile.[85] Yet while operative interference did predispose statistically to infection, *a majority of infected mothers had nonetheless not undergone operations.* It was doubtless an indictment of Mecklenburg's doctors and midwives that one third of the mothers who perished there of infection in 1904 had been tormented with instruments. Yet two thirds of those deceased mothers had delivered spontaneously![86]

THE EXAMINING HAND

A second major source of infection was the examining hand of the doctor or the midwife. Even though most mothers did not undergo obstetrical operations, most were examined vaginally, and by an unwashed hand. The doctors would come straight from their scarlet fever cases to the laboring mother's bedside, or the midwives would rush directly from the stables.* The first thing either birth attendant would do, as we saw in

---

* Carl Müller described the Lötschental's local midwife Marjosa: "She neither washed her hands before the delivery nor pulled on rubber gloves. Once she came—I saw it with my own eyes—directly from the stable."[87]

chapter 4, would be to poke a hand into the mother's vagina and see which part of the infant was presenting, whether the waters had broken, and how dilated the mother's cervix was. "Given that the majority of internal exams is quite unnecessary, and done only with the intent of satisfying one's own curiosity or the curiosity of the mother and her relatives," said an East Prussian doctor, "the number of infections and deaths which are attributable solely to internal exams by midwives becomes all the sadder."[88] Charlotte Douglas and Peter McKinlay, criticizing the Scottish medical profession as a whole for impatience, said, "The impressions of haste are intensified in that numerous vaginal examinations were made. Midwives particularly offended in this respect."[89]

SEPTIC ENVIRONMENT

A third major source of infection was simply exposure to a septic environment. In a home visited with scarlet fever or in a stinking lying-in hospital, the mother could escape internal examination, suffer no instrumental interference, pass through delivery her perineum untorn—and *still* become infected. It was because invasive bacteria to which she had no immunity would infiltrate her vagina as she touched herself, or rubbed against the toilet stool, or brushed against the midwife's woolen jacket. This is why, said Franz Unterberger, more mothers die of sepsis in Mecklenburg in winter than in summer: the midwives' woolen clothing promotes contagion from case to case.[90]

Several maternal mortality surveys in the early 1920s concluded that exposure to a septic environment was the source of about a quarter of all fatal infections. Janet Campbell, in a study of 256 sepsis deaths from all over England in 1921 and 1922, found that in 25 percent no intervention had occurred, not even a manual examination.[91] In 1925 in Baltimore's Johns Hopkins Hospital doctors came to the same conclusion: "We found 24 percent of the women presenting febrile puerperia had had spontaneous labour, had not been examined vaginally, had not had a torn perineum, and therefore had been subjected to no manipulation or repair. And the question which arises, is How did they get their infection?"[92] "Infections due to Streptococcus hemolyticus group A," said the Australian Arthur Hill a quarter of a century later, "are apt to appear 'out of a clear sky.' In many such cases during labour there has been no manipulation, no instrumentation, not even a vaginal examination. The 'clear sky' from which infection descended has been air contaminated with spray, droplets or dust."[93]

No more septic environment can be imagined than that of the maternity hospital before the advent of antisepsis late in the nineteenth century. Here is the Paris Hôtel Dieu in 1788. "One judges the dirtiness of a ward by its odor," Jacques-René Tenon advised his readers. "To really get an idea of what smell is, one should turn up here in the morning, at wound-dressing time." Of course, this was inevitable, he said, when they were obliged to place the huge beds every-which way, "with little alleys and dim passageways among them, where the walls are covered with spittle, the floor covered by the filth that drains from the mattresses and from the commodes when they're emptied, as well as with the pus and blood that pour down from wounds or bloodlettings." Tenon went on to explain that infected and healthy mothers were placed side by side in the same bed, in the same stinking room as the terminal venereal-disease cases, in wards right on top of the hospital's morgue. And the hospital's dirty laundry was heaped in a chest at the end of the delivery room, "fermenting there and increasing the corruption." Thus, "in no place in Europe, in no city, in no village, in no hospital, nowhere is the loss of new mothers comparable to that of the Hôtel Dieu of Paris."[94] The mortality in the Hôtel Dieu at that time was about one mother in ten!

It is the spectacular insalubrity of these institutions that made the mortality rate of their patients so terrible. We saw in the last chapter how hospital death rates peaked toward the middle of the nineteenth century. In 1866, Léon LeFort discovered that only 7 percent of these maternal deaths had been preceded by an obstetric operation. The others were all spontaneous deliveries.[95] To give one example: of 157 mothers infected in 1861 in Vienna's General Hospital, only 13 percent had had forceps or other operations.[96] We know from Ignaz Semmelweis's work that in precisely this hospital puerperal sepsis had been carried by contaminated hands. But even after 1847, when Semmelweis had required all the medical students to wash their hands in chloride of lime before making internal exams (thus enormously reducing the maternal death rate), a substantial quantity of mothers in that hospital continued to die.[97] They, like so many other women giving birth in Europe's maternity hospitals before 1875, were simply falling victim to the general contamination of the surroundings.

Thus, mothers in hospital were slaughtered by two kinds of organism: (1) fecal germs, to which one might become "immune" if one lived with them for long enough, but which were highly pathogenic to these new mothers, exposed for the first time to *others'* feces; (2) highly virulent micro-organisms to which no one ever becomes immune because they exist in so many variants; group A streptococcus, for example, has over fifty different strains, and even if one becomes immune to one or two of them through a previous infection, one is not immune to the others.

Home environments, too, were highly septic. Mothers who birthed in peasant huts or in the basements of worker tenements were surrounded by the most appalling filth. And highly contagious pathogens could easily turn up at home. The Scottish study found that in eleven of sixty-eight deaths from spontaneous deliveries where the source of the infection could be identified, the mothers had been in contact with outsiders carrying hemolytic streptococcus in their throats: eight of them midwives, three relatives. Thirteen of those sixty-eight mothers had been infected by other members of the family who were "septic": that is, three children had chronic middle-ear infections; one patient's mother had erysipelas; and so on. Fourteen of the mothers had been in contact with scarlet fever, in eight cases carried by another member of the family.[98] Thus, a lot of highly invasive pathogens circulated in people's homes in the years before the Second World War. But mortality in these homes was much less than in hospitals because the sheer volume of contamination was so much less in the former. A mother's child may have had a strep infection on his finger, but no one was pouring buckets of pus across her kitchen floor.

There is, however, another reason why the death rate from sepsis was so much lower at home than in hospital. Many mothers had probably become more or less immune to their own dirt. Gustav Zinke, a Cincinnati doctor commenting in 1918 on maternal mortality, said "people who live under unsanitary conditions, like those who from the time of birth are accustomed to poor food and impure air and water, acquire a certain immunity from diseases to which others, who have always enjoyed the best of sanitary surroundings, wholesome food, pure drinking water, and fresh air, would readily fall victims."[99] Of the eighty-one deliveries conducted by a "well-trained midwife" in the early 1920s in Hull, twenty-two women were classed as "very dirty," and perhaps another third as "moderate" or "unfavourable." Yet none of the mothers died. And there were no cases of "puerperal infection or umbilical sepsis. . . . An examination of the temperature charts showed almost complete absence of morbidity and all patients made a good recovery."[100]

So it is likely that working-class and peasant women acquired some immunity to their own fecal bacteria from a long series of "subclinical" infections (that is, infections without symptoms). Middle-class women, on the other hand, lived in more hygienic surroundings and had probably not developed these immunities, and thus, ironically, were more at risk to infection in childbirth. This, at least, is the most apparent explanation for the puzzling tendency of the poor to die from infection *less often* than the better-off. Numerous observers have commented on this tendency in the past. "It is remarkable," one doctor said about Prague, "that childbed fever affects mostly the women of the pampered classes. Years' long experience teaches that it strikes scarcely 1 percent of the births of the poor, while 3 percent of our ladies succumb."[101] In England, the lower the social class, the lower the rate of sepsis mortality:

	Number of Deaths from Puerperal Sepsis per 1,000 Live Births, England, 1930–32:
"Professional and managerial"	1.45
Skilled workers	1.33
Semi-skilled	1.21
Unskilled	1.16
Average	1.29[102]

The 1932 Scottish study of infection after normal delivery wanted to see if there was a relation to overcrowding. Those mothers living in the "least overcrowded" third of the scale had the highest rate of infections.[103]

Thus, we can see why home births ended less often in infection than did hospital births: (1) mothers were more immune to the germs in their immediate environment by virtue of long contact with them; and (2) homes had lesser concentrations of the virulent hemolytic streptococci to which no one becomes immune. Home-birthing mothers were, however, just as much at risk as hospital mothers to the other major sources of infection: internal exams and infection as a result of trauma.

A doubter might ask, Was it not because hospital mothers tended largely to be lower-class young women, harried by circumstance from pillar to post, that they became infected more often? Was it not, in other words, because their *resistance* to infection was lower? I cannot answer Yes to either of these questions. There was probably no general difference in the physical ability of home and hospital mothers to resist disease. Of course, many of the hospital mothers were enervated by their poverty, but so were many home-birthing mothers tired, hungry, and poor—and, in addition, they had the added drain on their general health which long histories of previous childbearing and childrearing would have caused. The length of a fatal illness may be taken as an index of the patient's ability to resist it. The duration of fatal infections turns out to be almost exactly the same in the hospital as at home. In my 200-year sample of childbirth sepsis (see appendix, pages 297–300), the average duration of hospital infections ending fatally was 13.5 days, of home infections 12.2 days. Among fatal infections in an 1861 epidemic in Vienna's General Hospital, the average lasted 12.3 days.[104] It thus seems unlikely that any particular group of mothers was especially resistant to these terrible infections.*

The Great Decline in Death from Infection: Home versus Hospital

Between 1870 and 1939 the risk of dying from puerperal fever declined steadily and dramatically. While hospital birth was roughly six times more dangerous than home birth in the 1860s, by the 1920s and 1930s hospitals and homes were equally safe, at least in regard to the risk of infection.

Because these findings contradict completely the conventional wisdom on both the timing of the decline and on the relative risk of home versus hospital in the twentieth century, I feel I should say a few words about how they were derived, and about why observers have been so long misled by the official statistics on infection deaths.

First, when did the great decline actually take place? The conventional wisdom has conceded that the revolution of asepsis made a great difference in hospital death risks in the 1880s and 1890s, but maintains that thereafter overall infection mortality remained high as a result of "meddlesome midwifery." Further, it is claimed that the doctors' inexperience and their fretful impatience with the natural process of labor made them intervene in home and hospital births far more often than necessary.† This meddlesomeness, it is thought, actually *increased* the mortality from sepsis in home deliveries from the 1880s to the 1930s.‡ The conventional wisdom

---

* Several authorities dismiss patient resistance altogether as a factor in the severity of group A streptococcus and *Clostridium welchii* infections, and emphasize instead the virulence of the invading strain.[105]

† Grace Meigs, for example, wrote in 1917, "In private practice it is doubtful whether the results are materially better to-day than they were before the introduction of antiseptic methods, for the reason that the doctrines of asepsis have not yet permeated the rank and file of medical men, much less of midwives."[106] Eardley Holland spoke of an "unfavourable change in the methods of obstetric practice," in keeping maternal mortality in Britain high.[107]

‡ Cullingworth, for example, said: "The death rate has not only diminished, but, in some districts, has actually increased during the past few years."[108] Francis B. Smith argues, indeed, that "the stability of the maternal death rate throughout the century suggests that antisepsis and improvements in obstetrics made little difference. . . . The resort to instruments might have maintained the rate during the last third of the [19th] century and into the 1930s."[109] Ann Oakley claims that "male medicine" brought about "a deterioration in the mortality record of women in childbirth," and finds it ominous that maternal mortality was high in areas where a doctor was "paid more for instrumental deliveries."[110]

argues, finally, that at all points in time home deliveries have been safer than hospital deliveries.* In light of my findings, none of these assertions is true.

How could other observers have been so misguided about the true nature of the decline in infection risks over the last century? The answer is that they relied on published, nation-level statistics. Because those statistics were crammed with abortion deaths, they gave a false picture of full-term sepsis mortality. (See table 8.A in the supplementary tables, page 315.) Now, medical observers in past decades were not incompetent. They knew that the flood of abortion deaths was interfering in some way with the reporting of regular maternal deaths; and they urged their national statistics offices to separate abortion sepsis deaths from full-term sepsis deaths. These were separated in various places, but so overwhelming was the torrent of abortion fatalities that many still ended up in general "puerperal sepsis," put there by local doctors anxious to circumvent scandal or to avoid offending the family. Observers, trusting these official statistics, have believed for decades that normal obstetrical mortality did not improve in the first four decades of the twentieth century, and that a mother birthing in 1935 remained as much at risk of infection as a mother birthing in 1885.

As to why many people have long thought home birth safer, we must recall the disabilities with which hospitals saddled themselves in reporting their maternal sepsis. Most notably, they included women who had been infected outside and who were admitted into hospital already acutely ill. A number of hospitals also included abortion deaths in their published annual totals, both abortion and full-term deaths being technically "puerperal." Finally, one must be careful to disentangle sepsis deaths in caesarean deliveries from sepsis deaths in other kinds of deliveries. Because home-birthing mothers were rarely at risk of being sectioned on their kitchen tables, it is unfair to the hospitals to include caesarean deaths in the comparison. (In any event, not all that many women died from caesareans compared with the total number of women giving birth in hospitals; for more on this subject, see chapter 7.)

Once we collect statistics free of these various defects, a remarkably different picture of the history of infection death emerges: the aseptic revolution appears immediately and dramatically in both home and hospital deliveries. By the First World War it generally would be fair to say that the only women dying of obstetric infection in hospitals on both

---

* This view of history is common among advocates of home birth today.[111] Doctors in the past believed the reverse.

sides of the Atlantic, aside from the occasional caesarean fatality, were abortion victims.* Nor were many more women dying at home.

Why didn't the decline begin in 1847, the year in which Semmelweis first published his famous finding that washing one's hands in some disinfectant solution enormously reduced maternal sepsis? Almost nobody listened to him. Physicians could not accept the notion that they themselves were inflicting upon mothers this "private pestilence," as Oliver Wendell Holmes called it. So throughout the 1850s and 1860s, childbed sepsis climbed even higher, as the hospitals grew larger, crowded with victims of all kinds of bacterial maladies, and thus became increasingly sewers of cross-infection.[113]

The real breakthrough came in 1867, when Joseph Lister described how the infection mortality from compound fractures had been greatly reduced when he first used phenol (carbolic acid) to wash the skin around the wound. His article, published in the *Lancet*, established the basis of antisepsis: killing germs before they could infect.[114] The Germans and the French began adopting Listerian ideas for obstetrics around 1874. First in the Anglo-Saxon world was Lombe Atthill, "master" of the Rotunda Hospital in Dublin, who around 1875 started "to insist upon the nurses and students washing their hands with carbolic soap, and rinsing them in basins containing a solution of carbolic acid."[115] †

In the next ten years maternity hospitals all over Western society began following this lead. Indeed, an important date in the official histories of these institutions is usually when antisepsis was first adopted. In 1877, the New England Hospital for Women started to use phenol.[118] Two years later, the York Road Lying-In Hospital in London followed and, within a short space of time, had virtually no more sepsis deaths *at all!* ‡ In the Amsterdam Maternity Hospital antisepsis was adopted in 1880, with the death of the old director, a Semmelweis foe, and the appointment of a convert.[120] In 1883, Henry Garrigues began using bichloride of mercury ("sublimate") at the New York Maternity Hospital.[121] The Berne Maternity Hospital adopted bichloride of mercury a year later.[122] And so on. When Catharine Macfarlane, a young American physician, visited

* I have seen nothing to contradict Hermann Fehling's general statement that by the 1920s "only about 5 percent of new mothers even had fever. . . . The febrile cases in our clinics are nowadays the gravely ill women with septic abortions, who are admitted from outside."[112]

† I have omitted recounting all the dubious attempts to "disinfect" the uterus itself once infection had taken hold, as well as efforts at "prophylactic" disinfection with strong douches—all of which did more harm than good.

Rudolf Dohrn calls 1874 the *Wendepunkt* [turning point] for antisepsis in Germany.[116] In 1874, F. Siredey began an antiseptic regime at Paris's Lariboisière hospital.[117]

‡ Their sepsis death rate for 1880 to 1884 was 6.0 per 1,000 deliveries; for 1885 to 1889, 0.9 per 1,000. In the 1890s they had only 1 possible sepsis fatality, a "sudden death, probably cerebral apoplexy," in 1897.[119]

TABLE 6.1
*Number of Full-Term Sepsis
Deaths per 1,000 Deliveries
(1860–1939)*

Year	Hospital	Home
1860–69	31.1	5.7
1870–79	21.6	4.5
1880–89	9.0	3.5
1890–99	2.6	2.1
1900–1909	1.2	1.4
1910–19	2.3	1.3
1920–29	0.9	1.3
1930–39	0.7	0.7

Sources: See supplementary notes,
pages 304–10.

Ernst Bumm's Maternity Clinic in Berlin, she found the following sign on the wall over each scrubbing stand:

Hot water, soap and brush, five minutes.

Clean nails.

Hot water, soap and brush, three minutes.

Rub dry with sterile towel.

Alcohol, five minutes.

Bichloride, three minutes.

After this regime, the doctor would be permitted to examine the mother, provided that he or she wore "short rubber gloves." Macfarlane added that "for intrauterine manipulations or for abdominal operations, rubber cuffs reaching from wrist to elbow are worn in addition to the gloves."[123]

By this time the doctrine of "asepsis," which means "germ free," had augmented that of "antisepsis." There was no way to sterilize the hands, but germs around them could be prevented from reaching the mother's uterus. So the wearing of gloves began in leading clinics around 1898.[124] To stop streptococci in the nose and throat from spraying the mother, people started putting on masks. Boiling of instruments, gauze, bed linen, and the like also became routine.[125] Not surprisingly, therefore, hospital sepsis had fallen to a negligible level by the turn of the century. Table 6.1 shows that, by the decade from 1900 to 1909, a mother ran *more* risk of a fatal infection if she gave birth at home than she would in the hospital.*

Yet sepsis mortality at home had been declining as well—down almost

* On the basis of different data, von Winckel arrived at somewhat the same results.[126]

75 percent from 1860–69 to 1900–1909. By the 1930s sepsis mortality rates in home and hospital were identical.

I don't think any important difference existed between the general practitioners and the midwives in their readiness to adopt asepsis, despite the yards of commentary—both pro-doctor and pro-midwife—that have been published on this subject. Of course, a lot of established midwives were reluctant to disrupt age-old routines by scrubbing, brushing, and demanding that great cauldrons of water be put on the boil. Not until 1931, for example, did the supervised midwives in the home delivery service of Queen Charlotte's Maternity Hospital in London begin wearing masks and gloves.[127]

Before judging the midwives, the reader should keep in mind the practical obstacles to making home births as "sterile" as hospital births. "In almost all midwife schools," wrote Alois Valenta in 1888, "the students find a ready-made antiseptic setup. There is an expensive wash basin with glistening vessels which contain various strengths of carbolic acid or bichloride solution and such. The students need only walk up and scrub themselves meticulously before and after each internal exam." You urbanites, he continued, just can't imagine what real conditions in the countryside are like. In some provinces "there isn't even enough clean water. And conditions in regard to wash basins, dry towels, underwear and bed linen just can't be comprehended by people in the cities."[128]

Yet the average general practitioner was also a mite slow to conform to the new asepsis. Most of the generation trained after the 1880s were probably conscientious in conforming to the hand-washing and instrument-boiling rules; otherwise, sepsis in home deliveries would not have dropped so much. But the medical literature of the years 1880 to 1930 is filled with horror stores. "We have the incompetent in our own ranks," said Frank Jackson in 1906. "I was asked once by a physician in one of our New England cities to attend a case of labor, until he could arrive." So Jackson went and found that the woman was progressing nicely, her waters not yet having burst. "When the physician arrived about an hour later, I acquainted him with my findings, and with the remark that it was time the membranes had ruptured, he wet his hands at the faucet, and with this careful (?) preparation he ruptured the membranes with his finger nail. I do not know whether the woman became septic or not, but I know that if she did, that man was criminally guilty."[129]

In this chapter I have battered the reader with statistics and bacteria in order to make three larger points. One is how common some serious infection was in the lives of traditional women. A second point is to emphasize the nefariousness of their infections, a hazard to which men were not at all exposed. A third point is to show that it was around 1900 that the rate of infection became dramatically reduced, rather than in the late 1930s as heretofore thought. I emphasize the timing because precisely at the turn of the century other terrible risks associated with womanhood also began to vanish, setting the stage for a new epoch in relations between men and women.

Postscript: Who Was More Dangerous—Doctor or Midwife?

I cannot leave this chapter without touching upon an intriguing historical debate: Who was more likely to bring infection to a new mother—a male doctor or a midwife? The doctors have damned the midwives as filthy, ill-kempt slovens. The defenders of the midwives have blasted the doctors for bringing to the mother's bedside germs contracted at the autopsy table.

The first step in resolving this controversy is to destroy the myth that it was only the doctors who caused "epidemics" of puerperal infection. De la Motte described the first midwife-initiated epidemic on record. In the spring of 1713 a midwife in Caen asked him to deliver a mother, saying she couldn't do it herself because of the "large number of women who had died among those she had delivered in the last two months."[130] In August Hirsch's sample of puerperal fever epidemics in domestic deliveries, infection was spread by a doctor in sixteen cases, by a midwife in eleven.[131] Over the period between 1875 and 1888 there were in Hamburg sixteen midwives who had each four or more sepsis deaths to her name; these deaths add up to one third of all midwife fatalities in the city. Many of them occurred in small "epidemics," such as the sepsis deaths of Midwife K., who began practicing in 1880. Three of her clients died of infection in the fall of 1883. In the next few years she had seven more sepsis deaths, and then, in June of 1892, caused a small epidemic, in which six of her patients died; after this she committed suicide.[132] *

In isolated deaths as well, in contrast to epidemics, midwives were also heavily implicated. In my own sample of infection cases over two hundred years, male doctors handled the delivery in thirty-five domestic cases; midwives alone in twenty-nine. Janet Campbell and Peter McKinlay's investigation of maternal deaths in Scotland between 1929 and 1933

---

* The 169 sepsis deaths exclude those in which doctors were later summoned. One of Midwife K.'s deaths, however, involved a forceps delivery. Note that there were surely many midwives in Hamburg who had no maternal deaths at all. The point here is that midwife-initiated epidemics *did* occur, not that they were necessarily frequent.

assigned the guilt in septic spontaneous deliveries thirty-three times to doctors, twenty-one times to midwives.[133]

The difficulty in making more systematic comparisons is that, in the era of traditional midwifery, doctors were called in mainly for complications, and did few "booked" deliveries themselves. In those complicated labors the midwife might already have infected the mothers with previous attempts at delivery; or the operation that the doctor had been summoned to carry out sufficed in itself to infect her. Thus, in the Düsseldorf district, the midwife-alone cases had an infection rate of four mothers for every thousand deliveries; the midwife-plus-doctor cases thirty-seven per one thousand.[134] Yet when the doctor infected the mother, as found by another study in East Prussia around the same time, it was usually the result of an obstetric operation (only three deaths of the doctors' fifty-five being attributable to an internal exam). When the midwife infected the mother, in two thirds of the cases it was from an internal exam.[135]

An Austrian study found sepsis deaths high in both small hamlets and big cities, and medium or low elsewhere, as this table shows:

The Number of Sepsis Deaths in Austria per One Hundred Thousand Deliveries, 1898–1902	
In communities of:	
Smaller than 500 population	220
501–2000	194
2001–5000	173
5001–10,000	161
10,000–20,000	174
More than 20,000	228
Average	192

The author's explanation was that sepsis mortality was high in small communities because the poorly trained midwives did more internal examinations. Mortality then fell off somewhat as towns got larger and the midwives in them were presumably better trained. Mortality in the big cities was high, he thought, because the doctors there operated too much.[136]

When doctors and midwives both did substantial numbers of booked deliveries, the returns are mixed. Sometimes the midwives come off better. A study of maternal sepsis deaths between 1922 and 1923 in New York State found that, whereas midwives did 10 percent of all deliveries, they were responsible for only 2 percent of the deaths.[137] On the other hand in Glasgow around the same time, the doctors did better than the midwives: when the doctor was present from the beginning of labor, there were, just before the First World War, only four notified cases of puerperal fever per one thousand deliveries. When a neighbor or a midwife was present from the beginning, the rate was seven per one thousand.[138]

Let me conclude this deluge of data by comparing the infection mortality of trained midwives in a London home-delivery service with the infection mortality of a English small-town doctor around the same time. The midwives of the Eastern District of the Royal Maternity Charity, who did home deliveries, reported 11 sepsis deaths from 1828 to 1829 (if I correctly interpret the various cases of "scarlatina," "intestinal irritation," and the like) in the course of 4,600 deliveries—a rate of 2.4 deaths per 1,000.[139] The midwives of the Western District of that same charity (also home deliveries) had a sepsis mortality rate of 4 per 1,000 a few years later.[140] Mr. G. Rigden, a small-town doctor with a thriving midwifery practice in Canterbury around this time, had a sepsis mortality of 2.1 per 1,000.[141] Thus, let us not make too much of sepsis rates that appear to favor, by only a small margin, *either* kind of practitioner. I think the chances that a doctor would infect a mother in a routine domestic delivery were roughly about the same as that a midwife would infect her. Only doctors were permitted, in most places, to handle difficult impacted labors; and of course, they would have to intervene instrumentally to deliver the mother. As she lay there torn, exhausted, and hemorrhaging, she would clearly be at greater risk of infection.

The point is that both doctors and midwives were about equally septic. The doctors treated other infectious diseases and presumably bore away with them great splotches of pus and infected blood on their frock coats. But the midwives, too, dealt with infected people. They had been the only medical personnel available for centuries in some of these remote communities. "In the isolated villages of Alsfeld County," wrote Dr. Wengler in 1917, "it is difficult, indeed often impossible for the midwife to avoid contact with infectious matter outside of her professional domain. People often ask her so urgently to help out with medical care that she is obliged to. For example, in one village where the incidence of puerperal fever is striking, I learned that day after day the midwife regularly bandaged the suppurating leg wound of an old woman. After I admonished her, the puerperal fever ceased."[142] "I'll concede," wrote another doctor, "that it's possible for the midwife to avoid contact with infectious material in her private life if she is financially so well off that she doesn't need to do housework, field work, or care for stable animals, and is able to afford help for other family members who fall sick." And then there are the infected mothers, he continued: "You can't expect the midwife to examine every vaginal discharge she encounters in order to determine whether it's infectious."[143]

Indeed not. She had to treat them all. The problem was the exploring hand, not the gender of the birth attendant.

CHAPTER 7

The Rise of the Birth Experience

CONSIDER the viewpoint of the mother who is about to give birth. From 1930 on the following scenario had become possible. Because of birth control she was more likely to have wanted the pregnancy than she would have a hundred years earlier. Anesthesia, for better or worse, meant that she would not have to suffer against her will from the pangs of birth. She could also decide how long she wanted to labor, for there would be no medical reason for curtailing the length of her delivery. And if she finally became exhausted, she could call for help, and her child would be born surgically. In other words, by 1930 the technical means existed for letting the mother herself control every aspect of the birth process.

Yet "woman-controlled" birth never happened. And the reason is that in the 1930s the doctors shifted their own concern from keeping the mother alive and undamaged to producing a healthy baby. Before 1930 little medical attention had been given to "perinatology," the care of the infant just before and just after its birth. As we have seen, from the sixteenth century to the beginning of the twentieth, birth attendants were preoccupied with sparing the mother the agonies of prolonged labor and, after 1880, with sparing her as well from infection. But by the first quarter of the twentieth century these objectives had been accomplished.

Caesarean births had begun to replace such dangerous vaginal procedures as version, high-forceps, and embryotomy. And few women now died of childbed fever. Then in the 1930s—for reasons some people will find heinous, others laudable—doctors suddenly attached a high priority to reducing the number of stillborn children and to ensuring that live ones emerged from their mothers in prime condition, neither traumatized in the birth canal nor brain-damaged from lack of oxygen. Doctors increased their own interventions because they started to realize that the "natural" process of birth often produces a damaged infant at the end. To minimize this risk, they would impose, rightly or wrongly, their own medical judgment upon the mother's wishes for control.

I have described the extent to which traditional mothers were deprived of meaningful autonomy in birthing, partly because of the midwives' adherence to the ironclad dictates of custom, partly because it is meaningless to talk of autonomy at all when a woman is vulnerable to the randomness of infection and obstructed labor, and to an unending stream of unwanted pregnancies. Ironically, the 1980s would find women again virtually without autonomy in giving birth. Every stage in delivery would be minutely regulated by protocols and medical conventions. Yet what a difference! In return for surrendering their autonomy, women today receive pink, brisk babies. *Nobody dies.* And the "birth experience" is valued as a basic part of womanhood.

This chapter traces the rise of that "birth experience." The phrase is intended to convey the spontaneous joy in yet another positive aspect of their womanhood which many women discover in giving birth. Historically, that kind of joy is new. We first watch it crystallize in the course of the nineteenth century. We then observe how certain "dark sides" in home delivery nudged both women and doctors toward the view that the pleasantest birth would take place in hospital. We finally watch the whole scenario of birth transformed by "the discovery of the fetus."

A New Sensibility

If the ideas I have proposed elsewhere are correct, some time late in the eighteenth or early in the nineteenth century the sensibilities of women began to change. Their emotional allegiance began to shift from the "women's group" to the nuclear family. In the wake of this shift came a new sense of maternalism toward their children and a new attitude of companionship toward their husbands, both replacing the rather austere emotional stand-off of the traditional family.

My views on this subject have been vigorously criticized by other scholars; and in any event, the purpose of this book is not to rehash these views.[1] I do, however, believe that this new sensibility of women began to show up in the domain of childbearing as well. Middle-class women in particular began after 1850 to limit the number of pregnancies. Stillbirth started to be perceived as a calamity rather than as a blessing in disguise. And women began to concern themselves with the "quality" of the birth experience itself, demanding now a gentleness and tenderness that previously had been absent. As the birth experience came to be seen as a projection of larger sentimental relationships within the family, a new emotionality was created in the lying-in room—just as traditional births had projected the unsentimentality of village life and the emotional remoteness between men and women. In this demand for change by women themselves is to be found an important part of the rise of the modern "birth experience."

SENSITIVE WOMEN AND DOCTORS

One sign of this new sentimentality was women's insistence that they be delivered by male doctors, rather than by female midwives. In traditional Europe women looked with alarm upon male birth attendants, necessary though it may have been to engage them in emergencies. When in the eighteenth century mothers appeared at Marseilles Maternity Hospital to be delivered, they would ask for the resident midwives, not for the surgeons. "Even today," wrote one of the hospital's doctors in 1889, "women of certain classes and in certain places, prefer this."[2] A Bordeaux official wrote in 1785 of women in the county of Foix: "It is part of their values always to prefer the midwives to the surgeons of the cities, regardless how skilled they are reputed to be. We do not believe we will be able to overcome this prejudice."[3] Why were doctors in Fulda so seldom called to make deliveries there? asked Joseph Schneider in 1806. "Because our women are not accustomed to male attendants and fail to call upon them until the most desperate crisis is at hand, leaving no possibility but delivery through instruments."[4] The only way childbirth in the countryside could be improved, said Adams Walther in 1884, was to train more female doctors. The midwives were incapable of handling emergencies, and "the women want[ed] to be treated by other women."[5] Thus, before the twentieth century women generally avoided male doctors.

This attitude began to change in the middle of the eighteenth century, however, when middle- and upper-class women in the cities began to insist upon man midwives and doctors. One historian believes the vogue began in France when in 1663 a surgeon was called to the court of Louis XIV to deliver in secret one of his mistresses, Louise de la Vallière. "The social vogue of the man midwife then spread rapidly in the aristocracy and the *grande bourgeoisie*," writes Jacques Gélis.[6] By 1786, when the Royal Academy of Medicine in Paris did a survey, man midwives (called *chirurgiens-accoucheurs*) were to be found in cities all over northern France and in both cities and the small towns of most of the rest of the country.[7] In Chambéry in the east, for example, "not so long ago our women would not have permitted a male surgeon to approach them in birth," wrote Joseph Daquin in 1787, the implication being that now they did.[8]

In German cities middle-class women began in the nineteenth century to engage man midwives and doctors for normal deliveries. "Frequent is the tendency," scolded Gmünd's Doctor F. J. Werfer in 1813, "for prosperous or would-be prosperous women to take an *accoucheur* [man midwife] for their delivery." Impatient to leave, these men would then intervene inappropriately with version or forceps. And if they did not, their patients, "seeking to be relieved of their long exertions and pains," would insist on an operative delivery.[9] This sounds a note we shall later hear again: the mothers themselves demanding that their agony be cut short by the instruments they knew the doctors had with them.

There was also a question of fashion. "It is striking," wrote a Landau doctor in 1831, "how the midwives are used less and less each year. Now that women have gotten over their previous prejudices about modesty, the man midwife has become fashionable for simple, natural deliveries."[10] Of Berlin a few years later: "Prosperous mothers almost always call a man midwife to attend them; the less well-off content themselves with a midwife or a so-called handy-woman [*Wickelfrau*], if they do not deliver in the clinic."[11]

The reason these well-to-do German women were placing themselves in the hands of male doctors was that the men knew how to handle emergencies, and the traditional midwives did not. Wrote a doctor from Halle in 1812, "You must realize that on the average women have less confidence in midwives than in doctors, if the doctor has become known as humane and skillful."[12] Interesting is the word "humane" in this context: it suggests a sensibility that I have not encountered in any discussion of childbirth before late in the eighteenth century. Again in Danzig toward 1840, women of the upper classes were said to prefer male birth attendants, "because in case of trouble one would have to be called anyway."[13] By the early twentieth century this middle-class preference for males had established itself all over Central Europe. Wrote a doctor from Leiden in 1912: "Perhaps I might say that here in the Netherlands most patients prefer a doctor for their confinement, if their finances allow it, and not a midwife."[14] "Precisely the more sensitive mother will avoid the midwife when she perceives that physical feats are expected from her that could more easily be mastered by the women of the people."[15] "Sensitive" women, of course, would prefer a male from whom they could anticipate an equal measure of sensitivity: a middle-class doctor.

The rush to engage a man midwife probably began earliest, however, in England. Already in 1736, John Douglas wrote with exasperation of the proliferation of male midwives in London: "Is it not evident . . . that the Doctor or Apothecary Midmen are sometimes as ignorant as the lowest class of midwomen?" The problem, he conceded, was that the midwives were not trained, and that the doctors, who refused to train them, were.[16] Scholars have now documented how complete, by the end of the eighteenth century, was the triumph of man midwives among the upper classes of London and of the cities of colonial America.[17]

Over the nineteenth century much of the obstetrics among the popular classes as well as the middle class slipped from the midwives to the doctors. Even in working-class cities like Glasgow, doctors were by the First World War attending almost half the births.[18]* An 1895 survey of a widespread sampling of "agricultural localities" in England found that three quarters of all mothers had booked a doctor in advance, while only 3 percent had expressly booked a midwife.[20]† In the 1860s in London's poor-ish East End, "30 to 50 percent" of deliveries were midwife-attended; in the better-to-do West End only "2 percent or less" were. In Edinburgh in those years midwives attended births "to but a trifling extent."[22]‡ And in England as a whole in 1892 midwives were present at only about half of all births.[24]

Midwives lost most ground of all, however, in the United States. Around 1910 they were still attending around half of all deliveries,[25] but mainly among groups outside the mainstream of American society: southern blacks and immigrants. In Mississippi toward the First World War, for example, midwives delivered 88 percent of black women, 16 percent of white.[26] The same roughly was true for North Carolina.§ Of the poor white mothers whom Margaret Hagood interviewed when she traveled through the South in the 1930s, 85 percent had doctors in attendance.[28] Most of the midwives were black. Among the Poles in Wisconsin "the opinion is not uncommon that a mother should be able practically to deliver herself, and that a physician is not only superfluous but even

---

* Of the 112,000 births from 1908 to 1912, 48 percent were "medically attended from the beginning."[19]

† Of 779 deliveries in "agricultural localities in many counties," 629 mothers had booked a general practitioner.[21]

‡ In New South Wales in 1914, doctors attended 58 percent of births; by 1935–36, 80 percent.[23]

§ "The negro mothers were almost invariably dependent upon the midwife."[27]

undesirable." Yet among native American mothers in Wisconsin only 16 percent took midwives.[29] Practicing in a German community in Minnesota, Dr. O. C. Strickler said in 1916 that "formerly, say about thirty years ago, about all our obstetric work was done by midwives, and the only time physicians were called in, was in cases of operative obstetrics. I find there has been a wonderful change in that regard. . . . The people are asking in advance for medical assistance."[30] Even in a city filled with immigrants like Chicago, 50 percent of deliveries were being done by doctors by the First World War.[31] The proportion in New York City was even higher (38 percent of births delivered by midwives in 1914).[32] Thus in the Anglo-Saxon world as a whole by 1914, general practitioners had clearly seized a substantial chunk, if not most, of obstetric practice from the midwives, the largest inroad being among the middle and the upper classes. This erosion probably occurred because mothers wanted to be confined in gentler circumstances, having as birth attendants people with whom they felt more in common culturally than in terms of gender.

Then a remarkable thing happened. In every place save the United States and Canada, the midwives staged a comeback. Whereas in the United States the percentage of midwife deliveries fell from around 50 percent in 1901 to one half of 1 percent in 1970, it rose in Britain over that period from 50 percent to 76 percent![33] While North American midwives ended up being virtually outlawed, those in Britain and the Continent came back to perform the great majority of normal deliveries. Figures for other countries are less dramatic than in Britain. Yet in 1976 in the Netherlands, for example, four births in every ten (of both home and hospital deliveries) were midwife-assisted.[34] The Netherlands had in that year about 800 midwives; West Germany had 5,500; Italy, 18,000; the Soviet Union, 330,000.[35] So the midwives have not lost out in Europe. Britain has even a shortage now, the midwifery divisions of Manchester hospitals being short-staffed by "at least 16 percent."[36]

But if, as I claim, the initial sapping of midwife strength in the nineteenth century demonstrated a new sensibility toward childbearing, why does the midwives' resurgence not demonstrate the loss of this new sensibility? The answer is that these modern midwives are highly trained, practicing for the most part in hospitals and under close supervision. The only thing they have in common with Europe's traditional midwives is that they are female. In 1970 almost nine tenths of Britain's births occurred in hospitals, the majority midwife-supervised. Of the midwife births in 1976 in Holland 42 percent took place in hospitals. In Scandinavia in the 1970s, almost all normal births were conducted by midwives, yet the great majority happened in hospitals. Finland in 1973 had only eight home deliveries.[37] Of France's nine thousand midwives, only 28 percent now do home deliveries; the others work in hospitals.[38] So while European women today continue for the most part to be delivered by other women, the circumstances have changed completely from the days of the traditional "handywoman." The presence of a male doctor at one's bedside now brings no particular reassurance; a hundred years ago it did.

BIRTHING IN BED

Another indication of women's desire for gentler, more sentimental births was the shift to the bed, from the birthing stool and the straw pallet. I last spoke of births taking place on the midwife's stool, dangling from a rope, or kneeling before a bench. The nineteenth-century bourgeoisie preferred the bed, and the doctors listened and gave up their own complicated birthing chairs.[39] As one Berlin doctor said in 1836, "Stools make deliveries harder rather than easier. Their arrival alarms the mother; they occasion prolapse, chills, and other accidents." Another doctor complained, "Stools are nothing more than protection against getting the bedding dirty and therefore are preferred mainly by the stingy or the impecunious." A recent student has concluded that if, by the 1840s, doctors everywhere were delivering their patients in bed, it was because the old midwives' stool was "uncomfortable, looked repellent, and put women into a panic. It had become an ominous symbol of pain in birth."[40] Thus, in even a small town like Memel, by the 1840s "normal deliveries among the upper classes take place pretty generally in the family bed."[41]

It was, however, in England that birthing in bed first established itself among the middle and the upper classes, probably toward the middle of the eighteenth century with the advent of the man midwives.* Do not think that putting women in bed somehow made it easier for "males to interfere in labor," because the position the English and the Americans wanted the woman to take was that of lying on her left side, her knees drawn up to her chest, her back to the physician. Edward Rigby said in 1844 that this position had been used in England for "about a century," before which time doctors had preferred mothers on their backs.[43] I return later to how birthing positions have changed in the twentieth century. Here I note that birthing in *bed*, in whatever position, originated among the middle classes.

RELIEF OF PAIN

Finally, births have become tamed with relief for pain. Today people debate whether it really hurts to have a baby, or whether the pain comes mainly from fear, and thus from the woman's inability to relax and bear

---

* Harvey Graham says that it started to become customary with John Leake in the 1770s.[42]

down properly.[44] As a man I am unable to comment on this debate; but I do know that women in past times often resented birth pangs so much that they considered them as part of "God's punishment for women."[45] A French village midwife told Yvonne Verdier, "In those days they used to scream. Wow, did they scream!" The midwives took it lightly: "Oh, I'm not going to get in a bother the moment I hear you yelling." Or, "As long as the mother doesn't say she's going to die, the kid's not yet ready." The old women said, "Go on and cry so loud the whole village hears you."[46] So these mothers thought they were in pain.

The perception of pain is determined to some extent by cultural expectations. If it's bad form to cry out, then women will try not to. "If you yell too loud and too much you will kill the baby," said the poor white women of the American South.[47] And the Victorians generally had the notion that it was bad form to "flinch." In villages a woman might ask the midwife after a first birth, "I didn't flinch, did I? Oh, I do hope I didn't flinch."[48] Similarly, a sharp remark from the doctor might embarrass the mother enough to shut her up. "Unseemly screaming in labor," wrote Doctor Otto Spiegelberg, "may often be at once checked by a few decided words."[49]

But let us say the woman was sensitive and decided it really did hurt. What kind of relief could she get for that pain before the mid-nineteenth century? None, or virtually none.[50] Women used to try and get drunk in labor to cut the pain. Midwife Marjosa in the Lötschental remembered tales of fearful excesses with alcohol"; she herself wasn't against a glass of schnaps or two for an exhausted mother. "But how can the mother cooperate in pressing down if she is drunk?" Marjosa asked.[51] Alcohol, in fact, is not an analgesic, for it does not block pain.

Then in 1847 two drugs, ether and chloroform, were used for the first time in obstetrics.[52]* They induce unconsciousness, and an unconscious mother, of course, is no longer able to press down with her voluntary muscles to help the birth. But the involuntary muscles of her uterus will continue to act, and she will awaken surprised to see her baby in front of her. In the hundred years after the discovery of ether and chloroform, it was mothers who desperately snatched these anesthetics from the hands of unwilling doctors and midwives.

The demand for ether and chloroform among women was irresistible. Word started to get around soon. One year after chloroform was discovered, the following scenario was already taking place: "The [labor] pains were most severe, and were becoming unsupportable; but they appeared to do no good. . . . I felt in despair," wrote the doctor. Then "after

---

* It is, however, possible that Harvard's Walter Channing had used ether earlier in obstetrics.

many hours of suffering" he gave his patient chloroform, and she was peacefully delivered.[53] The Edinburgh doctor who discovered chloroform, James Simpson, wrote later: "Women who were delivered before the discovery of anesthetics have ceased to lament that they were born in an unhappy era."[54] By the early twentieth century doctors were arguing that they had to give chloroform and ether, or they would lose their patients to someone who would. "The abolition of pain and fatigue will always create a great demand for service," said a Montreal doctor in 1930. "The novice must emulate his competitor or starve."[55] An American doctor seven years later thundered against the ubiquity of pain killers in obstetrics. Eardley Holland, visiting from London, replied to him at that meeting of the American Gynecological Society, "I agree with Dr. Kosmak about analgesics, but we have got to give them, for if we do not nobody will come near us."[56]

Indeed, physicians probably let patients' wishes get the better of good sense. Both ether and chloroform cause all kinds of problems in their administration, some of them fatal. The drugs were often implicated in various studies of maternal mortality. For example, the anesthetic was considered the "direct cause of death in 20 cases" in New York City between 1930 and 1932. The committee responsible for assessing these fatalities noted that "anesthesia during labor and delivery is a problem of the most pressing importance, more so in the United States than in any other country. This has come about to a large extent through pressure from the lay public." Who in particular? Middle-class women in big cities, said the authors. "The accoucheur may disregard these demands only at great risk to his own practice."[57] A similar committee on maternal deaths in England observed in 1937, "The increased sensibility to pain and discomfort has led to the movement to secure for women of all classes the relief from pain in childbirth which was formerly accepted as part of the course of nature."[58] So women were demanding that something be done.

The attraction of chloroform especially was its ease of administration. "The patient's face is anointed with cold cream or Vaseline and a damp towel is placed over her eyes. The mask is adjusted to fit her face and the chloroform bottle is adjusted to drop moderately freely," wrote a West Virginia doctor of a typical home delivery.[59] Or one could just put a handkerchief over the mother's face and trickle drops onto it from time to time.

Thus did some kind of anesthetic become well-nigh universal in childbearing by the 1920s. "An anesthetist is considered desirable for most, if not all, cases," said England's Doctor Janet Campbell in 1924.[60] And Dr. F. E. Leavitt, who circulated in 1916 a questionnaire among eighty-four rural practitioners in Minnesota, said "There is no procedure in obstetrics that is practiced with such uniformity as the administration of chloroform and ether. Everyone of those replying use one or the other in labor."[61]

Yet because of the dangers of ether and chloroform, the reader might well ask, How could substances of such high risk have been responsible for the kind of "release from vulnerability" that I argue took place for women circa the period 1900–1925? The answer is that these substances were replaced. Starting around 1900 a number of other less dangerous analgesics and anesthetics came along, ultimately displacing ether and chloroform entirely. In 1902 one researcher began to experiment with a mixture of scopolamine and morphine, later called "twilight sleep," which merely induced in patients forgetfulness of pain, not complete unconsciousness. In 1906, Carl Joseph Gauss of Freiburg published the results of his research with twilight sleep in some five hundred births, and a huge vogue for this mixture began, above all in the Anglo-Saxon world, which lasted for the next thirty years.[62] There were many problems with scopolamine-morphine narcosis which it is unnecessary to go into here; but just as it was falling into disuse, nitrous oxide came along. Although it had already been revived in 1922 after years of oblivion, it required at that point the presence of a skilled anesthetist. Then in 1933 someone invented a device for administering it so simple that midwives could use it in home deliveries; indeed, mothers could give it to themselves as they felt the need. From 1939 on such synthetic narcotics as meperidine hydrochloride (Demerol, called "pethidine" in England) began to catch on; they had the advantage of blocking pain at the beginning of labor without slowing contractions or fatally depressing the infant.[63]

I wish to emphasize how unenthusiastically, before the Second World War, most doctors viewed the diffusion of these drugs, how much the whole demand for relief from birth pangs came from women, rather than from the medical profession. When James Simpson introduced chloroform in the late 1840s he encountered heavy resistance, some of it for medical reasons, some on the biblical ground that, to pay for Eve's handiwork, women were doomed to endure the pangs of labor.[64] Charles Waller of St. Thomas's Hospital in London, for example, wrote in 1858 that, during instrumental deliveries, women could easily be injured if they were completely insensible to pain. And "in natural labours no reason exists for the employment of a remedy, the efficacy of which is at least doubtful, and its action often hurtful."[65] This medical hostility to women "in revolt against the normal processes of labor" continued, despite the clamoring of the patients.[66] The simple fact, said British obstetrician James Young, is that "the induction of anesthesia in response to the dictates of humanity tends inevitably toward the risk that the doctor, in the higher interests of his patient, may be compelled to hasten the delivery of the child."[67] In other words, the more you anesthetize them, the more you intervene. "The patient may brag about having had the baby in her sleep," said George Kosmak at an obstetrical meeting in 1947, "but what about the effect on the baby?"[68]

This medical resistance to pain killers, of which these are merely a few examples, has persisted from 1847 to the present. Since the Second World War it has been an undercurrent, in the face of official insistence that "relief from pain should be one of the main objects of any modern maternity service."[69] And I quote these doctors only to make the point that anesthesia should be seen as part of women's rejection of the traditional birth, rather than as a result of doctors' efforts to impose something undesired on them. Representing the viewpoint that anesthesia was some kind of sinister doctors' plot against women are Richard Wertz and Dorothy Wertz who argue that, "What was at issue was not the patient's consciousness or the degree of anesthetization but control of birth."[70]

Thus, in terms of choosing a birth attendant, delivering in bed, and demanding pain relief, these new female sensibilities appear early in time. But to give women the safe, gentle births they were asking required more than simply putting them on their sides in the big family bed and blotting them out during labor. A number of ominous problems continued to frustrate the demand for a new kind of birth experience, and only in the first quarter of the twentieth century were most of these overcome.

The Dark Side of Home Delivery

From this point on I concentrate on Britain and the United States. Just as in previous centuries Germany and France had provided models for the rest of the world, after the First World War leadership in obstetrics was taken over by the Anglo-Saxons. The rest of the world would follow behind. We can, therefore, grasp the larger story of what has happened to women everywhere in the last sixty years by focusing on a few key places.

Even though in 1920 a mother probably would neither die of a post-delivery infection nor suffer much pain, several unpleasant things might nonetheless happen, especially if she gave birth at home. The biggest problems were the poor training of the G.P.'s and an abuse of forceps. How these problems arose, and their chief consequence—the displacement of normal deliveries from home to hospital—are the subjects of the next two sections.

POORLY TRAINED DOCTORS

We have already seen to what extent home deliveries were being done by doctors rather than by midwives by 1920. A particular sore spot was that most of these physicians were not well trained to do obstetrics and became skilled to the extent that they learned on the job, through trial and error. Keep in mind the doctors' long tradition of not involving themselves with obstetrics. Country doctors had once limited themselves to prescribing opium and lancing boils and had little practical understanding of childbirth. The problem arose with the enormous expansion of medical schools late in the nineteenth century, when their young graduates began to settle in small communities and establish for themselves general practices. For these young doctors, obstetrics mattered a good deal, but the average medical education in those days poorly qualified them to do it. As "an occupation degrading to a gentleman," midwifery was not taught in Oxford or Cambridge before the 1840s. And even later students had too little opportunity, in practice, to watch at births. Edinburgh, for example, had over one thousand students in the 1870s but only seven thousand births in "the rank of life that made them available to undergraduates."[71] A typical student in a large London hospital in the 1890s would attend just one labor in his week-long obstetrics rotation. He was, as historian F. B. Smith retells the story: "not permitted to touch the patient. After the child was delivered and the patient taken away, he never saw her or the child again. He and his colleagues asked to be shown the obstetrics instruments: the consultant refused, saying that their request was 'most irregular'; he sent them to obtain 'special permission,' which was refused. [The student] and his friends at the end of the week were certified as having attended the whole number of deliveries that occurred in the hospital during that week. He was thereby fully qualified in the words of his certificate "to undertake anything required in obstetrics."[72]

Things were no better in the United States. When in 1911, J. W. Williams surveyed the heads of obstetrics departments in forty-three medical schools, several replied that they had "accepted the professorship merely because it was offered to them but had no special training or liking for it"; one said "he had never seen a woman delivered before assuming his professorship." The schools with smaller lying-in hospitals were among themselves able to offer "only 553 cases for the instruction of 575 students," half of the deliveries occurring when students were not around. "It is apparent that each student on an average has an opportunity to see only one woman delivered." "Do you consider the ordinary graduate from your school is competent to practice obstetrics?" asked Williams. One quarter answered "no," and many of the "yes's" were qualified, as in "Well, yes, in a way; that is, some of them."[73] Also, the emphasis in obstetrical instruction then lay more on the heroic rescue than on the normal delivery. "We can all recall our student days when the professor who gave spectacular clinics was more popular" than the unostentatious. The speaker, a medical conservative named Rudolph Holmes from Chicago, blasted the "pyrotechnic exhibition which characterized the older arena. . . . A clinic which gives a student 18 major obstetric operations in his two weeks' practical training has misappropriated the student's time."[74]

In practice these young G.P.'s could scarcely help but do disastrously. Many had "never seen the forceps applied until they use them themselves in general practice."[75] Stanley Warren of Portland, Maine, described his first forceps delivery, a forty-three-year-old Irish woman with her first child: "Labor commenced in the early morning of Tuesday, January 1, 1875, and progressed very slowly until the next Sunday afternoon[!]. Then, under the direction of an older friend, I applied Simpson's forceps at the brim [of the pelvis], but it required the combined strength of both of us upon the instrument to extract the child."[76] J. S. Templeton of Pinckneyville, Illinois, remembered how, in doing a version, he had fractured an infant's leg early in his practice: "[I] was alone, and had to superintend the giving of the chloroform and deliver the child at the same time, and . . . while bringing down the feet a leg was broken about the middle third of the femur. . . . This is one fracture bill that was never collected, not even charged."[77] A maternal mortality committee in Rochdale found in 1936 that "the problem of the doctor presented the greatest difficulty. The training he received was lamentably inadequate at most schools, and the average man went into practice with no real practical experience. . . . In spite of everything that so many authorities had said concerning droplet infection it was rare to find a doctor who would wear a mask."[78]

Some of these men improved with experience. Some simply never had enough experience because, in a city like Manchester in the 1930s, there were 650 practitioners who in total attended only 900 booked cases a year, "with an additional 2,413 cases on the formal request of midwives. . . . Obviously experience in obstetrics was not available in sufficient amount to maintain skilled practice."[79] As more British midwives became formally trained, even fewer births went to G.P.'s. A maternal mortality committee in Wales said in 1934, "Twenty or thirty years ago, it was not uncommon for a doctor to attend 100 confinements or more a year. Now normal cases are delivered mostly by midwives. . . . The result is that the doctor not infrequently lacks the background of straightforward cases with which to compare the abnormal case."[80] This, then, was one part of the dark side of home delivery in the 1920s and 1930s: incompetent attendants.

A related abuse in home deliveries was giving the mother pituitrin, a uterine-stimulating drug. Discovered in 1906 by Edinburgh's Henry Hallett Dale, it started to be used obstetrically after 1909, when another British doctor named Blair Bell wrote about it.[81]* It would, in fact, accelerate slow labors, literally "blasting the baby through the birth canal."[84] Although pituitrin had the unfortunate side effect of occasionally rupturing the uterus, it came to be widely used alongside forceps. In Hermann Fehling's Strasbourg clinic, pituitrin reduced forceps deliveries by a third.[85] Dr. G. H. Luedtke of Fairmont, Minnesota, told how "one dose of pituitrin finished the work in from five to ten minutes. . . . Forceps deliveries are becoming very rare with the proper use of pituitrin." Indeed, in his practice he used it about half the time.[86]

Thus, "meddlesome midwifery" at home was becoming a major problem. A maternal mortality review committee studied "manipulative interference" in the thirty-five thousand births in Wales in 1934. Obviously some of the operations were necessary; but in home births *with no complications*, doctors had nonetheless interfered in 31 percent (in only 10 percent of such hospital births, by comparison).† Now, contrast the doctors' 31 percent with the midwives' 3 percent rate of interference in normal deliveries, and you will acquire some understanding of why the medical profession as a whole was concerned about the "orgy of intervention" in those years.[88] Bear in mind that all these interventions were still being done on the *mother's* behalf. Up to now, almost nobody was seriously concerned about the fetus.

ABUSE OF FORCEPS

A second problem in home delivery was overuse of forceps, especially among urban practitioners in the Anglo-Saxon world, where some men prided themselves on being "forceps fiends." Glasgow's Dr. Alexander Miller, for example, used forceps 8 percent to 10 percent of the time in the early days of his practice—25 percent by the time he wrote in 1899.[89] In the Redditch area forceps use rose from 4 percent in the 1890s to 20 percent in the 1920s; and among the doctors' *booked* cases between 1922

---

* Pituitary extract did not become widely known in obstetrics until recommended by J. Hofbauer in 1911.[82] This extract from the posterior pituitary gland of domestic animals has a rather nasty history of sending mothers into profound shock as well as of rupturing uteri. The sixteenth edition of *Williams Obstetrics* states, "Oxytocin should have long since completely replaced pituitrin in all hospitals."[83]

† Of 2,238 instances of "manipulative interference" by doctors, 2,177 were "forceps and other forms of interference not specified."[87]

and 1926, almost half the deliveries were instrumental.[90]* The activities of these men were widely criticized and represent part of the profession's motivation for shepherding mothers into hospitals, where such abuses could be controlled.

Not merely were too many forceps deliveries being done at home. They were being done incompetently. Many doctors, in fact, failed to deliver the baby with forceps, and ultimately the mother would be transported to the hospital with the diagnosis "FFO"—failed forceps outside. It was the large number of FFOs that sounded the death knell of home deliveries in general.

Let me review. In those days the textbooks said three conditions must be fulfilled before a doctor could apply the forceps: that the mother's cervix be fully dilated, that the infant's head come first, and that the head be fully engaged in the pelvis.[95] In an FFO either the mother's cervix was not quite open—and the doctor, in his haste to be finished, started yanking away; or some malpresentation existed for which the forceps was inappropriate. One study of the reasons for failure in 558 cases found that in perhaps one third the mother's pelvis was too small, usually from rickets; in a further third, failure came from the child's emerging from its mother face up ("persistent occiput-posterior"); in a final third, as the report diplomatically stated, "it was apparent that anxiety to relieve suffering had prompted an attempt to assist delivery before sufficient dilatation of the soft passages."[96] Another study found that the proper rules for forceps had been followed in only four of one hundred failed cases.[97]

There were terrible stories: "A doctor who may handle a new-born infant with gentle care may think nothing of . . . putting his foot against the bed and, as I have many times been told, pulling with all his might."[98] James Hendry confessed in 1928 that "I have myself had the mortification of performing caesarean section in a 'failed forceps' case, and delivering a child with a fractured skull and both cheeks very badly torn by the forceps."[99] Here is one without anesthetic: "Delivery was difficult. The forceps slipped five times and caused severe hemorrhage. The perineum was torn to the rectum." The mother was sent the same day to the hospital and died there.[100] In another case done without anesthetic, the mother "awakened the neighbourhood with her screams," and died shortly after her admission to hospital.[101]

---

* Note that these high frequencies were not typical of the medical profession as a whole. In trained-midwife deliveries with medical backup in 1926 in England, forceps were used in only 6 percent.[91] In Hamburg from 1901 to 1935, forceps were applied in home and hospital deliveries combined only 3 percent to 4 percent of the time.[92] Rates in Kansas (5 percent) and Iowa (4 percent) were also quite low.[93] In Chicago's Maternity Center, only 6 percent of births in the home-delivery service were instrument-assisted, 1932–43.[94]

In fact, one out of every ten mothers in an FFO died later in hospital.
Two thirds of the children were killed by the procedure.[102] The amazing
thing is the frequency of "failed forceps" cases in those years. In 1931,
a big maternity hospital in Glasgow received seventy-six of them; one
in Newcastle, forty-four; one in Edinburgh, twenty-four; and so on.[103]
These tragic home deliveries inevitably provoked an outcry among the
public and within the medical profession. "Hardly a week passes without
some reference in the lay press to conferences on maternal mortality,
to questions in Parliament on the same subject. . . . Obstetrics is made
to appear the Cinderella among the ashes," said Hendry in 1928, adding
that the public had started to feel "there is danger in the doctor."[104]
The leaders of the profession, too, were furious at the abuse of forceps
in private practice. "It is a pathetic and humiliating sight to see a healthy
young woman dying in childbed, with her little wedding presents as yet
untarnished about her, because the medical attendant has thought it right
to risk the production of injuries in a first and normal labour."[105] Comments of this nature are found throughout the literature. Jellett, for example, raged in 1929 against "turning a physiological process in a healthy
woman into a death trap."[106]

The red thread running through "failed forceps" was the impatience
and haste of the general practitioner. Yet "impatience" has several dimensions, not all of which are necessarily reducible to medical callousness.
Of course these men felt themselves rushed by "the multiple calls of
general practice."[107] "For heaven's sake let's get the forceps on and be
finished with it," said one doctor.[108] But many physicians felt a deeper
resentment—unprofessional, of course, but nonetheless quite human—
at being called to home deliveries at all. "Midwifery, in fact, does not
pay," said Victor Bonney in 1919, "except in so far as it serves as an
introduction to other forms of practice; a pernicious thing, for underpaid
work can never be the best work."[109] The doctor received "the pitiful
fee of one guinea for spending the night in such a place as has been
described, and then making ten visits free and paying for the cab and
the chloroform out of his own pocket."[110] The fees were low to begin
with, and then in England the midwives could grab for themselves the
easy deliveries, leaving the local G.P. with the middle-class mothers and
the tough emergency cases. "What happens when a nurse [midwife] is
imported? She manages the thirty normal cases without help, and the
doctor is £60 out of pocket"—on the assumption that in those days he
charged £2 per delivery.[111] The doctor actually got about as much for a
tonsilectomy as for a delivery—hence, the temptation to "hasten delivery
by every available means."[112] However anxiously G.P.'s might have com-
peted with midwives in Britain fifty years previously, by the 1930s the

former were ready to give up home deliveries—"a small part and the least attractive part of their practice," as the Welsh maternal mortality survey put it in 1937.[113]

Even in the United States, where few midwives troubled mainline medical practice, doctors became increasingly sour about doing home deliveries after the First World War. Thus, two doctors in Litchfield, Minnesota: "Obstetrics is the hardest work we have; much night work, long trips, long hours, and the poorest compensation." Dr. Workman, of Tracy, Minnesota, said, "I am trying to get out of obstetric work. I cannot afford to give time for fees paid."[114] Thus, if the work was rushed and sloppy, if tears of the perineum were not repaired because they were not looked for very carefully, and if the forceps was applied with the mother's cervix only half dilated, the reason was partly that by the 1920s and 1930s much medical ill will had developed about attending home deliveries.

There is, however, another dimension to the doctors' prematurity in applying forceps: pressures from the mother herself and from the relatives standing around. Remember what communal events home births were, the bystanders commenting freely to the doctor. When from their viewpoint the mother had suffered enough, they would urge him to action. The doctor, called in an emergency, would find this scene: "The woman is crying she can endure no longer. The husband implores the doctor to do something. The midwife, who perhaps has already been on the scene for 48 hours, is also worn out and exhausted. Day breaks. The older children, who sleep in the same room, are about to awake and there's no other place to put them. And even the doctor is oppressed by the thought of how much work is piling up for him at home. In these situations you are pressured to act even against your will—and how often does it happen, to the disadvantage of the mother." For the rural doctor, said the writer, "waiting is a real art."[115] W. J. Sinclair found the "gossips" exasperating; he meant those who "claim the privilege of offering well-meant but ignorant suggestions concerning the 'exhausted' condition of some vigorous young woman in the first hours of normal labour."[116] Doctor Janet Campbell warned in 1924, "The medical attendant may not find it altogether easy to resist the demands of his patient for speedy relief."[117] In long drawn-out first stages of labor only some clinical experience would permit the doctor to "resist the importunities of the patient and her friends" for its curtailment.[118] Which is precisely why the flood of junior physicians with little experience was pernicious for the patients. Ironically, the new lease on life that English midwives obtained with the 1902 Midwives Act probably made the problem worse, for they were even more subject to the relatives' importuning. Thus, deliveries by the "Queen's Institute Nurses" in the early 1930s had a forceps rate more than twice that of several big London hospitals: "The midwives are compelled by the patient or her relatives to summon the doctor (in many instances unnecessarily) to terminate the labour."[119]

American doctors, too, felt the kiss of the bystanders' lash. Attending a mother in her second confinement, a Pinckneyville, Illinois, doctor let her labor for about five days: "The child was smaller than the first one, but I cannot help feeling that in the first case we were too much in a hurry, and though abused by the neighbor women I felt repaid for the time and trouble of waiting it out this time."[120] So the neighbors did not always stand about in reverential postures. Moreover, their opinion mattered in the doctor's future success in that town. Said a Tennessee practitioner, "There is usually present one or more experienced women who know, or think they know, every detail as to the proper management of child-bed cases. Hence, the impression made . . . will make or break a doctor's reputation."[121] With fifty years of hindsight it is pointless for us to try and attach blame, to insist that the relatives or the doctors' own impatience and spinelessness were at fault for the "meddlesome midwifery" of the 1920s and 1930s. The point is that these various pressures to intervene at home could all be easily neutralized if a mother were to give birth in the hospital.

The Shift from Home to Hospital

Before 1900 only unwed mothers and poor women gave birth in the hospital. Of Kansas it was said around the time of the First World War, "the hospital seems to be generally regarded as a last resort."[122] In Wisconsin in those years hospital birth was "almost never done."[123] Around 1920 fewer than 10 percent of births in Chicago occurred in hospital.[124] But by the 1980s hospital births had become the rule in every country in Western society except the Netherlands; and by 1976 even there, two out of every three mothers were giving birth in the hospital. Whereas in Germany virtually no married women had babies in the hospital before the 1920s, by the 1970s 98 percent of them would deliver there (see table 7.1). Detroit's hospital confinement rate zoomed from around 5 percent in 1908 to 94 percent in 1945. In the United States as a whole, 99 percent of all mothers would deliver in the hospital by the end of the 1970s, and nine British mothers out of every ten.[125] As I write these lines, home deliveries are a thing of the past.

Why? What could have motivated these millions of women to abandon the folkloric coziness of a home delivery for a brusque hospital ward?

TABLE 7.1

The Percentage of Hospital Births, Germany and the United States (in the Nineteenth and Twentieth Centuries)

Year	Percentage
Germany	
1877	less than 1%
1891	1
1924	9
1936	27
1952	46
1962	72
1970	95
1973	98
United States	
1935	37
1945	79
1955	94
1977	99

SOURCES: See notes to tables, pages 380.

Let's examine things from the viewpoint of each of the three participants: the doctors, the midwives, and the mothers.

Because we today have little notion of the homes of working-class people in the 1920s, we poorly understand the reluctance of doctors to do deliveries in them. "You find a bed which has been slept on by the husband, wife or one or two children; it has frequently been soaked with urine, the sheets are dirty, and the patient's garments soiled; she has not had a bath. Instead of sterile dressings you have a few old rags or the discharges are allowed to soak into a nightdress which is not changed for days."[126] By contrast, the doctors practically wept with pleasure when they thought about how nice hospitals were. Adolf Weber, an Alsfeld doctor with many years' experience in farmhouse and hospital deliveries, said that in the latter, "The mother lies in a well-aired, disinfected room; light and sunshine stream unhindered through a high window, and you can make it light as day electrically too. She is well bathed and freshly clothed, on linen sheets of blinding whiteness. . . . You have a staff of assistants, who respond to every signal."[127] This theme of light recurs repeatedly. In hospital one could *see* what one was doing. "Only those who have to repair a perineum in a cottar's house, in a cottar's bed, with the poor light and help at hand, can realize the joy."[128] The stories go on and on.

Part of the medical enthusiasm for hospitals rested on the incorrect belief that sepsis was higher in home deliveries, and that sepsis death rates had been increasing. In chapter 6, I noted that view was the product of misleading statistics. So Victor Bonney's influential plea in 1919 for conducting labor as a "surgical operation," staining the baby's head "violet green" with antiseptics, and generally treating pregnancy as a "life-endangering tumor" to be "got rid of as soon as possible" rested on false assumptions.[129]

But the theme that appears most often in the doctors' discourse is that hospitalizing mothers would reduce the number of dangerous procedures at home and curb the operative mania of the local G.P.s. In the hospital there would be no relatives to demand premature intervention. A Swiss doctor said that waiting for the mother to deliver spontaneously "went much more easily in a maternity hospital, where you can reflect in calm and with a correct picture of the clinical situation, and judge all courses of action, than at home," with the relatives screaming at you.[130] A Minnesota doctor said he liked the hospital because "it enabled him to get away from the fool family."[131] "Why does the harassed general practitioner do those things which he should not do, and leave undone the things he should do?" asked Lapthorn Smith after Bonney had given his 1919 talk. "Would it not be far better that all these women should be sent into a hospital for confinement?"[132]

Accordingly, by the late 1930s the leaders of the profession aimed at delivering most mothers in the hospital. Thus, the English report on maternal mortality in 1937: "A reduction in the group of deaths following abnormal labour will be effected only when general practitioners realise that they must not, except in a grave emergency, attempt in the patient's home difficult obstetric operations which would tax the skill of experienced obstetricians in well equipped hospitals."[133] And Edwin Daily of the Children's Bureau of the U.S. Government was explicit when addressing the annual meeting of the American Obstetrical Society in 1944: "*All* maternity patients should have care during labor and during the first 10 days after delivery in hospitals"[134] (italics in original).

Nor did the midwives universally set themselves against hospital delivery. It was the hospital that saved their profession. Midwife Alice Gregory, for example, helped found around 1900 a maternity hospital in Woolwich, England, which would serve as a training school for midwives. (Gregory was scathingly contemptuous of traditional midwives, "who have always been led to believe that neither they nor the patient can get on without *plenty* of brandy and gin."[135]) German midwife Lisbeth Burger wrote in 1936, "I can understand that women want to go to the hospital. There everything's all set. They spare themselves work, upset, and money. And other things enter in if the apartment's too cramped and small. But it is so impersonal."[136] A midwife who practiced in the slums of Berlin spoke of "those holes in the wall, as hot as the lead rooves of Venice in summer, suffocating with the heat of the oven in winter. . . . A clever woman would do better to go to a clinic, for the calm and comfort that offer family harmony the best guarantee."[137]*

The shift of middle-class women to hospitals for delivery is perhaps the most important development in our story during the 1920s and 1930s. Morris Vogel writes that during these years hospitals "moved to the center of medical practice," not just in obstetrics but across the board. Whereas mothers birthing in Boston's hospitals during the 1870s had been mainly poor or unmarried, by the 1920s only 3 percent were unmarried. The Massachusetts General Hospital opened a private maternity ward in 1917, and shortly thereafter was obliged to set aside an entire floor for deliveries. In 1915 the trustees of the Boston Lying-In Hospital said, "There are hundreds, of limited means, who are able and anxious to pay moderately for a bed in a semi-private ward, and with the rapid growth of the apartment house population, the number is fast multiplying."[138] "The class of cases coming into the hospital has changed very much within the last twenty years," wrote Emma L. Call of the New England Hospital in 1908. "They are now mostly married women in fairly comfortable circumstances, while formerly they were largely of the unmarried class."[139] In truth, the demand for hospital births among the modestly well-off was huge.

One can understand why women who lived in hovels might prefer the calmness of the clinic. But since it was the collective decision of middle-class women that promoted the move to the hospital for the average birth, what was their motivation? Was it, as some writers have argued, that the doctors mercilessly drummed into the heads of women their male-chauvinistic desires for control?† Or did the rush to the hospital take place as part of women's larger desire to tame the birth experience? A thousand circumstances enter into a collective change of mind of this magnitude: life in cramped apartments in big cities; the bitter poverty in Europe, just after the First World War, which caused health insurance funds to start paying for hospital births; the diffusion of the medical understanding that first mothers are slightly more at risk for complications than are mothers who have borne more children.[141] Yet, in the 1920s, rustic mothers in England were flooding into "cottage hospitals," and

---

* It is unclear to what extent a doctor who collaborated may be speaking here.

† "Clinics sought to socialize their patients to obey routines and to trust the staff by making weight control a means of obedience training during repeated prenatal visits. . . . Doctors found that the scales were a convenient means of social control over the lives of patients."[140]

American middle-class women who knew no ruinous inflation were rushing into maternity suites, so there must have been some underlying factor.

Caesarean Birth: The Final Push toward the Hospital

That underlying factor was women's heightened expectations, in the early twentieth century, of safe delivery. Traditional mothers accepted obstetric risks with the same fatalistic resignation that villagers displayed toward all risks they felt themselves unable to control, such as hail, plague, and war. The modern temper, on the other hand, insisted upon action in the face of adversity. By the 1920s the most effective way of cutting through adversity in childbirth was caesarean delivery. And because the margin of safety it supplied was available only in a hospital, to have that margin women started choosing hospital deliveries.

Before 1800 caesareans had been operations of desperation, performed on undelivered mothers only as they lay dying, in order to save the infant. Thus, there are reports of priests becoming specialists in abdominal delivery.[142] The old midwife ordinances contained instructions for ascertaining whether the mother was dead so that the infant could be cut out of her: "If she does not respond to penetrating odors, is ice-cold, without pulse, looks collapsed and pale as death, and if her breath leaves no traces on a mirror," she was thought dead, and the operation could begin.[143] Other anomalous circumstances, too, might merit an abdominal delivery: for instance, when the town authorities of Medingen cut a woman's child out of her in 1350 before burning her at the stake because she had "stolen three unblessed pieces of communion bread to sell them to the Jews." (The child survived to be baptized.)[144] Some hint of an operative tradition persisted among the common people, for now and again there are tales of farmers, sowgelders, and midwives doing caesareans successfully. In Tyrone County, Ireland, for example, Mary Donally, "an illiterate woman, but eminent among the common people for extracting dead births," was called to a woman who could not be delivered by other means. Mrs. Donally took a sharp razor and made an incision a bit to the side of the midline. "She held the lips of the wound together with her hand, till one went a mile and returned with silk and the common needles which tailors used. With these she joined the lips in the manner of the stitch employed ordinarily for the harelip, and dressed the wound with whites of eggs."[145]

With the revival of scientific medicine in the eighteenth century however, caesareans started to be attempted by doctors.[146] Mireille Laget concluded, "It is likely that the operation became less and less exceptional during the eighteenth century."[147] Yet even though increasing, abdominal deliveries in the eighteenth century must have been few, for Jacques-René Tenon, writing in 1788, was aware of only seventy-nine successful ones in all of Europe since 1500.[148]

So few were done because of the terrible mortality that clung to the operation. "Caesarean" was synonymous with "death sentence." Of 80 caesareans in Britain before 1858, only 29 percent of the women survived. Of 120 performed in the United States between 1852 and 1880, 58 percent of the mothers died.[149] The year 1794 saw the first successful abdominal delivery in the United States.[150] But thereafter, as everywhere, American doctors avoided it because it was just too forbidding.

Why? In theory the technique is simple. The surgeon makes a vertical incision in the midline of the belly, cutting the connective tissue between the major muscles of the abdominal wall; he or she then slices through the fatty layers of "fascia," pushes the bladder down and out of the way, and finds the huge pregnant uterus bulging forth in the abdomen. Today a surgeon makes a crosswise incision far down in the uterus near the pelvic bone (a "low cervical" section), slips a hand under the child's head and gently lifts it out, cuts the cord, and manually removes the placenta. Then everything is stitched up again, one layer at a time, and the operation is done in thirty to forty minutes.

In those days, however, infection could seize hold of the open abdomen; the mother might go into shock from the pain. Worst of all, once the child was removed, the surgeon might omit to stitch up the uterus, on the grounds that stitches would just be pulled out again anyway as the uterus returned to normal size. Thus, when mothers did not perish from sepsis in the filthy cities and hospitals (rural caesareans were in the nineteenth-century United States twice as successful as urban ones),[151] they would die of internal bleeding.

The invention of anesthesia (1847) and the enunciation of antiseptic principles in surgery (1867) opened the way for abdominal delivery. But the final breakthrough did not come until the early 1880s, when a couple of German doctors spelled out clearly the surgical technique toward which many others had been groping for some time: the surgeon would carefully approximate the edges of the uterine incision and firmly stitch them together. From that moment on, caesarean delivery became a serious possibility.[152]*

For a long time hospitals continued to rely on other emergency operations, such as high-forceps, infant destruction (craniotomy), or cutting through the pubic bone, rather than attempt caesarean delivery. Dublin's

---

* A number of American surgeons had already sutured the uterus before the Germans adopted the technique.[153]

TABLE 7.2

Caesarean Deliveries in the United States
(1890s–1979)*

Year	Frequency (percentage of all hospital deliveries)	Mortality (in percentages)
1890s–1900s	—	12.1
1900–09	1.0	—
1910–19	1.9	5.5
1920–29	2.9	7.6
1930–39	3.2	4.4
1940–49	2.8	.9
1950–59	3.7	.4
1960–69	6.8	".1"
1970–79	12.8	".02"

* After 1960 the caesarean mortality rate fell so low that authors stopped publishing series on the subject. Thus the Frigoletto and Williams series for 1960 to 1969 contained no deaths at all. I have put in quotation marks the .1 per 100 death rate from Rhode Island. The Frigoletto series for 1970 to 1978 contained no deaths, and the Rhode Island death rate had sunk to .04 per 100 abdominal deliveries; hence, a death rate of ".02." Rates this low have little meaning, and the main point is that fatalities in caesarean deliveries are extremely rare.

SOURCES: See notes to tables, pages 381–82.

Rotunda Hospital did its first successful caesarean in 1889; the Boston Lying-In in 1894; the Saint-Antoine Hospital in Paris, in 1896; the Lille Charité, in 1897.[154] Then the pace quickened. As many as 1 percent of all births in big U.S. hospitals were caesarean in between 1900 and 1909; 3 percent by the beginning of the Second World War (table 7.2). At the Rotunda in Dublin, too, the rate was plus 2 percent by the 1940s.[155]

It is important to note that increases in caesareans were matched by a decline in other kinds of obstetric operation, so that before the 1930s there was little *overall* increase in the amount of operative interference. In fact, we can chart the history of caesareans by noting at what point they drove various older operations out of existence. If the mother's pelvis is terribly contracted, said Detroit's J. H. Carstens in 1894, caesarean delivery should be done, rather than removing the infant in pieces (evisceration).[156] As caesareans advanced in Baden, podalic version retreated.[157] In 1925, Hermann Fehling noted how caesareans had reduced the use of high-forceps in Germany.[158]* At the Preston Retreat Hospital

* High-forceps means applying the instrument to the child's head before it has engaged in the pelvis. Great traction is then exerted by means of a special lever on the forceps; hence, the "Tarnier axis-traction forceps."

in Philadelphia, the use of high-forceps declined from 3.3 per 100 births in 1905–11 to .4 per 100 in 1912–17, as caesareans doubled in frequency over that time.[159] The last time a pubic bone was sawed through at New York's Sloane Hospital to help enlarge a mother's pelvis ("pubiotomy") was in 1902; the last cutting of the two pubic bones at their junction ("symphysiotomy") occurred in 1908.[160] While the use of high-forceps and version in Chicago's Michael Reese Hospital fell from 3.6 percent in 1925 to 1.1 in 1931, caesareans almost quadrupled. Accordingly, the total number of operations over that period increased scarcely at all.[161] In four large New York hospitals the total operative delivery rate declined slightly from 1933 to 1948, but the caesarean's share of that total climbed from 38 percent to 70 percent.[162]

I have dwelt at length upon these operations to reinforce the point that the coming of the caesarean did not cause more "intervention in childbirth." Instead, it effected a shift from old-style operations to an abdominal procedure far less damaging to the mother. Remember, after all, what risks of mutilation craniotomies entailed, how often uteri were ruptured in version, and how many women required months to walk normally again after their pubic bones had been sawed through. This lessened risk is reflected in a steady decline in maternal mortality in caesarean birth: from 12 percent in the 1890s to 4 percent by the 1930s (table 7.2).

It is therefore interesting to note how many *doctors* opposed what was obviously in the interests of their patients. My focus is the women, and not conflicts of medical opinion. Yet I cannot forbear mentioning that, in Britain particularly, long after infant-destruction operations and pubic-bone operations had been rejected elsewhere, they were preferred over caesareans. Why? Was a delay in labor feared? Do a "prophylactic pubiotomy" they counseled in the Rotunda Hospital in 1912![163] Dublin obstetrician Henry Jellett thundered in 1929 against "the glamour and spurious fame" of the caesarean and preferred to destroy the infant if the mother's birth canal were obstructed.[164] British textbooks continued to display a fondness for craniotomy for a while after their American counterparts had turned from it.* In a moment we shall see the importance of this earlier American repugnance to destroying the infant.

---

* Early editions of *Williams Obstetrics* were quite permissive about craniotomy; the second edition (1908) allowed it if the mother "possibly presents signs of infection" or "if the child is not in good condition."[165] But the editions of the 1930s and 1940s restricted it tightly, preferring caesarean-hysterectomy unless it was the mother's first birth.[166] The tenth edition in 1950 virtually banned craniotomy: "It is never employed today on living infants."[167] British textbooks, in contrast, showed a latitudinarian view until relatively recently. The Queen Charlotte's *Text-Book of Obstetrics* in 1936 weighed caesarean delivery and craniotomy evenly in the balance under "relative indications": "Should the fetal heart

The larger point to which this mini-history of caesarean birth has been building is that if the operation were to be done at all, it had to be in hospital. Of course, it was technically possible at home. In Iowa, for example, in the early 1930s, 43 caesareans were done at home (as opposed to 307 in hospital).[170] But it was harder to get a specialist to administer anesthesia at home; blood supplies were unavailable if the mother started hemorrhaging or went into shock, etcetera. The problems of home caesarean will be obvious to the reader. "If danger is to be foreseen," wrote a leading German obstetrician in 1927, "hospital delivery is to be preferred in order to keep open the possibility of caesarean."[171] And because one never knew when danger might strike, it made sense, said the people of the time, for most deliveries to take place in the hospital, because the operation for overcoming them—abdominal delivery—could best be done there.

The Discovery of the Fetus

Neither hospitalization nor the caesarean caused the great wave of intervention that marked obstetrics in the 1980s. As we have seen, mothers were put in the hospital to protect them from the forceps and the pituitrin fiends at home. And the availability of the caesarean before 1930 caused no increase in the overall amount of interference. It was, instead, the "discovery of the fetus" that has caused the massive increase in obstetric intervention of the last forty years.

Let's back up a moment. I have already established the first quarter of the twentieth century as the turning point in the diminution of death and mutilation in childbirth, as marking the end of the mother's "traditional" victimization. We have seen her to the threshold of the maternity hospital and its stiff linen sheets. But between the 1920s, when the traditional period ended, and today a further startling development has taken place. The "end of victimization" should have meant that women could more and more control their own deliveries. Instead they have come to control them less and less. This recent loss of control has occasioned much criticism today of the "male medical establishment." And while I do not pretend to judge whether this disappearance is good or bad, I should like to say a few words about how it happened.

---

be irregular and slow it is almost certain that the fetus will not survive delivery even by caesarean section; it should be considered already dead, and it is quite unjustifiable to submit the mother to the greater risk of caesarean section."[168] Thus, in Gilbert I. Strachan's *Textbook of Obstetrics*: "After repeated failures at forceps extraction, it may be justifiable to perforate a live fetus in view of the risks of caesarean section."[169] That view would have been denounced by the postwar Americans.

Before the 1930s, doctors had relatively little interest in the condition of the infant at birth. All the obstetric innovation we have witnessed from the eighteenth century on was directed toward sparing the mother. It is much easier for mothers to deliver small babies, said New York's James Voorhees in 1917, and so he created conditions which would keep them small. "After the sixth month the amount of carbohydrates in the woman's diet should be cut down. This I advise as a regular rule." He also urged that labor be induced before the mother reached term. "Nothing pleases me more in my obstetrical work than to have a baby born a week or two ahead of time. . . . Consequently it is not unusual for me to try to 'shake the apple off the tree' ahead of time by castor oil and quinine," or by starting labor with a rubber bag, as he went on to suggest.[172] These techniques were calculated to produce underweight, premature babies, easy for the mother to deliver but endangered after birth. Doctors then bothered little with the special medical problems of infancy. A historian of American pediatrics has written, "In 1900 there probably were not over fifty medical practitioners in the whole country who took a particular interest in this age group." At present there are more than twenty thousand pediatricians in the United States.[173]

So it became the rule to shorten deliveries for the *mother's* sake. An august Scottish practitioner bragged in 1925 about how he hastened births along, gently dilating the cervix and vagina (!) with his hand, giving pituitrin to "save the physician hours of weary waiting," then "guiding the head during its delivery" with forceps to "save" the perineum from tears. Not one word did he say about the health of the child in these deliveries.[174]

This lack of interest in "fetal outcomes" also kept the caesarean rate low. In 1929, when the overall mortality from caesarean delivery was only about 4 percent, London's East End Maternity Hospital refused to do them for placenta previa. "The fetal mortality in these cases was necessarily very high," said one doctor in defense. "It is probable that some of these infants might have been saved by caesarean section, but the important point is that, from the mother's point of view, operation was unnecessary."[175] Refusal to use the caesarean to save an infant in trouble created horrifying operating room scenes. A surgeon who had practiced in Berlin before the 1930s described infants who after craniotomy would come crying out of their mothers (because the medulla was still intact); the hospital staff would have to plunge the child into a bucket of water to silence it.[176] Thus, it is fair to say that before 1930 neonatal care had little priority in medicine (ironical, in view of the profession's steadfast opposition to abortion).

Then toward 1930 the fetus was "discovered." One cannot date this *prise de conscience* exactly, but certainly in the late 1920s and early 1930s there was a trend toward sparing the infant in delivery. Particularly in America "fetal indications" began to be accepted for obstetric operations, in addition to "maternal indications." In plain language, this means intervening in birth to help the child even if the mother is perfectly all right. In fact, the first reference I have seen to fetal indications for major operations came in 1901 from Frank Meriwether, a practitioner in Asheville, North Carolina, who urged caesarean delivery rather than craniotomy. Although some of his rhetoric recalled the old debates between priests and accoucheurs about whether the infant's life has precedence over the mother's, Meriwether pointed out that a caesarean would be better for *both* of them.[177]* The influential Chicago obstetrician Joseph DeLee lectured his conservative colleagues at a 1921 meeting of the American Gynecological Society. Normal labor could hurt a child, he said. "I claim that the powers of natural labor are dangerous and destructive in many instances to both mother and child, and that interference . . . can prevent a goodly portion of this danger." Forty of the "fifty healthy babies" who died under a British clinic's policy of non-intervention "might have been saved by the prophylactic forceps operation," he said.[178] "Prophylactic forceps" means applying the blades when the infant's head is in the mother's vagina, and what DeLee advocated in 1921 is now the accepted policy in the United States today.

As one might imagine, this policy of speeding normal labor to save an infant from stress was debated for many years. It would exceed the scope of this book to describe the endless arguments about whether stillbirths came from too much intervention (forceps injuries) or from too little (lack of oxygen owing to prolonged labor).[179] But by the 1941 meeting of the American Gynecological Society, mainstream opinion favored intervention on behalf of the fetus. "More babies and mothers will be injured by undue prolongation of labors that fail to progress than by timely operative interference."[180]

This new emphasis on "perinatology," which means the care of the infant in the last two months of pregnancy and the first week after birth, produced a number of changes in the management of labor, all of which are today the objects of lively discussion. It might be of interest simply to indicate how recent are the historical roots of today's average hospital delivery, in which the following events typically occur: the mother checks in; her pubic region is shaved; if she is at all "postdue," labor is induced and an "oxytocin drip" started at the same time; she is placed flat on her back, her feet in stirrups; as the infant's head appears in the vagina,

* Devout Catholic doctors, of course, had never accepted the legitimacy of a craniotomy on a living fetus.

she is given an episiotomy (see pages 171–72); then forceps are routinely applied if the head promises to be at all delayed in popping out. If complications occur that threaten to delay her progress, such as the child coming by the breech, she will be delivered abdominally. And at the end of what in the 1920s would have been damned as "this orgy of intervention," will appear a healthy baby. As I write these lines, Toronto, where I live, has a "perinatal" mortality rate of only thirteen per one thousand births, down 34 percent from 1970. And a maternal mortality rate of "nil." The same trend has happened in many other places.[181]* The following developments are, therefore, not necessarily pernicious:

Routinely shaving the mother's vulva. Before 1900 the preparation of the vaginal area received almost no attention; but by the turn of the century, doctors were sufficiently preoccupied with keeping germs away from the vagina to suggest numerous innovations, among them douching the vagina with a solution of phenol ("carbolic acid") and clipping or shaving the pubic hair.† Yet shaving in particular aroused so much resistance among women in those days that it remained more a medical wish than an actual practice. Said one doctor in 1906: "No vulvar orifice is absolutely sterile without shaving. In private practice shaving will not be permitted. In the hospital this precaution should be taken."[187] A London obstetrician would have liked to shave the vulva, but said, "This would be misunderstood and resented in private practice."[188] Hermann Fehling, looking back on that period in 1925, wrote of Germany that "private patients resisted the abduction of their hirsute adornment. Thus a certain circumspection was commanded us."[189] Nor before the 1930s was medical opinion unanimous about shaving. An Australian doctor called it "barbarous" in the *British Medical Journal.* And someone at a leading lying-in hospital in Berlin said, "We distance ourselves from the practice."[190]

But by the 1930s shaving had carried the day. Previous editions of the standard textbook, *Williams Obstetrics,* for example, had merely recommended cutting the pubic hair "if necessary," or had presented the choice between cutting or shaving. But the 1936 edition stated unambiguously, "Shave the external genital and pubic region."[191]‡ Shaving

---

* Perinatal mortality in France declined by 41 percent from 1970 to 1977; in the United States, by 33 percent.[182]

† In his *Text Book of Midwifery,* Spiegelberg, though enthusiastic in 1882 about antiseptic precautions such as douching, made no reference to preparing the pubic hair.[183] D. Lloyd Roberts, too, was silent about the pubic hair, saying only "The nurse should cleanse the external genitals."[184] The American Charles Jewett, however, said that "the vulvar hair may be clipped short."[185] J. W. Markoe noted that in home deliveries they merely clipped the pubic hair.[186]

‡ Pubic hair references are also found in the second, the fifth, and the seventh editions.[192] The fifth edition noted, moreover, that mothers whose pubic hair had not been shaved had a *lower* infection rate than the shaved group.[193]

became common policy in Britain and France as well during the 1920s and 1930s.[194]

How had women's resistance to shaving been overcome? I have seen no direct discussion linking shaving to neonatal well-being. But mothers of the time might have been persuaded that a healthy infant would best come from a nonseptic birth canal. Certainly their attendants saw shaving as a means of denying habitation to micro-organisms. It is, in any event, interesting that women's opposition to shaving was broken precisely at the moment when the welfare of the neonate was thrust so much into view. Today, however, as a result of a resurgence in women's resistance to shaving, doctors are backing away from it. The 1980 edition of *Williams Obstetrics* states unaggressively that "in many hospitals . . . shaving or clipping" is the practice.[195]*

Lying on one's back. What position exactly women occupied during the expulsive stage of labor would seem a minor point, except that it matters quite a bit to them while they are actually in labor. So I hope the reader will not lose patience if I dwell for a moment upon the strange history of delivery on one's side versus delivery on one's back.

Why would any doctor want to deliver a mother on her side? One advantage of the side, explained Glasgow's William Leishman in 1879, "is that she is not disturbed by seeing such preparations as may be neces-sary for her assistance or relief"—in other words, not witness the forceps being hauled out.[197] That sounds fairly sinister. Yet so many other doctors justify the side position as reducing "unnecessary exposure" that one is inclined to see some element of propriety here as well. Lying on the left side "is the established obstetric position in England," wrote W. S. Playfair in 1880, "and it would be useless to attempt to insist on any other, even if it were advisable."[198] Given the backwater that was Ameri-can medicine in the nineteenth century, it is not surprising that American doctors accepted this English practice. Said one of them in 1867, "It is the almost universal custom in this country and in England to direct the woman to lie upon her left side with the knees drawn up, a posture which is highly convenient to the practitioner, and productive of the least possible exposure." Furthermore, he said, bystanders receive "with something like astonishment and aversion" the direction that the woman turn on her back, seeming "to regard that attitude as, at the least, indelicate."[199] Initially, therefore, delivery in bed conformed to the moth-er's desire to safeguard whatever scraps of her modesty remained from the doctor's prying eyes.

Then another of these curious international divergences took place. Whereas the English have retained to this day the custom of delivering

---

* The twelfth edition (1961) was the last unreservedly to recommend shaving.[196]

women on their left sides, toward the 1930s Americans began insisting that women lie on their back, *with their feet up in stirrups!* This shift has been quite recent. Around the turn of the century, some American doctors actually preferred the side position.[200] In 1913 Chicago's Joseph DeLee felt either position acceptable. Indeed he argued that in some deliveries, because of the poor beds, the bad light, "and the general difficulty of maintaining asepsis, the lateral posture is preferred."[201]

How things had changed by the 1930s! DeLee gave up on side deliveries in 1929 "because of the difficulty of preserving asepsis and the inability of listening constantly to the fetal heart-tones."[202] Whereas a number of American textbooks accepted the side position around 1900, I am aware of none that did in the 1930s. Instead, in the 1930s the lithotomy position was chosen for normal deliveries. "Lithotomy" is the operation of incising the bladder to remove stones, and patients in this operation need to have their knees bent back toward their chests and held wide apart. This position is accomplished in obstetrics by strapping the mother's feet into stirrups at the end of the delivery table. The first edition of Williams's textbook to mention stirrups was published in 1936, shortly after the original author, John Whitridge Williams, had died. It shows stirrups both in hospital deliveries and *at home,* the stirrups clamped to the backs of two kitchen chairs.[203]

Why these innovations in the 1930s? It would, I think, be a mistake to attribute them to the doctors' growing avidity for intervention, because as we have seen, intervention had been going on for over a century already. The side position was perfectly compatible with obstetric operations. The clue to a preference for the "dorsal" position lies rather in DeLee's comments about listening to the fetal heart. A change in the child's heartbeat may signal the onset of distress. But it is difficult to listen with the mother on her side, turned with her back to the doctor. Listening is much easier if she is on her back.

What remains mysterious even today are two things: (1) The English adherence to side deliveries, when virtually everyone else has rejected them, the Germans and French always having been partial to the back.[204]* This preference seems to be another of these English quirks, like craniotomy and whipping schoolboys. (2) The American fondness for stirrups, when virtually the entire rest of the world is happy to let the mother lie semi-recumbent and push down with her feet against the delivery bed as she expels the child. Despite widespread unhappiness among women, American obstetricians today continue to strap the mother's legs

---

* Robert Percival, while preferring the dorsal position, noted in 1980 that "in this country [England] women are not infrequently delivered lying upon the left side, with the thighs partly flexed and the knees held apart by an assistant."[205]

apart, as though the practice were God-given, rather than an innovation of the last thirty years.[206]

Inducing labor by puncturing the bag of waters and then giving the mother an oxytocic solution to soften her cervix. The artificial induction of early labor has a long history as a means of protecting the *mother* from an overly large fetus.[207] I alluded to it a moment ago. But inducing labor started to be presented in the 1950s as a means of protecting the fetus itself. The operation was designed to elicit a fetus that, at forty weeks, was—like Baby Bear's porridge—neither too early, nor too late, but just right.

The 1930s and 1940s evidently did not see an increase in induction. Rates were already high before then, and would not again increase in the United States. The American incidence of 9 percent of births induced in 1967 was the same as the 1920s and 1930s.[208] What changed was the reasons for performing the operation. Several researchers dramatized in the early 1950s the hazards for the fetus of being "post-term," meaning the longer the pregnancy went on after forty weeks, the greater was the likelihood of the placenta's failing to supply the child with enough oxygen.* American obstetricians began therefore inducing less often for such tenebrous indications as the fear that the mother might start convulsing ("pre-eclampsia") and more for fetal reasons.† So from the viewpoint of American *mothers* little has changed in their encounter with induction: in the 1920s their doctors would have given them castor oil and quinine, plus a bag to dilate the cervix. Vexing and uncomfortable. Today their membranes are (painlessly) torn, and then a line containing oxytocin is put into their arms. Equally vexing, but supposedly for the benefit of the fetus.

I must add parenthetically that in Britain the course of events has been rather different. In the 1960s the British were already inducing 15 percent of all deliveries, as opposed to 9 percent in America. In 1970 the British rate was 27 percent; by 1972, 33 percent. In the mid-1970s some British hospitals had induction rates of 40 percent and 50 percent.[211] Whereas the Americans had managed to keep nonmedical indications more or less under control in inducing labor, the British tended much more to accept the convenience of the family or of the hospital staff. A manual for British midwives published in 1975 said flatly, "It is logical

* For example: "The oxygen supply to the human fetus in a clinically normal pregnancy falls gradually up to the 40th week and rapidly thereafter." They observed further that fetal deaths for which there is no apparent cause "are uncommon at 40 to 41 weeks, but by 43 weeks in primigravidae and in multigravidae they are the highest single cause of death."[209]

† *Williams Obstetrics* now accepts post-term pregnancies of forty-four weeks as the main indication for inducing labor (if the fetus is in no distress) and leans toward managing genuine pre-eclampsia with caesarean delivery.[210]

and humane that the expectant mother should share the benefit of induced labor now that it has proved a safe and effective procedure," and went on to talk about eliminating "unpredictability" and letting the husband "arrange to be on holiday."[212]

Episiotomy—the next intervention in birth. Although technically an episiotomy is an incision in the vulva, the term has—ever since Fielding Ould first described it in 1742—come to denote the cutting of the tissue at the base of the vagina in order to enlarge the vaginal outlet.* That band of tissue, which extends from the bottom of the vagina to the external rectal sphincter muscle, is known as the "central perineal body"; obstetricians call it the "perineum." Hence, episiotomy means taking a pair of scissors and making a big cut in the perineum.

Why would anyone want to do such a thing? Remember that a certain percentage of mothers tear their perineums as the infant's head comes bursting through. When the tear actually extends back to the anus, it can be very nasty, risking, for example, the creation of a fistulous opening between rectum and vagina, and making a jagged path of scar tissue which, unless properly stitched, would be the source of great discomfort. Now, this sort of disaster happens rarely. And serious tears of any kind are infrequent. In 16,000 births from 1911 to 1929 in Sursee County, Switzerland, only 9 percent of the mothers had appreciable tears.[214] In 10,000 deliveries in the Jena University Hospital just before the Second World War, only 6 percent of the mothers tore (seven times as many first mothers as multiparas).[215] The conservative doctors at the Chicago Maternity Center found in the early 1930s that 6 percent of mothers were likely to tear: the 3 percent on whom they did episiotomies, and an additional 3 percent who did not have the procedure.[216] † Thus, if no intervention took place, perhaps one woman in fifteen would have an unpleasant tear in need of repair.

It was considerably before 1930 that episiotomies came into vogue.‡ Their purpose in those days was to make it as easy as possible to sew up a tear that would have occurred naturally anyway. A neat man-made

---

* For the first midline episiotomy, Fasbender gives credit to G. P. Michaelis in 1810. What Ould describes, however, is clearly an incision in the midline: "There must be an incision towards the anus with a pair of crooked probe-sizars; introducing one blade between the head and the vagina . . . and the business is done at one pinch, by which the whole body will easily come forth."[213]

† Note that in Joseph DeLee's deliveries one tenth of all primiparas had lacerations in the perineal body severe enough to expose the external anal sphincter.[217]

‡ Dr. Anna Broomall did episiotomies in 30 percent of 200 deliveries in the 1870s.[218] Charles Jewett recommended the operation in 1907 to simplify the repair of a "posterior laceration."[219] On British conservatism, see, for example, Alfred L. Galabin: "In rare cases only, in which a laceration through the sphincter ani appears to be otherwise inevitable, this operation is advantageous."[220] Robert W. Johnstone said, "The operation of episiotomy is rarely necessary."[221]

incision is simpler to stitch than a jagged natural one. Doctors directed the incision to the side—a "medio-lateral" episiotomy—so that a spontaneous tear would not extend to the anus—a major disaster in home delivery. As one text pointed out, "It would require only three or four such tears to put the physician responsible for them pretty well out of business."[222] (Now, by contrast, the incision is usually made in the "midline," because medio-lateral episiotomies bleed more, are slower to heal, and are more uncomfortable to the mother.)

But only in the 1930s did the infant start to figure in the reasons for doing an episiotomy. As a result, the frequency of the operation increased significantly. The new logic was to spare the child a prolonged expulsive stage of labor. Enlarging the vaginal outlet would permit speedy forceps delivery of its head. When in 1937 an obstetrical surgeon justified the high frequency of episiotomies, he placed "fetal indications" first: "The fetus is to be protected from the effects of a prolonged second stage, particularly from certain injuries which may result when the head acts as a dilator" of the mother's soft parts.[223] Joseph DeLee's textbook mentions protecting the fetus for the first time in 1933. *Williams Obstetrics's* first reference appeared in 1950: the operation "spares the baby's head the necessity of serving as a battering ram."[224]

By the Second World War episiotomies were becoming routine for all first mothers, who tear more easily, and for all mothers who previously had an episiotomy, who presumably would need one again. In other words, sooner or later episiotomy would become routine for everyone. During 1933 to 1935, 53 percent of the fifty-six hundred women who delivered at the Chicago Lying-In Hospital had episiotomies, "to protect the perineum from serious laceration and also to protect the fetus from a sudden increase in intracranial pressure."[225] By 1941 episiotomies were "routine" in the Boston Lying-In Hospital, as in many others.[226]

By the 1970s a mother birthing anywhere in Western society would have a good chance of an episiotomy: 65 percent in Ontario, 64 percent in a Wuppertal hospital in Germany, 70 percent to 90 percent in an Inner London Hospital, 60 percent among first mothers around Brighton.[227] * Said a British midwife, "I am very sorry that some doctors and midwives have become so 'scissors-happy' lately." She went on, reflecting the views of many midwives, to say that if no fetal distress is present, there is "no need to hurry the birth of the baby."[229] I cannot pretend to comment on the question of when does the mother's interest in a pleasant birth experience outweigh the potential advantages to the

---

* One "Inner London" hospital, in early 1979, had "70–90 percent. . . . Two of the hospitals had a 90 percent episiotomy rate."[228]

child of moving swiftly through the vagina and into the world. It is clear, however, that in general the operation since the 1930s has been done in the expected interests of the child.

Forceps. Now the infant's head is in the vagina. The mother has just had an episiotomy, which tends to be a precondition for the next intervention: the delivery of the child's head with forceps. One third of all mothers birthing today in the United States will have forceps deliveries.[230]

Let's go back a moment. When forceps were first introduced in hospital deliveries late in the eighteenth century, they were sparingly used—once in every two hundred-odd deliveries in the big Paris maternity hospital, for example.* With anesthesia forceps use increased somewhat in hospitals, because the mother's inability to bear down does slow the delivery, and because she would be insensible to the pain of the forceps. Yet toward 1900 forceps in the hospital were used considerably less than at home.† By the 1920s only one woman in twenty would experience a forceps delivery in hospital.‡

Then in 1920 the Chicago obstetrician Joseph DeLee proposed the "prophylactic" use of forceps. The instrument was not to be restricted to the few emergency "fetal indications"—such as the umbilical cord falling out or the placenta separating prematurely—but was to be expanded to all cases where the infant's head was in the vagina but unable to exit because the muscles of the pelvic floor (the "perineum") were still too rigid. If it looked as though the head would not emerge in the next fifteen minutes, the attendant would first do an episiotomy, then apply forceps and tug it out. DeLee said that, in addition to saving the woman "the debilitating effects of . . . the physical labor of a prolonged second stage," prophylactic forceps would "save the babies' brains from injuries and from the immediate and remote effects of prolonged compression."[236] I dwell on this at length because DeLee's operation has become a cornerstone of American obstetrics today.

The operation did not catch on immediately.§ J. W. Williams assailed prophylactic forceps in the last edition of his textbook (1930) which

---

* From 1775 to 1777 in the Hôtel Dieu forceps were used .4 times per 100 births; half of the mothers survived.[231]

† One study of teaching hospitals in Central Europe in the 1880s and 1890s found forceps used 3.6 times in every 100 deliveries.[232] At Dublin's Rotunda the forceps rate was 3.0 percent from 1889 to 1896, 3.9 percent from 1910 to 1919.[233] In 1916 at Hartford General Hospital, 6.9 percent.[234]

‡ A 1929 U.S. nationwide sample of 207 general hospitals and 16 obstetric hospitals put forceps use at 17.9 percent.[235]

§ Many conservative obstetricians fulminated against it for years. See, for example, the clash between Joseph DeLee and Rudolph Holmes at the 1921 meeting of the American Gynecological Society: "The modern general trend in operative obstetrics has not benefited the woman or the unborn child," said Holmes.[237]

he personally was to write: "I am confident that the results would be disastrous were [DeLee's] suggestion generally adopted."[238] But during the 1930s it was generally adopted. By 1968 forceps were applied in 38 percent of U.S. hospital deliveries.[239] Note that in the British Isles the frequency remained much lower: 6 percent in Dublin in the 1920s, 11 percent in 1974.[240] Behind this massive American increase in "elective low forceps," as the operation is known today, lay a new concern with delivering the child as quickly as possible. At the White House Conference on childbirth hazards in 1933, one doctor noted, "Until comparatively recently forceps were used very infrequently and then only when the mother was unable to deliver herself, fetal indications not recognized." Now, of course, they were recognized.[241] The 1936 edition of *Williams Obstetrics* dropped the line criticizing DeLee, and the 1950 edition accepted "elective low forceps" without reservation: "The vast majority of forceps operations performed in this country today are elective low forceps," necessitated by "analgesic programs [that] interfere to a greater or lesser degree with the mother's bearing-down efforts."[242] But as I noted earlier, it was common practice for birthing women to be completely knocked out with ether or chloroform long before the 1930s. What changed in the 1930s was not the frequency of pain relief but the attitude toward the new-born infant.

Forceps use is now declining in American hospitals—down 11 percent from 1968 to 1975; down 7 percent in Ontario from 1975 to 1977.* The reason is not new callousness toward the infant but increasing reliance on caesarean births as the best way to end deliveries one fears might be taking too long.

Today one out of seven American mothers is spared the procedures mentioned above. She will have a caesarean birth.† Table 7.2 shows the stunning increase in abdominal delivery since the 1950s. Indeed, from the 1960s to 1970s, caesareans *doubled* in frequency: from 6.8 percent to 12.8 percent of births. Of Ontario mothers, 14 percent were delivered abdominally in 1978.[244] Although the frequency of caesareans in Britain has always been lower, the trend has been the same: in Oxford up from 6 percent in 1970 to 10 percent in 1974, for example.[245]

It was only in the 1960s and 1970s that caesareans increased, for previously doctors had tried other means to accelerate the birth. Then a consen-

* The current (16th edition) of *Williams Obstetrics*, has retreated to the viewpoint that the classic DeLee operation—episiotomy plus low forceps—should apply only to a "minority of nulliparous women."[243]

† Medical usage today avoids the term "caesarean section." "Section" means simply "incision." All this hospital talk about being "sectioned" is thought to be jarring to maternal sensibilities.

sus developed in the 1960s that the risks to both mother and child were *less* from caesareans than from less high-powered kinds of intervention. The 1956 edition of *Williams Obstetrics* was still rumbling gloomily about "the possibility of rupture of the uterine scar in future pregnancies." The 1966 edition said this whole notion "is now viewed by many conservative obstetricians with increasing skepticism." Instead, "the focus of obstetric thinking has been directed increasingly toward infant survival and the prevention of trauma to the child during birth."[246] By 1976 the president of an important obstetrical association could unambiguously state, "A change in attitude has occurred; formerly focus was on the mother and delivery, and now it is centered on fetal outcome." A participant from New York's Sloane Hospital added, "[The rise] is due to an increasing desire to spare the fetus any trouble whatever."[247] Thus, sparing the fetus trouble had triumphed.

Its triumph has drawn another victory in its wake: that of the obstetrician over the G.P. If in the last quarter of the twentieth century the average American woman is delivered by an obstetrician, rather than by a general practitioner or a midwife, the main reason is that only specialists trained in surgery can confidently open up her belly. Nobody else can do that. General practitioners once performed most of the caesareans in the United States, but in the 1930s the technique of the operation shifted from procedures they could easily handle to ones with which they had some difficulty. Before 1930 the "classical" caesarean dominated; and in making an incision in the upper part of the uterus, the doctor would slice through the protective layer of peritoneum, whose function is to shield the abdomen from infection. There were other problems with the classical operation, such as a tendency for the scar to rupture in a later delivery because it had been placed in the middle of the uterine muscle. Then several surgeons proposed around 1920 the "low cervical" operation—an incision down near the bladder, where the uterus consists mostly of connective tissue and little muscle. Moreover, cutting down there decreased the risk of infection spreading to the abdominal cavity in general. But the "low-flap" or "low-segment" operation was technically more difficult: the doctor had to free up the bladder, push it out of the way, and then carefully peel the peritoneum off the uterus, slice through it, and stitch it back together afterward. Because it took doctors in those days maybe ten or fifteen minutes longer to do it, and because one had to be quite familiar with the anatomy of that region to attempt it at all, many G.P.'s felt intimidated once the low-cervical caesarean became the "procedure of choice." Of those graduating from medical school in 1941, one man said, "Many will be general practitioners in the country. They or any good abdominal surgeon can do a classical operation easily. But if they try to do a low-flap operation, they may get into serious trouble."[248] *

There you have it. G.P.'s who attempted these high-powered procedures could indeed get into trouble. So within medicine, and among the public as a whole, pressures increased for women to seek out obstetricians trained in surgery for their attendance in childbed. By 1967 specialists attended 51 percent of all births in the United States.[249] In Britain, the midwives made the tremendous resurgence I have described (see pages 144–45); but supervising them would be, increasingly, specialists instead of general practitioners. The specialists' share of deliveries in Britain climbed from 13 percent in 1946 to 20 percent in 1970, and the G.P.s' sank from 11 percent to 3 percent.[250] In an out-of-the-way state like Iowa, the great majority of deliveries in the 1960s were attended by G.P.'s, almost half of whom were older than fifty. A University of Iowa specialist recommended that those who did fewer than twenty-five deliveries a year drop out of obstetrics altogether.[251] So much for the kindly old practitioner, who "knew how to sit and wait."[252]

The surge toward caesarean delivery, and the accompanying reliance on obstetricians, has had an enormous impact upon the lives of women, reducing significantly the areas of autonomy in birthing over which in the 1920s and 1930s they still had free choice. I cannot say whether the benefits to the infant from these obstetric operations are real or fanciful. I wish, however, to note how capriciously changes in views of what constitutes "medical progress" have affected the lives of birthing mothers. Until perhaps 1930 progress in technique represented a deliverance from the horrors of traditional childbirth and opened up the possibility of pleasure in the birth experience unconstrained by fear of death or mutilation. With the discovery of the fetus in the 1930s, modern medicine has snatched from women's hands whatever hopes of autonomy and control had previously glimmered.

---

* Both DeLee's *Principles of Obstetrics* and *Williams Obstetrics* have clear accounts of the evolution of the caesarean. Earlier editions discuss as well the relative advantages of the classical and the low-cervical approaches.

CHAPTER 8

Abortion

LET'S SAY a woman was pregnant but didn't want to be. If she wanted an abortion, was it easy to get one?

In this chapter I shall argue that since the dawn of time women have been able to get rid of unwanted pregnancies, mainly through abortive drugs. But because of the danger of some of these drugs, a woman had to be absolutely determined to end the pregnancy in order to persuade herself to use them. Thus, throughout most of recorded history, abortion was confined to women who were desperate. Then in the years 1880 to 1930 there was a major breakthrough, giving all women the possibility of reasonably safe abortions more or less at will. This new accessibility of abortion, I believe, helped lift from women's shoulders a major source of vulnerability: vulnerability to unwanted pregnancies.

Among the most desperate were unmarried women. It is hard for us to imagine with what dismay they in particular viewed pregnancy, for once they were found out, they would be fined, jailed, or humiliated by church courts, to say nothing of the reproaches which the community generally would heap upon them and their families. Madeleine Mercanton, for example, decided not to abort her illegitimate child, and secretly gave birth in Switzerland's Vaud Canton the night of 27 May 1756. Unfortunately the infant died shortly thereafter. Mercanton was thereupon charged with "having concealed her pregnancy" (a crime virtually everywhere in Europe), with having "denied giving birth," and with "having left the infant lying in its blood, neglecting to cut the umbilical cord.

In addition she is strongly suspect of having smothered the child." As a result she was sentenced to "having her right hand cut off and to decapitation."[1] In these circumstances one might understand why women like Mercanton were frantic to get abortions.

What happened after a woman learned she was pregnant? Dr. Egon Weinzierl asked unmarried mothers admitted to Prague's Women's Hospital just after the First World War, about how their families and employers had responded. A third of them reported terrible family quarrels, being thrown out of the house because the father was the local mayor, or being told, "If you want to come home, no kid." Of those who had had jobs, 42 percent were fired—"not at all infrequently with curses and humiliation, employers making fun of them and ridiculing them." Thirty of the five hundred women interviewed had attempted suicide.[2]

Married women squirmed as well under the burden of unwanted pregnancy. One Duisburg woman had written an abortionist that her period was supposed to come on 24 August, "but unfortunately it has not and it is now more than a week overdue. I just can't stand it that I'm once again going to be in this miserable situation." She already had three children. "For working people I think that's enough. So to keep this from happening again I implore you to send me reliable information as soon as possible."[3] Anarchist Emma Goldman worked toward the turn of the century as a midwife in the tenements of New York. Most of the poor women "lived in continual dread of conception," she wrote. "When they found themselves pregnant, their alarm and worry would result in determination to get rid of their expected offspring . . . jumping off tables, rolling on the floor, massaging the stomach, drinking nauseating concoctions, and using blunt instruments." But Goldman found this understandable, even though she refused to do abortions on them, because "each additional child was a curse, 'a curse of God,' as orthodox Jewish women and Irish Catholics repeatedly told me."[4] Thus if one wants to understand how women's historic experience with their bodies has changed, one must ask what access to abortion they had.

Traditional Methods of Abortion

To get rid of an unwanted pregnancy, a woman would move progressively from the least to the most dangerous procedures, stopping at whichever worked. The least dangerous rarely worked. Folklore called universally for "hot sitz baths," sometimes with mustard powder thrown in.[5] But the women who claimed they got abortions that way were probably not pregnant, or else lied about their true means. Professional abortionists never wasted time with hot baths.

Next on the ladder came external trauma to the uterus. One bound oneself as tight as possible to conceal the pregnancy and maybe to end it as well. Thus, plenty of village women would end up concealing pregnancies, going into labor near term, and then being accused of infanticide or dying unassisted in the delivery.* Binding was almost as ineffective as a sitz bath.

There were other kinds of trauma. The pregnant mistress of a sixteenth-century English priest "tightened her girdle and performed exercises with a rolling pin in order to destroy the fetus."[7] The literature is filled with tales of women who flung themselves from lofts and ladders, tumbled down stairs, and leaped off chairs. In Finland they would "throw themselves with head and feet downward for long periods on the top of the grain chest, slide on their stomachs down the stairs, jump off high places like the stove bench, lift and carry heavy objects—all in order to dislodge the fetus from the uterus.[8] In the early 1860s a peasant came before the assize court in the Loire-Inférieure department for having flung from a horse at full gallop a domestic servant whom he had impregnated. In fact, he threw her down twice; and when the pregnancy persisted, he tried applying loaves of steaming hot bread to her abdomen. This, too, failed, and the woman bore a healthy child at term.[9]

Of all the external violence that women applied to their bodies, the only technique likely to have been systematically successful was massage. Even today, in some Third World countries skilled midwives are able to induce abortion through abdominal massage.[10] This technique turned up occasionally in Europe as well. In one case a masseur, using two fingers, drilled through a woman's vaginal wall and into her peritoneum when she was in the third or fourth month of pregnancy.[11] Only because of this dismal accident did we find out about the incident. Presumably other pregnancies were massaged away more competently.

HERBAL CONCOCTIONS

After a pregnant woman had tried all these means and failed, she would probably have recourse to drugs. First let us discuss how widely used they were. By way of background, the reader should keep in mind that in both folklore and academic medicine drugs go right back to the ancient Greeks and Egyptians. The pharmacopoeias of Dioscorides and the Hippocratic school were copied and recopied throughout the Middle Ages and

---

* Johann Storch tells of a woman who, having concealed her pregnancy by binding herself, perished while giving birth unassisted in the washhouse.[6] The infanticide literature abounds with stories of women, mainly young servants, who successfully concealed the pregnancy through tight binding, then killed the child after its birth.

early modern period, so that an enormous amount of drug lore continues, in an unbroken stream, through two thousand years of Western history.[12] This tradition survived until the end of the nineteenth century, when "medical nihilism" toward drugs caused most of the traditional pharmacopoeia to be swept away.

So the typical villager, male or female, would constantly be dosing himself or herself with spring tonics, fall tonics, herbal teas for heart burn, teas to keep the uterus in place and prevent it from rising up toward the throat, decoctions for ulcer and cancer, and drugs to procure bowel movements. As evidence of the enormous variety of uses these potions could serve, a uroscopist was charged in 1729 with having prepared for a woman an abortifacient containing aloes, gentian root, and jalappa (all potentially abortive drugs); he got off by arguing that this potion could have been a valid stomach remedy, and that he didn't even know the woman was pregnant.[13] In fact, many of the drugs that peasants took for complaints like "hysteria" were also used for abortion and for everything else imaginable.[14]

Thus, every family had a medicine chest: "Every household in country or city has the most diverse plants dried and ready to use, especially chamomile, peppermint, lindenblossom, elder, wormwood, yarrow, coltsfoot, and others. People either collect these plants themselves and dry them, or buy them in the pharmacy or drugstore, from traveling salesmen, or at the fairs."[15] For our purposes it is important that women in particular kept these medicine chests, and that drug lore in general, whether for obstetrical or general medical purposes, belonged to the realm of "women's culture."[16]

If any medical area existed in which village women aspired to special insight, it was the "anomalies of menstruation," a medical circumlocution for missed periods. Dr. J. Thomsen, commenting on a local abortion trial, wrote, "Because these drugs naturally belong to the secret areas of women's life, the village crones have seized upon this specialty, quite understandably, given their proclivity toward any kind of quackery. There are now, above all in the countryside, everywhere 'wise women' whose knowledge of menstruation remedies has won them some reknown."[17] Another physician wrote of the Frankenwald district, "Even today one is astonished at the supposed or actual knowledge that women, young and old, have of drugs that affect pregnancy, which they reveal in confidential discussion."[18]

Doctors as well had a hand in this "polypharmacy," for ever since ancient times academic medicine, under the influence of "humoral" theories, had considered it harmful for a woman to miss her period. All that nasty menstrual blood would build up inside her and cause an imbalance in the rest of the "humors" in her system, the theory went. Of course if pregnancy was the reason for missing a period, one should not intervene. But a period missed for other reasons called for active medical measures, for drugs called "emmenagogues" to restore the menses. Almost everything that had been written about emmenagogues until the 1930s was medical hocus-pocus, based on a complete misunderstanding of the body's endocrine system. In theory, there are drugs that can bring on a missed period in a non-pregnant uterus: the prostaglandins, or any "progesterone-antagonist" (progesterone being the hormone that maintains the rich uterine lining which falls away in menstruation).[19] But in the majority of cases a woman will miss a period because she is pregnant. "Everybody knows that if a healthy woman's menstrual periods cease, the cause in 999 cases out of 1000 is pregnancy," said Dr. F. J. McCann at a 1929 meeting in London of the Medico-Legal Society.[20] And most "emmenagogues," to the extent that they were pharmacologically active at all, were in reality abortifacients.

I dwell upon this medical interest in emmenagogues because it helped reinforce the popular tradition of uterine folklore. For every Frau Taentzlin, brandishing long lists of uterotonic drugs at her village clientele, was an academic herbalist, quoting Hippocrates and Soranus.[21] The Frenchman J.-B. Chomel, for example, wrote in 1737 that emmenagogues were herbs that "re-establish the evacuations natural to the female sex. One normally administers them to restore the menses to girls and to cure most of the illnesses that the suppression of the menses causes, such as chlorosis, jaundice, colics, migraines."[22] Because doctors had no way to determine whether a woman was pregnant before the fourth month, the old medical literature is filled with cautionary tales: the woman—knowing she was pregnant—complaining about the headaches that "menstrual suppression" had caused; the doctor alert to ensure that the woman was not pregnant before writing a prescription. Johann Storch, for example, suspected pregnancy when a servant woman came to see him. He tricked her by prescribing only a mild laxative, "which occupied her until her growing belly became so large that it could no longer be concealed" (thus ruling out an abortion).[23] This is another of those little ironies with which my tale is filled. Women historically were not all that concerned about irregular menstruation unless caused by pregnancy.* It was the doctors, operating under the influence of antique theories about "bad humors," that helped make available to them drugs for abortion.

Shoring up this peasant interest in drugs, finally, was centuries of empir-

---

* Otto Stoll, in connection with a survey of folk medicine practices in Switzerland, said, "On the whole, peasant women are fairly indifferent to anomalies in their 'periods' or 'menses.' "[24]

ical experience with potions that strengthen the contractions of the uterus in labor (oxytocics). A number of the world's plants do exert a selective effect on uterine muscle. Rupture of the uterus, for example, was in the 1950s the *leading* cause of maternal death in Uganda because witch doctors insisted on giving birthing mothers these enormously potent local herbs.[25]* Ergot, as we shall see in a moment, has a long folkloric history of obstetrical use. The Egyptians in 2200 B.C. were rubbing saffron oil on the bellies of parturient women to overcome difficult labor.[26] Traditional Europeans were firmly convinced that, because the infant was thought to help in its own delivery, a mother would need special chemical help to deliver a stillborn fetus. Thus, a fifteenth-century English "leechbook" had recipes "for the deliverance of a dead child" involving savory, wine and hyssop.[27] And the seventeenth-century man midwife Percivall Willughby sought to facilitate the labor of Goodwife Forman of Spoondon, who had "suffered much," by giving her "a decoction of germander, pennyroyal and calamint, boiled in a posset drink, the which I tinctured with saffron; and to a draught I added a spoonful of the Earle of Chesterfield's powder, and two spoonfulls of oil of sweet almonds. This quickened her throws, and at last, brought forth the child."[28] Since time out of mind village midwives have given mothers infusions of herbs to strengthen contractions, "help expel the placenta," or stop post-delivery bleeding.[29] I shall not list all these in detail because the plant names themselves would have little meaning to most of today's readers. The point is that people could say to themselves, If these plants will help the uterus contract in childbirth, perhaps they will work earlier in the pregnancy as well for abortion.

Thus references abound to women dosing themselves with drugs for abortion. "Potions were widely known and used to contrive sterility and abortion," writes one medievalist.[30] Virtually every writer on obstetrics I have read commented on the popularity of these drugs. Thus de la Motte in eighteenth-century Normandy: "There are some totally perverse young women who, far from seeking out drugs to help them complete their pregnancy happily, desire nothing so much as to rid themselves of a child, not only at the expense of their health but of their life as well, and who find sufficient iniquitous individuals to give them these pernicious drugs."[31] Dr. Edward Moore, medical officer of Bethnal Green, noted in 1862 that over the past decade he had attended 217 cases of abortion among paupers, "mostly produced by herb pills and various drastic purgatives, not always, I think, unintentional."[32] These writers were witnessing the results of thousands of years of folk experience with abortions. Over

* Thirty-four percent of all maternal deaths from 1952 to 1959 in Uganda were due to ruptured uteri.

that time, certain lessons did trickle down about plants that might activate the smooth muscle of the uterus, or interfere with the implantation of the young embryo, or impede the sperm's fertilization of the ovum— but nobody had any notion of how they worked. Nor do we have much today. But it is striking how the same plants considered "good to bring on the menses" recur in societies thousands of miles apart and with no contact with one another. The same names recur in Peru, Bavaria, India, and China.[33]* "Folk culture has brought together with astonishingly reliable empiricism," wrote Zurich's J. R. Spinner in 1920, "the appropriate drugs for the practice of criminal abortion, drugs that under some circumstances can produce an abortion."[35]

Drugs for Abortion

What were these drugs? How did they work? And were they safe?

The following list of four drugs has been culled from a file that includes around 120 which received at least one mention as "good" for abortion or for delayed menstruation in the clinical or folkloric literature of past times. Dozens more could be added if I included all those cited in early-modern "herbals" as suitable for bringing on the period or for "driving out stillborn children." But these four are mentioned far more often than the others, and it is fair to think them the most often used as well.

To avoid swamping the reader with detail, I shall not linger upon their various chemical ingredients. Yet I might point out that the "active principle" in one of them is a chemical called an "alkaloid," and in the other three a "volatile oil." Thus, volatile oils, or "essential oils" as they are sometimes called, stand out as by far the most important chemical agent in the procurement of abortion, supplying the active principle of numerous other abortion plants not included in this "hit parade," such as pennyroyal, sage, thyme, and rosemary. The volatile oils evaporate, or "volatilize," when heated, as opposed to the "fatty oils" which do not. Because the volatile oils include strongly aromatic components, they represent the "essences" or odiferous constituents of many plants, and thus are often used in the perfume industry. Taken orally, these drugs come in two principal forms: (1) a homemade tea from the dried leaves, twigs, seeds, or roots of the natural plants; (2) a store-bought "oil" distilled by steam (or extracted with some solvent such as alcohol) from the plant by a chemist; the volatile oil is usually the main ingredient of this oleaginous mixture.

---

* The World Health Organization is currently attempting to learn more about the potential abortifacient qualities of some of these indigenous plants.[34]

Ergot. Among these abortifacient drugs, ergot remains the best known today because several of its components, such as the alkaloid ergometrine, are still used medically to staunch uterine bleeding in childbirth, for example, or to control migraine. "Ergot" itself is the popular name for the fungus *Claviceps purpurea,* a hard, black, spurlike growth protruding from stalks of infected grain, especially rye. One doctor recalled how as a thirteen-year-old he used to walk in summer through the fields near Ansbach, collecting basketfuls of this "natural curiosity, not having the slightest notion of the meaning of the drug." Thus "every peasant maiden" had the opportunity to procure some for herself.[36] Since the days of Hippocrates, ergot has been known to act upon the uterus. Adam Lonicer mentioned it in his 1582 herbal as a "proven remedy for the tremors and pains of the uterus."[37] And the professional midwives of Germany seem to have used it since time out of mind to strengthen contractions in labor or help the uterus expel the placenta.[38] Ergot was, for example, outlawed among the midwives of Hanover in 1778.[39] It is the only oral drug for "bringing on the flowers" in the previously mentioned fifteenth-century English leechbook.[40] So even though academic medicine did not systematically explore its obstetrical uses until the early nineteenth century, ergot has for a long time possessed an "oxytocic" reputation.

Similarly, ergot has had a long career as an abortive.[41] Lithuanian midwives told a folklore investigator that they knew of it for abortion.[42] Among the village *matrones* of France, ergot was called "uterus powder"; in Germany, sometimes "infant's death" (*Kindesmord*).[43] The major problem with ergot, however, is that it acts on the uterus only late in pregnancy. And women who want to abort usually try to find something that works in the second or third month. The earliest gestation terminated by ergot of which I am aware came at the fourth month, and that was a pregnancy already threatened by bleeding, which might spontaneously have ended even without the ergot.[44] Dr. James Whitehead succeeded, on three out of four occasions, in inducing abortion at five months in a woman with a severely contracted pelvis.[45] And an American doctor claimed that while "ergot is too difficult to be obtained by the negroes for them to do much mischief with it," he knew of three white women who had taken it at three to four months of pregnancy; two of them aborted.[46]*

Ruta graveolens (Rue). On the list of abortive drugs, rue unquestion-

---

* Note that ergot failed to abort a one-month pregnancy reported by O. Vago in 1969; the uterus underwent a tetanic contraction but the pregnancy persisted and resulted in a live birth at the end of the eighth month.[47] Louis S. Goodman and Alfred Gilman said that "even an immature uterus is stimulated" by ergot alkaloids, though the sensitivity varies "especially with the degree of maturity and the stage of gestation. . . . The gravid uterus, however, is very sensitive."[48]

ably is number two. Indeed, a nineteenth-century French doctor called it "just as powerful as savin, and more reliable."[49] (See pages 186–87.) It may be traced from classical times, through the medieval herbals and the midwives' kits of the seventeenth century, to a solid reputation as an abortive drug in the folklore of traditional Europe.[50]* There is widespread opinion in the older pharmacological literature that rue oil exercises a direct influence on the uterus. After a series of experiments on guinea-pig and cat uteri, Jean Renaux concluded in 1941 that rue produced abortion not through its general toxicity but as a "direct consequence of the stimulation of the uterine muscle."[52] He and collaborators thus affirmed earlier findings on rue and challenged the negative results that other researchers had obtained two years earlier.† Dr. Hélie of Nantes provided, in 1878, the first clinical findings on rue in women. A young girl of sixteen came into his office "and asked about the means of provoking an abortion. She seemed to me three to four months pregnant. I tried in vain to detour her from her plan.

"Because you won't do me this favor," she said, "I'll go elsewhere and come back and tell you about it after I succeed."

In fact she returned two weeks later. She was no longer pregnant. She told Dr. Hélie that, "according to the advice of a woman," she had "taken three fresh roots of rue, about the size of a finger, sliced them up and boiled them in a liter and a half of water, down to about three cupfulls, which she drank that evening all at once." There followed "a horrible stomach pain, vomiting, and nausea," and forty-eight hours later she aborted. Hélie told several similar stories and was convinced, in contrast to the conventional wisdom of his time, that the drug acted directly on the uterus.[54]

Thus did women from India, to Hungary, to New Zealand drink rue tea or take oil of rue for abortion. Even in the American South before the Civil War, elderly black women said, "It is more effectual than tansy to procure abortion."[55] Authorities at the Botanical Garden in Brest finally had to put their rue plant behind glass.[56] And when in Germany in the 1920s rue finally disappeared from peasant gardens, its reputation still clung as being "only for lovers."[57]

Tanacetum vulgare (Tansy Oil). Tansy oil is on the list mainly because it was the most popular abortion drug in the United States. Its most

---

* According to Ernest Guenther, "Oil of rue is distilled in France from pure *Ruta graveolens*, elsewhere from the poor cousins *R. montana* and *R. bracteosa*." Its active principles, which may or may not be responsible for producing abortions, are two ketones: methyl nonyl ketone and methyl heptyl ketone.[51]

† Patoir et al., found that in general the abortions produced in animals were not without grave side effects and that the abortive dose was nearly a fatal one. None of the four female animals dosed with rue aborted: they died before term or after delivering at term.[53]

potent ingredient was "thujone"; and even though official pharmacology has maintained that tansy oil is a deadly poison, it was nonetheless widely used.[58] For example, Southern slave women took tansy, "commonly cultivated in our gardens," for abortion.[59] It was known as an emmenagogue among the Spanish New Mexicans and the Maritime Indians.[60] Dr. John Metcalf reported a woman "who had drunk freely of tansy tea for some days before the occurrence of labour."[61]* Another doctor said that "tansy is a tradition among American women for its certainty as an abortifacient."[62] A specialist declared it in the 1930s the "favorite remedy" for abortion in rural America.† It was known in India.[64] Et cetera. In sum, women have taken tansy since at least the days of Saint Hildegarde of Bingen in the twelfth century.[65] So it must have some efficacy.

Juniperus sabina (Savin). The reputation of the volatile oils as abortifacients will rise or fall with that of oil of savin, because of all the plants containing these oils, the evergreen bush *Juniperus sabina* was by far the most widely used for abortion. Its active principle is the hydrocarbon volatile oil "sabinene," and it has been shown to induce uterine contractions experimentally in animals.[66]‡

Its use for abortion goes back to the ancient Romans, reappearing then in Hieronymus Bock's 1565 herbal: "So do the young hussies get hold of powdered savin, or drink some of it. Thus many children fail to survive. For this business we need a tough inquisitor or magistrate."[68] At the end of the eighteenth century a Göttingen professor wrote: "When I traveled through the countryside in Swabia and saw a savin bush in a farmer's garden, it confirmed what I had in many cases already suspected, that the garden belonged to the barber or the midwife of the village. And to what purpose had they so carefully planted the savin bush? If you look at these bushes and shrubs you'll see them deformed and without tops, because they've been raided so often, and even at times stolen."[69] "Everywhere I went in the farms of Franconia," reported another observer toward the end of the nineteenth century, "I saw [the savin bush] and whenever I was able to get information, it had been planted by one of the female members of the family."[70]

Those women who couldn't plant it in their own yards stole from the public botanical gardens. "This is the reason why its cultivation in public gardens here and there was forbidden, or the plants removed. The gardeners have a long tale to tell about this, and I know gardens where

---

* Note, however, that advanced tuberculosis might have caused her abortion.
† This was Frederick Taussig, who believed it "relatively harmless, with only an occasional death reported, but also invariably useless unless other measures are also employed or the patient is unusually predisposed to abortion."[63]
‡ Patoir, however, concludes on the basis of guinea pig and rabbit experiments that it is toxic, not abortive.[67]

the savin tree had to be protected by a fence from the 'public.' "[71] The Franconian government warned about planting savin in 1791; the Austrian government forbade it in 1807.[72] Many later ordinances also restricted the sale and planting of savin.

Augustus Granville described a woman who in 1818 appeared at his Westminster Dispensary in London with "amenorrhea" (a missed period), several months overdue. She had been vomiting. Granville prescribed savin and reported that "a trifling appearance of the menses occurred in about a fortnight after this."[73] One student concluded from a study of cases that attempted savin abortions were "usually crowned with success."[74] Yet in the medical literature poisoning cases far outweigh those in which the mother suffered no grave side effects. Of course, women who had successfully carried out a "criminal" abortion would not broadcast the news to their doctors. Yet it is striking that so many savin cases ended fatally for the mother. In Sweden, for example, between 1851 and 1900, fifteen pregnant women died from *aetheroleum sabinae* in what were officially reported as "suicides."[75] In thirteen of the thirty-two cases that Lewin located in the literature, the mother died; and in eleven of those thirty-two she failed to abort, whether dying or not.[76] Rudolph Lex, after reviewing reported cases, concluded that "when abortion does happen, almost without exception it is tied to the death of the mother."[77]

Thus, there is a problem in writing the history of abortion: Whether to give greater credence to the doctors who reported the poisoning cases they attended, or to the medical folklorists such as Dr. N. Kronfeld who emphasized the commonality of drugs like savin: "In the Alpine lands its criminal use is as common as reciting the alphabet."[78] The problem that haunted herbal abortion was its unreliability. If we, for a moment, accept the hypothesis that a relatively safe abortive dose did exist for many of these drugs, what were the women doing wrong to end up horribly poisoned? The numerous reports about the uselessness of abortive drugs, together with the equally numerous reports about their dreadful toxicity, can only be explained in terms of the difficulty in finding a standard, reliable dose. This difficulty had several components:

· The amount of natural volatile oil in these plants could vary sharply from year to year, depending on whether the season had been rainy or dry. It would vary with the month in which the plant was harvested, the active ingredients normally reaching their maximum presence about budding time.* It would vary with soil conditions, with the plant part used in distilling, and with the technique of extracting the oil.[80] So one

---

* The amount of apiol and myristicin, the two phenol ethers in parsley which seem implicated in abortion, changes greatly across the growth cycle of the plant.[79]

could never really know how potent an oil was. (This, moreover, was a problem that plagued pharmacists and eventually helped lead to the discontinuation of the volatiles for medical use).

· The presence of active ingredients could depend on the length of time a plant was stored. Ergot, for example, loses its potency as it is kept on the shelf. The active principles in the volatiles certainly diminished the longer they were cooked, and those peasant women who boiled the leaves of parsley or savin for hours on end, probably cooked away much of the volatile oil.[81]

· Indeed the recipes that circulated in the women's subculture varied considerably, some midwives urging the mother to drink two or three glasses of the decoction in an afternoon, others counseling that it be consumed over a period of days. Still other circumstances affected how much of the active ingredients actually reached the gut, in order to be absorbed in the circulation. For example, young servant women taking Eastern white cedar (*Thuja occidentalis*) for abortion were said to drink too much at a time, vomiting it up because it tasted so foul, and thus getting no effect. But they were trapped because they had to prepare it secretly and were unable to take a series of smaller doses.[82]

Given these circumstances, herbal abortion probably appeared capricious to many women. The outcome, as far as they were concerned, was unforseeable: one cooked up a batch of savin twigs for three hours, and then one would either go into horrible convulsions, abort with a slight feeling of nausea, or feel no effect at all, the pregnancy continuing. Such randomness made any systematic use of drugs for fertility control probably out of the question for most married women. Yet the vast number of folkloric and medical references to their use suggests that herbal abortion was nonetheless a considerable factor in "miscarriage." A woman could interrupt one pregnancy with a tea of saffron, and another pregnancy, five years later, with some store-bought pennyroyal oil, and end up with six live births out of a somewhat larger number of conceptions. Only at the beginning of the twentieth century would more reliable drugs, such as quinine and apiol, become widely available to give herbal abortion an important role in reducing fertility.

Abortion with Instruments in Traditional Society

If drugs didn't work, the woman might well complete the pregnancy because, before the second half of the nineteenth century, instrumental abortion would not have been a realistic possibility. Instruments intervene directly in the uterus, either to scrape the embryo from the uterine wall early in pregnancy, or to stimulate mechanically the uterus to begin contracting later in pregnancy, or to puncture the sac of waters which envelops the child. Such abortions were little done. For example, among those incarcerated in the Bastille as professional abortionists late in the seventeenth century, most worked with drugs, not with instruments.[83] A Strasbourg ordinance of 1605, which prohibited midwives from doing abortions, mentioned only "bloodletting, purgatives, and other drugs." Nothing was said about instruments, and presumably midwives did not use them in abortions.[84] When, indeed, women themselves or abortionists did intervene vaginally, it seems to have been toward the end of the pregnancy, when the fetus would be large and easy to get at. Thus, one of the few references to vaginal interference with pregnancy I have seen stemmed from Dr. Coutèle of Albi in 1808: "[The abortionist] arrives at the woman's house under the pretext of dilating her passages, and gives her a douche calculated to commence premature labor. Or the abortionist tries to burst the pouch of waters before it has completely formed. From the time one's finger can touch it, the child's head receives a series of murderous attempts, and people refer vulgarly to these lesions made with the fingernails as *Détados*, when they are seen at birth."[85]

But most evidence suggests that women had little access to instrumental abortions at any stage of pregnancy. Dr. Munaret explained that when women approached him for abortions, he would feign to go along, and give them "certain pills calculated to dissolve the fetus [*germe*], on the express condition that the woman employ no other means, external or internal, and that she have the patience to await their action. For I never neglected to add that my pills are very slow to *work*, that several months might be required, et cetera." Thus, by the time it became apparent to the woman that Dr. Munaret's "secret pills" were not going to work, the fetus would be "too big and strong" to be aborted. "Is this not a perfect result? Saving a child from death and its mother from crime"?[86] The implication is that these tricked women would not have access to the more certain techniques of vaginal intervention.

One reason for this traditional timidity is the uncertainty in village culture about the anatomy of the uterus and about what transpired inside it. The birth attendants' confusion about the mechanism of labor which I described earlier, turns up in a general folkloric disorientation about the insides of the body. A tailor's apprentice in Germany wanted to give his sweetheart an abortion; and after trampling on her belly had proven fruitless, he took his large cloth shears, inserted them in the vagina, and tried to cut the fetus's "life thread" [*Lebensfaden*]; he succeeded only in mutilating the vagina.[87] "Abortion through vaginal intervention must be rare among the peasants," wrote Otto Stoll in his survey of folk practices in Switzerland, "because second parties are required who are familiar with the anatomy of the birth canal."[88]

It would be unfair to the doctors to call their knowledge of pelvic anatomy rudimentary. But they as well had relatively little experience with vaginal procedures of any kind and, when called upon to do them, performed clumsily. The simplest way of all to terminate a pregnancy is simply to press down on the abdomen with one hand, and with a finger of the other to press through the cervix and feel about inside the uterus until one encounters the conceptus, then simply pull it away. Men skilled in obstetrics, such as Guillaume de la Motte, could do that easily.[89] But before the fetus got to be a couple of inches long, even that was quite difficult. At the end of the first month, the embryo is only about a quarter of an inch long and, at nine weeks, only an inch and a quarter (the amniotic sac at that point being about two inches long);[90] so only after a couple of months will the fetus be accessible even to primitive vaginal intervention. (As you will shortly see, not until the 1890s would curetting for abortion begin.) One august medical authority said in 1821 that dilating the cervix and then inserting a metal instrument "is quite difficult to do in practice."[91] He was referring to the "diabolic and incredible villany" of the abortionist, but the implication was that these procedures were challenging for *anyone*.

Indeed! Dr. Henry Oldham tried in 1849 to perform a therapeutic abortion on a woman whose vagina had been scarred shut. First he gave her ergot; nothing happened. Then he tried rotating a uterine sound (probe) in her uterus; no result. Then he attempted to terminate the pregnancy with electroshock; "no uterine action." Then finally a week later, after her pregnancy had advanced to the fourth month, he was able to "pass a common male sound into the uterus, and by a little manipulation it was distinctly felt to penetrate the amniotic bag." Seven days after that she finally aborted.[92] Or consider the "adroitness" of a French doctor, who in 1857 impregnated his domestic servant. A potion of savin and rue which he gave her produced nothing but "colic, vomiting, headaches, deafness, and convulsions." So he waited for three months and then, with the aid of a speculum, tried to introduce a rubber sound into her uterus. Three times he pushed it in, and three times she cried out in pain. "But no blood flowed out, only a bit of water." Moreover, the child continued to move about. Miss N. refused to submit herself to a new attempt, and gave birth at term on 7 October.[93] Thus even doctors found abortions difficult to effect.

An even more forbidding obstacle to instrumental abortion, however, was the risk of infection. An unclean knitting needle can infect a mother at three months' gestation just as easily as can an ungloved hand at nine. And the occasional references to septic abortion suggest that post-abortal abscesses and fevers must have loomed awesomely to the women in village culture. "Madam M., a widow of thirty-six, came to see me in 1810 for the dull, severe pain she was feeling in her pelvis," wrote Dr. Martin. Finally she revealed the whole history. "Around a year ago I had the misfortune to become pregnant, and wishing to safeguard myself from shame and from the rebukes of my family, I took a number of useless drugs to get an abortion." Then someone steered her to an abortionist who "introduced into my uterus a pointed rod that caused me intense pain." She aborted, "but since that time I have not ceased to suffer, and I have fallen into the state of languour in which you see me."[94] She obviously had a pelvic infection from the abortion. Septic abortions in those days were, however, so rare as virtually to constitute medical curiosities. Joubert, in his 1766 article on "Miscarriage" for Diderot's *Encyclopedia*, cites one in Nürnberg in 1714![95] How far we are, at this point, from the early twentieth century, when one hospital pathologist said that he usually saw a fatal abortion *about once every ten days.*[96]*

The First Abortion Revolution

The increase in abortions after 1970 was dramatic but, in terms of the experience of average women, not as dramatic as the *first* great increase in induced abortion toward the end of the nineteenth century. Abortion changed in those years from a desperate expedient of unmarried servants and child-weary forty-two-year-olds to a common means of birth control. Because the procurement of abortion then was strictly illegal for any reason except saving the mother's life, most abortions transpired in secret. Thus, it is difficult to document changes in their frequency. There are a number of indications, however, of a significant rise in induced abortions after 1880.

We have, for example, reports from doctors and midwives called to attend abortions because complications had developed. This is the best index of all, yet remains far below the real mark because most aborting

* Note the naïveté of James C. Mohr's argument that around 1828 in the United States "childbirth was just as subject to shock and infection as abortion." He infers from the fact that "contemporary writers did not stress the great dangers of an abortion induced by mechanical means" that such abortions were relatively safe.[97] It seems to me more likely that if early American doctors said little about septic abortions, it was because few instrumental abortions were being done.

TABLE 8.1

The Number of Abortions (Spontaneous and
Induced) per 1,000 Women, Ages 15 to 45
(1901–27)

Reports from Doctors, Midwives, and Hospitals	
Malmö (Sweden)	
1901–9	3
1910–19	6
1920–27	8
Magdeburg	
1912	20
1923	23
1927	18

Reports from Health Insurance Funds (per 1,000 female members of childbearing age)	
Leipzig	
1887–1905	9
Berlin	
1915	13
1927	33

SOURCES: See notes to tables, page 382.

women called no one to attend them.* Table 8.1 suggests nonetheless a big rise in those communities for which suitable data are available.

Many more women were admitted to the hospital for "incomplete" abortions—which is to say, abortions where some of the products of conception remain in the womb. No such women turned up at Zurich's Women's Hospital from 1888 to 1891; between 1908 and 1911, 27 did.[99] The annual number of abortions treated in Vienna's hospitals climbed from 400 in 1892 to 4,500 in 1912, not including the additional thousands of women seen for abortion in outpatient departments. One local doctor recommended transforming some of the city's barracklike obstetrical wards into incomplete-abortion clinics.[100] An Oslo hospital treated 31 women for abortion in 1913; 357, in 1929. It is true that in these years Oslo

---

* Thus the "maternal mortality committee" for Wales concluded, "From inquiries made among doctors and nurses it would appear that abortion per se is not a common reason for calling in their services, and as a rule it is only where the condition of the woman gives rise to concern that their attendance is requested. It would be difficult to obtain statistics of the number of natural abortions, and there would always be a certain number . . . which are not revealed except to the woman's intimate friends."[98]

women began going more often to the hospital for all complaints; for example, admissions doubled for appendicitis. But the abortion rise was *ten*fold.[101] And in a community like London's suburb of Camberwell, overall hospital admissions for women remained the same, while abortion admissions rose more than 40 percent in the 1920s.[102] Whereas 117 women were treated for abortion in 1921 in Sheffield's City General Hospital, almost triple that number were a decade later.[103] Everywhere hospitals were raking in the septic and incomplete abortions. Said Dr. P. Balard of Paris, "There are each year almost as many interrupted pregnancies as completed ones."[104]

In some cities after 1900 there were more abortion patients in the maternity wards than there were full-term mothers! In the Kiel area, for example, abortion patients rose from 19 percent of total obstetric patients in 1921 to 61 percent in 1927.[105]* "You won't give me an abortion?" said women in Breslau to their doctors. "Then I'll just go to Berlin."[108]

Many of these abortions were spontaneous.† Is there any way we can estimate the number of *induced* abortions‡ as opposed to spontaneous abortions, or miscarriages? The problem with abortions done at home, whether by skilled abortionists or by women themselves, was infection. Sticking something into the uterus introduces contamination. A woman's temperature rises. Severely infected women may get peritonitis or pelvic

---

* Kiel is the most extreme case I have seen. Yet abortions in Germany as a whole increased from 3 percent of all obstetric admissions in 1902–04 to 9 percent in 1920–22.[106] By 1904 there were twenty-three abortions per one hundred obstetric admissions in Paris's Lariboisière hospital.[107]

† According to Ralph Benson, "About 12 percent of all pregnancies terminate in spontaneous abortion."[109] This figure does not include the very early abortions, most of which the woman is not even aware of, and which constitute, according to two authorities, as much as 75 percent of all conceptions.[110]

‡ Women in the past were often reluctant to admit that their miscarriages had been illegally procured. Yet several studies suggest that before the Second World War the great majority of abortions after the second month were, in fact, induced rather than spontaneous. In a Leningrad hospital, for example, 1,368 abortion patients who had miscarried at least once, were asked if their earlier abortion had been induced (they ran no risk of prosecution because abortion in the Soviet Union by that time had been legalized); 92 percent confessed a previous induction.[111] Lengthy interviews among abortion patients in a Stockholm hospital from 1920 to 1921 revealed that *all* the febrile abortions had been induced.[112] Of one hundred abortions treated in the hospital, seventy-eight had been induced, according to a paper Dr. Blondel gave to the Société d'obstétrique de Paris in 1902.[113] Of abortions in Magdeburg, from 1925 to 1927, 16 percent were the result of accidents, job hazards, and legal induced abortion; the other 84 percent were in the category of *Ursachen die Jedermann kennt* (causes known to all).[114] Three established authorities offered the opinion that the infected abortions were induced.[115]

A complicating factor is that drug abortions also sometimes touch off fever. Of thirty women who confessed to drug abortions in the Oslo Civic Hospital from 1920 to 1929, eighteen were febrile.[116]

TABLE 8.2

The Number of Septic Abortions* per 100 Abortions Treated in a Hospital (1901–39)

1901–9	25
1910–19	32
1920–29	33
1930–39	38

* Therapeutic abortions are excluded; "septic" means any abortion patient with a fever over 37.5–38.5°C.
NOTE: These are composite data from many studies.
SOURCES: See notes to tables, pages 382–83.

abscesses. Yet overall, relatively few abortions resulted in infection.* Infected abortions interest us mainly as an index of the total number being done. It is, for example, significant that in Malmö, Sweden, only 3 percent to 4 percent of abortions among first mothers involved fever (most being spontaneous), and that 20 percent to 25 percent of abortions among multiparous mothers were febrile: mothers of established families were having induced abortions more often than were just-married women.[119] Of 82 abortion patients, who were in a Kiel hospital in the 1930s, and whose abortions were clearly induced, over three quarters had a high fever.[120] It was around 1903 that the number of febrile abortions began rising in Kiel.[121] But, as table 8.2 shows, in many other places also septic abortions increased during the first quarter of the twentieth century.

A consequence of this onrush of infected abortions is that, as we saw in chapter 6, the whole phenomenon of "puerperal fever" after 1900 became shifted from full-term deliveries to abortions (see supplementary notes). In completed pregnancies, "childbed fever" once afflicted women as a result of the microbes on the birth attendant's exploring hand. After 1900 "maternal sepsis" came essentially to denote an infected abortion. It is a minor tragedy of women's history that this shift in "maternal mortality" was not noted at the time, for one of the arguments that destroyed home delivery was that sepsis would be much less in hospital.

Inevitably, so much septic abortion would lead to a terrible increase in post-abortion fatalities. For example, 37 women died after abortion in 1885 in Berlin; 73 in 1896.[122] In Hamburg there were 41 abortion deaths in 1907; 229, in 1922.[123] By the late 1920s an estimated 8,000

---

* Of 198,000 notified miscarriages (*Fehlgeburten*) in 1936 in Germany, for example, 12,600 (6 percent) were febrile.[117] Of 6,871 miscarriages notified in Magdeburg in a special study from 1924 to 1927 (for which the clinical course was known) 443 were febrile (6 percent).[118]

women died *annually* of abortion in Germany.[124] Many additional deaths were unreported, classified instead as "sausage poisoning," a "middle-ear infection," or "appendicitis."[125] An inquiry in New South Wales into "the death of a young woman from 'myocarditis' revealed that a post-mortem had demonstrated a knitting-needle was in the peritoneum." One should, reflected Dr. Dunstan Brewer, consider every death in women between the ages of fifteen and forty-five to be an abortion death unless proved otherwise.[126] Autopsies in Halle and Breslau during the late 1920s revealed *eight times more* abortion deaths than in the official figures for the previous period. These deaths had been concealed under diagnoses of "peritonitis," "heart attack," and so forth.[127] Thus did the great majority of abortions "escape the coroner's court."[128]

The cause of death in most abortions was sepsis: 67 percent in Switzerland in the 1890s, 85 percent in England in the early 1930s, 86 percent in Philadelphia between 1931 and 1933.[129] Of 74 abortion deaths in Sheffield between 1921 and 1930, 72 were from infection.[130] There is no reason why a spontaneous abortion should become infected. But with syringes, catheters, and curettes poking into women, there was something of a chance of major complications—general blood poisoning, the dissemination of air emboli throughout the bloodstream, shock, and collapse.[131]

Let us, however, not become so riveted upon these terrible complications as to forget that the average abortion was fairly safe. What happened was that *so many* women were getting abortions that the small mortality rate accompanying the procedure became translated into a large absolute number of deaths. Let us say that a million women a year have abortions and that the mortality rate is one tenth of 1 percent: that means one thousand abortion deaths a year—a horrifying number, but a minimal risk for the average woman. Of course, those women admitted to the hospital with incomplete or septic abortions had a poor prognosis (1 percent to 10 percent of them dying, according to various statistics).[132] But the death rate was far less for the uncomplicated abortions, which comprised the vast majority. It is impossible to estimate the true mortality rate for abortion. But the death rate in Magdeburg for those abortions seen by doctors and midwives at home (plus those treated in hospital) was only 1.3 percent. The same figure prevailed for Austria.[133]*

Moreover, as sterile conditions became more common in the performance of abortion, the mortality rate dropped, sinking dramatically in the late 1930s with the "sulfa" drugs.[134] One Danzig doctor said in 1931 that the death rate from illegal abortions treated in his clinic had been declining "because of the greater participation of the medical profession

* Excluding Vienna, whose death rate was .6 per 100 women treated for miscarriage.

in illegal abortions and because of the improvement in knowledge of surgery and anatomy . . . among the unofficial abortionists."[135] Thus, as more doctors did abortions, fewer women became infected.*

What was the likelihood of the average woman having an induced abortion in the years from 1900 to 1940? Considerable. Among married women around the First World War, perhaps one pregnancy in three terminated in miscarriage. Since only a small portion of these miscarriages were likely to have been spontaneous (see second note on page 193), Max Hirsch's estimate seems fair that among urban women one pregnancy in four was ended through an illegal abortion.[142]†

Whatever the defects of these clinical data, there certainly was an increase in the number of women who said they had ever had a "miscarriage" (a term that includes spontaneous and induced abortions): up from 12 percent in Berlin in 1882–85 to 36 percent in 1915–16;[144]‡ up from 8 percent in Vienna in 1907 to 20 percent in 1920–24;[148] up from 7 percent in Amsterdam in 1883–84 to 24 percent in 1943;[149] and so forth.[150] Of course, these figures must be taken with some grains of salt because many of the women doubtless concealed some illegal abortions and forgot about some spontaneous ones early in pregnancy (or didn't even realize they had been pregnant). On the other hand, perhaps one woman in ten who believed she had had an abortion turned out not even to have been pregnant.[151] Another problem is that these data lump together women interviewed in many different settings, such as lying-in hospitals, eye-

---

* It is difficult to pin down statistically, yet I have the general impression that after 1900 doctors were increasingly willing to do "criminal" abortions, or abortions for "social indications" (that is, without urgent medical reason but done at the woman's request), which in those days the medical profession saw as tantamount to criminal. Many individual doctors asserted it was happening. In the United States, for example, John A. Lyons said in 1907, "I am informed there exists in the city of Chicago a regularly organized union of physicians who do nothing but this kind of work [criminal abortion]."[136] Likewise, Frank H. Jackson in 1909: "To our disgrace the men who are performing most of the abortions in this State [Maine] are not outcasts from their profession . . . they are often pointed out as honest, hard-working physicians."[137] And especially the comments by Dr. Edward Weiss of Pittsburgh on a 1922 paper by H. Wellington Yates:[138] "Physicians who will go to almost any limit to secure a good result in other cases, will produce an abortion on the slightest provocation."[139] Max Nassauer of Munich raged in 1919 against the *Abschaum der Ärzte* (the scum of the medical profession) who did abortions.[140] Adolphe Pinard of Paris said in a 1917 meeting of the Société Générale des Prisons, "We all know doctors who do abortions."[141]

† Hirsch ventured "23 percent" as a global figure.[143]

‡ Other data for Berlin based on personal interviews or insurance claims are to be found in an article by Bleichröder: of 3,767 conceptions among 1,000 married women admitted to hospital as general medical patients, 1,209 ended in abortion.[145] Dr. C. Hamburger interviewed over 2,000 married eye patients, heavily working-class in origin, in 1908 and 1913 and found the share of pregnancies ending in abortion to be 17 percent for both years.[146] On the basis of extensive personal-history data, Karl Freudenberg estimated that the frequency of abortion in general among married women rose in Berlin from 9 percent in 1909 to 37 percent in 1921. In 1909, 4 percent of pregnancies ended in illegal abortions; in 1921, 31 percent.[147]

clinics, general medical practices and birth-control clinics. Accordingly, differences may reflect more the nature of the sample population rather than change over time in the over-all likelihood of an abortion. But there does seem to have been an increase from perhaps 10 percent to 25 percent of pregnancies ending in abortion. That may not sound very dramatic. Yet if 8 percent to 10 percent of all pregnancies end spontaneously (excluding the numerous very early abortions), the real change in induced abortion would be from about 2 percent of all pregnancies toward 1850 to 15 percent in 1940. This represents a substantial change indeed.

The people of the time would not have disagreed with this assessment. One could fill volumes with observers' impressions in the 1920s and 1930s that "criminal" abortion had become epidemic. I shall spare the reader these, however, and note only that the midwives in particular complained long and bitterly about abortion. Lisbeth Burger said that in her little Silesian town "in the months after the Great War and throughout the inflation time, the abortion disease raged like the plague through all groups of people, in city and countryside, among poor and rich, old and young, among married and single. When I am called, it is mostly to miscarriages. Normal births have become a rarity."[152]* British midwives reported in the 1930s that abortion had become so common that mothers would ask the midwife if the baby was "all right," since they had taken so many drugs to end the pregnancy. "It is a common thing," said one midwife, responding to a questionnaire on abortion, "when patients come to book, for them to say they are booking as they could not get rid of it." "Not one family in twenty welcomes the advent of a third child," said another midwife.[153] Nothing like these quotes exists for the years before 1870. Of course, these English midwives had not done a scientific study, but they knew their patients were relying on abortion as a means of birth control.

The New Techniques of Instrumental Abortion

The motives that caused women to seek out all these abortions lie beyond the scope of this book; they are to be found in the larger history of the family and sexuality. What I wish to address here is the extent to which medical progress made possible the abortion revolution. Was it accomplished with traditional techniques, in the hands of women who now suddenly wanted to limit their family size?[154] Or was it the result of new techniques floating into the hands of women who had always

* The climate in which she published her book was, of course, extremely hostile to abortion.

wanted to curb their fertility but had not known how to go about it? I shall argue for the second, because I believe that women had always resented the vulnerability to which unwanted pregnancy subjected them.

Let me be systematic, treating the new techniques for abortion in the order of their historical appearance:

METHODS OF PUNCTURING

Least innovative of the techniques was puncturing the amniotic sac with a sharp object. Such folkloric abortive devices as goose quills are as old as time. But at the beginning of the nineteenth century new medical techniques started to make these simple punctures less haphazard: doctors began putting pointed wires inside hollow catheters.* This technique, invented to initiate premature labor, decreased some of the damage that could be caused by a naked needle tip, wavering about inside the uterus. By mid-century this had become the standard medical technique of inducing labor, while remaining risky before the discovery of asepsis.† This technique, like all the others I shall describe, was soon taken over by abortionists. "Who could have thought," wrote W. Schütte in 1855, medical officer of Wolfenbüttel, that medical progress "could be perverted to such antisocial ends."[157] Yet compared with the techniques I am about to discuss, simple puncture remained unimportant.

The abortion revolution began with Charles Goodyear's discovery in 1839 of the vulcanization of rubber. As rubber catheters began to circulate after 1850, abortionists needed no longer to seek a bulls-eye with a pointed object, and thus to risk perforating the uterus in searching for the conceptus. They could simply rotate a blunt catheter in the uterus until they hit the fetus. Thus Washington's Dr. James F. Scott described in 1895 what he imagined to be the typical criminal abortion: "A dirty catheter is clumsily passed into the womb and stirred around till the ovum is ruptured. The vagina is stuffed with cotton, and the woman, having paid her fee, is told to depart."[158] Already in 1865 Paris's Dr. E. Ferdut mentioned scraping with a solid rubber catheter as a criminal means of terminating pregnancy early.[159] Frederic Griffith, on a trip to Paris, was able to persuade a market woman selling catheters and the like to show him a few. These particular devices were of metal rather than rubber, yet they were used as follows: "It is recommended that a woman can best perform the operation unassisted, and verily I believe that the average Frenchwoman can locate her uterine os [the outside entrance to the cervix] as certainly as she can touch the tip of her nose." She would press down on the abdomen with one hand and, with the instrument in the

* Heinrich Fasbender said that England's Robert Lee was the first to use this procedure.[155]
† W. Schütte described it in 1855 as the procedure of choice.[156]

other, gradually dilate her cervix "by a rotary onward motion . . . until the sensation of rupture occurs and the escape of bloody fluid proves the success of the operation."[160] If blood did not appear at once, the woman would move into the procedure to which I now come.

SYRINGES

The injection of fluid into the uterus became popular at some point in the second half of the nineteenth century. It works on the principle that, even early in pregnancy, the uterus can be induced to contract if its walls are irritated. A stream of water shot at high pressure from a syringe will do this, so that simple mechanical irritation appears to produce the abortion. Among the new techniques for abortion, syringing was probably the most popular, and would remain so right until the Second World War. It is, par excellence, the accomplishment of nineteenth-century technology.

Syringes had been used medically since the ancient Greeks, and Hippocrates mentioned one fashioned from a pig's bladder.[161] A German surgery textbook from 1531 depicts what is evidently a rectal or an aural syringe— as it has a short nozzle—made of metal.[162] And the early nineteenth century would see the elaboration of a huge variety of enema syringes, most of metal or glass.[163] But their diffusion required rubber, for the brass and pewter ones used by doctors and midwives would have been far too expensive. Moreover, they lacked the long pointed nozzles required to fit into the uterus.

During the nineteenth century these requirements started to be met. The two basic types of domestic syringe were: (1) a water bag connected by a rubber tube to a thin nozzle of metal, bone, or hard rubber; halfway along the tube would be a bulb, which could be squeezed to eject water from the nozzle at high pressure; (2) a rubber bulb with a threaded aperture, onto which a short nozzle could be screwed (for vaginal or rectal douches), or a long, curved nozzle for uterine douches. Either type could forcefully squirt water into the uterus and produce an abortion by irritation (or perhaps by actually detaching the placenta from the uterine wall). Medical interest in syringing in order to induce premature labor became steadily livelier during the century. Jacob Friedrich Schwieghäuser recommended it obstetrically for the first time in 1825. In 1846 a Hamburg doctor named Cohen suggested a *Clysopompe* (syringe type 1) with a tin nozzle, filled with hot water, for inducing labor. In that same year Franz Kiwisch recommended starting labor by injecting a steady stream of water against the cervix.[164] These techniques started to be used. By 1867, J. Lazarewitch was able to report twelve cases of labor successfully induced by uterine injections.[165]

Injections were not slow to be picked up outside of medicine. In 1865, Dr. Ferdut called "Professor Kiwisch's procedure" newly popular among abortionists (referring to *intra*uterine injections).[166] Ambroise Tardieu quoted the testimony of a woman who was tried in 1867 for having sought an abortion: "[The abortionist] had in her hand a syringe which was armed with a long cannula. I asked her if she was going to jam it into my belly. She said, 'Don't worry, not any more than that much,' and pointed to the first phalanx of her little finger. In addition to the syringe she brought a gray bottle with a whitish liquid. . . . The woman made me stand up against a wall with my legs apart, knelt before me, sought out the opening of the uterus with one hand and with the other introduced the cannula, guiding it along her finger which remained in my vagina. She made two injections, a few minutes apart." To tell if a second were needed, the abortionist looked into a bowl, into which the water draining from the uterus was flowing. "If the water had been accompanied by a bit of blood, the second injection would not have been necessary. That evening towards nine I had my miscarriage, losing a great deal of blood."[167]

In the last quarter of the nineteenth century the syringe would be the procedure of choice of professional abortionists. All one required was a "large rubber bulb and a thin cannula";[168] a speculum, for visualizing the cervix, was optional, as many abortionists could easily insert the cannula by touch. (Only a few of the midwives doing syringe abortions in Thuringia, in fact, used speculae.)[169] The abortion patient would sit between two chairs in a darkened room, "so that she can see nothing."[170] One midwife, tried in 1892, had done at least seventy-two successful syringe abortions without a speculum, using one hand alone.[171]*

Although syringes continued for a short while after 1900 to be popular among professionals, the device began increasingly to be taken up by pregnant women themselves for use on their own. "The uterine syringe is used among abortionists less often" than other means, wrote a Königsberg doctor in 1915. "The mothers themselves employ it frequently, often without the help of second parties."[172] Among women treated in the early 1920s in a Hamburg hospital for complications resulting from syringe abortions, twenty-four had injected themselves; twelve had been injected by professionals.[173] In Vienna self-syringing started only around 1908.[174] Indeed, in Berlin only toward 1900 had the rubber bulbs gone on sale to the public.[175]

Why women were so late in seizing the syringe is not entirely clear,

* The abortionist had caused one death. The doctor thought it likely that the injections were more vaginal than uterine, given the person's technique; yet in numerous other instances, using just such one-handed technique, abortionists were able to locate the external os of the cervix and insert the nozzle of the syringe.

given the advantages it offered over most drugs. Whereas in the Mönchen-Gladbach district the syringe failed for only 1.3 percent of the women prosecuted for abortion, drugs had failed 15 percent of the time.[176] Of thirty-four women who had used instruments on themselves and were treated for abortion in a Nancy hospital, twenty-six had successfully aborted.[177]

Thus, given the efficacy of syringe abortion, it is understandable that women were prepared to endure discomfort to have one. Mlle. X of Nancy called the doctor urgently one Sunday afternoon because of violent pains in her abdomen. Her story went back to a missed period, which she'd "awaited impatiently for a month, requesting then some advice from a friend knowledgeable in these matters, who had told her that at the slightest delay in the menses, she should give herself an intrauterine injection." A second period was missed. "Mlle. X decided to abort herself. That Sunday at 1:00 P.M. her mother, with whom she lived, went out of the house for a few hours. Following the advice of her friend, she squatted above the toilet seat and introduced her left index finger into her vagina. Having found the cervix, she pushed a cannula into it which she had previously boiled, then attached the other end to a litle glass syringe and pressed the plunger. Immediately she felt a violent pain in her abdomen." Et cetera.[178]

The reader's heart may have missed a couple of beats in reading the preceding accounts. Rightly so. Syringe abortion was not without its risks. Mlle. X boiled the cannula. And many professional abortionists practiced "rigorous asepsis."[179] But stories abound of professionals who would hastily shove in an unsterilized cannula.[180] Thus, a woman poking an object into her uterus risked, at a minimum, infection. What percentage of women became seriously infected is impossible to say because we do not know how many had abortions in the first place.

In addition to infection, mothers risked *perforation* in instrumental abortion. The medical literature bulges with ghoulish tales of women whose intestines came spilling out because of a perforation in their vaginal wall.[181] I shall not dwell on this but merely point out that syringing one's uterus did require considerable dexterity—as is demonstrated by the fact that midwives, who among all women should have been most dextrous in manipulating their birth canals, sometimes had perforations from aborting themselves.[182]

Even if she guided the cannula properly, avoiding perforations of the vaginal fornices and the uterus, a woman might still press too hard on the plunger or bulb of the syringe. At that point several nasty things could happen: the high pressure might squeeze the water through the fallopian tubes into the peritoneum, causing peritonitis if the water were unsterilized. Or if, inadvertently, air bubbles had gotten into the bulb of the syringe, they might pass into a woman's veins, whence they would travel to the heart and lungs, causing death from "air embolism."[183] Or pressing too hard could just make her extremely uncomfortable. For example, a woman who had moved to Duisburg, Germany from Austria later needed an abortion. She got a local "professional" to syringe her. But apparently the local woman had pressed too hard, and the Austrian had suffered much. When, after recovering, she spotted her abortionist on the street, she called out, "There's that goddamn woman who nearly killed me. You'd never get that in Austria. But just come up here and look what happens."[184]

Despite these risks, by the first quarter of the twentieth century injections had become the most popular form of self-abortion. Rubber-bulb douches had turned into household articles. When a factory worker in Lüdenscheid wanted to abort his twenty-three-year-old wife, he bought a "Piccadilly" douche—and uterine nozzle—from a workmate. Commented the doctor who later treated the woman for a perforation: "That a factory worker may buy these sophisticated abortion instruments from fellow workers, who act more or less as manufacturers' representatives, shows clearly how deeply the knowledge of these procedures has already sunk into the broadest classes of the population. Thus we should not be surprised at the universal increase in miscarriages, especially at the infected ones."[185] An Elberfeld gynecologist stormed against the proliferation of rubber douches on the market. "It is now customary that women are able to procure abortions independently and privately with these devices, which they keep in their night tables like any other domestic object. Earlier, abortion was not something one did at home. It lay in the dirty hands of a few professional criminals. But today, owing to this instrument and its epidemic diffusion among the population, abortion has become the fashion; indeed, it has made itself right at home."[186]

In France one could buy the cannulas at drugstores, herbalists, and in the marketplace; in Germany, even at the hairdresser's.[187] "The technique of abortion has nowadays become so simple," said a councillor of Rouen's appellate court, "that it is no longer necessary to have recourse to professionals. It suffices to have an understanding girl friend and to procure . . . the famous cannula. I have always been struck at how easy they are to obtain." One woman had got hers after her lover had written on a slip of paper to the druggist "special cannula."[188]

In Germany traveling salesmen sold the syringes at five marks apiece. One could find them in drugstore windows. And if working-class women could not afford their own, neighbors would own one jointly. "A colleague of mine often treated two neighbor women in short succession for incomplete abortion. When asked about this remarkable coincidence, they admitted to owning jointly a uterine syringe, which they used alternately as they became pregnant."[189]

Various studies confirmed the paramountcy of the syringe over other instrumental techniques. Of thirty-six instrumental abortions treated at Zurich's women's hospital in 1888–95, twenty-nine were syringe; ditto for two thirds of those abortions seen in Nancy's hospital just after the First World War; 85 percent of the instrumental abortions treated in Königsberg's hospital had been done with a uterine or a vaginal syringe. In Essen, 61 percent of all instrumental-abortion cases brought to trial in the 1930s had involved injections, usually with soapy water.[190] Elsewhere in the world the syringe reigned less supreme; it was unimportant, for example, in Oslo in the 1920s. Thirty of fifty-one women treated in 1935 in a London hospital said they had used *vaginal* douches; none mentioned a uterine syringe.[191] It is unclear whether the numerous syringes advertised late in the nineteenth century in the United States served for abortion as well as contraception.[192]* But I have seen few direct references to syringe abortion in the United States and am inclined to think that injections were more a West European device.

DILATATION PLUS CATHETER

Before discussing the next technique, let me remind readers that before 1900 doctors did not know how to do an instrumental abortion in the first two months of pregnancy, the embryo being so small that they had no adequate way to grasp it. From around the eighth to the sixteenth weeks of pregnancy a doctor could, to be sure, push a finger through the cervix and remove the embryo with it. But before the eighth week the conceptus was too small, after the sixteenth week too large, simply to be pulled away. Of course, an injection could have been attempted at any point, but most doctors felt uneasy about them in legal, therapeutic abortion because they saw so many infections from the illegal ones.†
The crucial areas in which progress remained to be made, therefore, were safe abortions in very early pregnancy and in the middle of pregnancy.

As it happened, the next advance touched the latter: abortions at midterm. The technique involved opening up the cervix and then inserting a thin, solid catheter to irritate the uterine walls, thereby precipitating

---

* James C. Mohr refers to "Chamberlain's Utero-Vaginal Syringe," marketed by Parke Davis of Detroit. But its popularity is unclear.[193]

† Hunter Robb of Western Reserve University was among the few obstetrics writers even to mention syringe abortions for therapeutic purposes. He described the procedure, then added, "The method is not to be recommended. Septic infection has often been observed . . . thrombosis and embolism. . . . The advantages offered by it are that it is not only prompt in its action, but also very certain."[194]

labor. Dilatation-plus catheter was soon taken up by the professional abortionists, who apparently were starting to become uneasy about the potential complications of syringe abortion. But the abortionists added their own twist. They began to content themselves with merely establishing uterine *bleeding* through dilatation-plus-catheter techniques. Then the woman—now able to offer a legitimate reason for being "scraped out"— would go to a regular physician. She was bleeding, and the pregnancy was obviously over. It was important that she remove the catheter before she went to the doctor, and for this purpose abortionists would attach a string to it which permitted her to pull it out.[195] These catheters soon became familiar tools of the trade. Elizabeth Crowell, a nurse, said in 1906 after checking the bags of five Buffalo midwives, "In one bag I found the usual instrument for criminal operations, the wired gum catheter." Women in Portland, Oregon were able to buy catheters for abortion in drugstores and apparently inserted them unassisted.[196] And so on.

Often merely dilating the cervix suffices for an abortion; one does not have to insert a catheter. Keep in mind how smoothly this technique flowed from larger currents of "medical progress." Early in the nineteenth century doctors turned their minds to inducing labor in women who should not give birth at full term, such as women with contracted pelvises. So how does one dilate the cervix without lacerating the patient? In 1820 sponge tents were first proposed for the job. These were difficult to insert in a tightly closed cervix, however, so later in the century were introduced tents made of seaweed from the Laminaria genus or of the bark of the American slippery elm tree. Put in the cervix in a tight roll, the tent would absorb mucus and gently expand.[197] The rubber bag that Stéphane Tarnier invented in 1862 functioned along these lines, dilating the cervix as water was pumped into it. All these devices took form as part of a larger obstetrical interest in inducing premature labor.

But they were aptly suited for midterm abortion as well. In the 1860s one doctor used laminaria tents successfully on a woman with a contracted pelvis who was three months pregnant. "I hasten to submit," he wrote, "this single instance of its use, believing no time should be lost in communicating for the benefit of the profession and help of the malformed female, this simple and cleanly mode of procuring necessary abortion."[198] By 1878, Tarnier's rubber bags had passed from the hands of the doctors into those of the professional abortionists.[199]

By the 1920s and 1930s laminaria abortions were commonplace. A number of patients hospitalized with complications in Berlin said that doctors using laminaria tents had induced the abortion, seldom using injections or catheters.[200] A Ministry of Health study of maternal mortality in Wales in the early 1930s called slippery elm bark "a very popular abortifacient."[201] Seven of fifty-one abortions treated in a London hospital in 1935 involved slippery elm.[202] And the Ministry of Health's Inter-Departmental Committee on Abortion said in 1939, "A considerable body of evidence was submitted to us showing that slippery elm bark enjoys a particular popularity as an instrumental means. . . . Its use in this way is so well-known that some shops, we were informed, refuse to sell it, except in powder form, or sell it only in sticks too small for the purpose." Of eighty-four abortion deaths from sepsis which the committee studied, "seven had been preceded by the use of slippery elm bark."[203]

In the 1970s I questioned the elderly pharmacists of Ontario about whether they had dispensed drugs for abortion during the 1930s. Slippery elm was often mentioned. One man said that when women he knew asked for slippery elm, he would sell it to them straight. If he didn't know them, he would first grind it up—as if they required it only for cough syrup. "You should have seen some of the expressions on those women's faces," he said.

THE "D-AND-C"

Let's assume a woman wanted an abortion within a few weeks of discovering she was pregnant. The technique I've just described—dilatation plus catheter—might well not work early in the pregnancy. Only after around the fourth month does the simple widening of the cervix disrupt anything much inside the uterus. And as for inserting a foreign object early in pregnancy, hospital pathologists today occasionally see full-term placentas with IUDs inside them.

After 1900 a new operation came along to make possible early abortion: the "D-and-C," which stands for "dilatation and curettage." In this operation, the uterus is opened with metal dilators or seaweed tents, and then its insides are scraped out with a curette.

The story begins in 1843, when a French gynecologist named Joseph Récamier invented the uterine curette. Curettes, or sharp little knives, had always been around in medicine, but Récamier attached a handle to his so that it could scrape "fungous growths" from the uterine walls.[204] The device attracted little attention until several lighter and more flexible versions began appearing in the 1860s and 1870s; and after 1867 the principles of surgical cleanliness began to diffuse as well so that one could poke a curette into the uterus and not risk infecting the woman.[205] Doctors would curette, among other reasons, to remove the remains of incomplete abortions. But not until the 1890s was the curette used to perform a *legal* abortion.[206] Only in the years before the First World

War did doctors generally awaken to the curette's potential in terminating pregnancies of five to six weeks.[207]*

Behind the scenes a tense tug-of-war had already begun between doctors and women desirous of abortions. Dr. R. Herman of Haine-Saint-Pierre in Belgium counseled his colleagues in 1896: "On the subject of curettage, beware of pregnant women. I know other doctors who have been taken in by them"—that is, tricked into doing a D-and-C because the patient complained of periodic bleeding or of other symptoms that might justify curetting a nonpregnant uterus.[209] By the First World War many practitioners found themselves doing a little *pas de deux*, in which their patients didn't ask for abortion, and the doctors didn't say they were going to do one, but in which early pregnancies were nonetheless interrupted by curettement. "Well, you certainly have a nasty cough there," a doctor would say, suggesting tuberculosis as a legitimate indication for abortion.[210] "A catarrh at the apex of the lung, or a bit of turbulence at the apex of the heart, or some kind of highly subjective nervousness must cease to be considered warrants for the termination of any pregnancy the woman wants to get rid of," said another doctor.[211] In the view of a Viennese practitioner, word had "gotten around among the laity" that uterine interventions had become quite safe as a result of asepsis. "Women today no longer rely on the chemical action of abortifacient drugs but immediately demand intervention with instruments. Very often the abortionist [meaning the doctor] and the patient meet each other halfway. The woman only alludes to her distressed condition and the co-operative doctor or midwife avoids hearing a full confession, perhaps half-consciously prepared to assume that she is pregnant. The doctor immediately thereupon undertakes some instrumental manipulation, without explaining to her the purpose, dilating, manipulating a sound, poking, scraping, wiping out, et cetera."[212] Thus with neither doctor nor patient criminally complicit, curettement made possible early medical abortions—assuming the woman could find a doctor willing to be her partner in this ballet. How many doctors went along is unclear, but *somebody* was doing all the abortions I described in the previous section.

Inevitably the D-and-C spread beyond medical circles to the professional abortionists, although here, too, the record is cloudy. Performed competently the D-and-C would have produced little in the way of morbidity or mortality, and thus would not appear in hospital and judicial records, the usual sources. So it is quite possible that in the first half of the twentieth century the D-and-C became the chief means of instrumental

---

* Not until the 1950 edition does the major American obstetrics textbook, *Williams Obstetrics*, mention the D-and-C for abortion.[208] All previous editions had preferred manual abortion with the surgeon's index finger, or dilatation with a tampon, to produce an abortion.

abortion, while leaving few historical traces. Already in 1878 a Parisian doctor was complaining that curettement had passed into the hands of professional abortionists: "The curette, which does such fine service for us in daily practice . . . is figuring quite specifically among the instruments used by criminal abortionists."[213] I have, however, seen few later references to nonmedical abortionists using curettes. Indeed one study of Essen in the 1930s maintained that only doctors used them for abortion.[214]

Throughout this section I have argued that the abortion revolution depended upon medical and technological innovation. There may indeed have been an increased willingness among women to seek out abortions, but that desire would have been frustrated without the discovery of asepsis, without the search for techniques to induce premature labor, without the rubber syringe bulbs and sterilizable rubber catheters we have seen, without the invention of the uterine curette and of the graduated dilators that opened the cervix. Thus I am bolstering the case that relatively safe medical abortion had descended from the technological heavens by the 1930s to make women less vulnerable to pregnancy. ("Relatively safe" means seeing things from the viewpoint of women in the 1780s, and not the 1980s.)

ABORTIONISTS VERSUS DOCTORS

I cannot resist tacking on a final question, in view of the hundred-year-old clichés about "butchers" and "back-street abortionists" which have punctuated public discussions of this subject. My impression is that the professional abortionists were fairly competent, and that the real "butchers" were the physicians, rushed, guilt-ridden, and unpracticed in abortion procedures. Several kinds of evidence back up this impression. It would be incompetent for a doctor, before performing an abortion, to fail to see if the woman has an "ectopic pregnancy." "Ectopic" means "outside the uterus"; and perhaps one pregnancy in every hundred implants itself in the uterine tube, on the wall of the intestine, or in some other site outside the uterus.* Attempting to abort such a pregnancy with intrauterine maneuvers invites disaster, as the manipulations might rupture the sac. It is therefore interesting to see how often doctors who were about to do abortions omitted this elementary check in women. A Kiev hospital, for example, treated 726 ectopic pregnancies between 1924 and 1932. The women had already attempted to get abortions in 51 of them, and two thirds of these attempts were made by doctors.[216] Perhaps the professional abortionists as well failed to check for ectopic pregnancies, but the cases in the literature fall to the burden of physicians. A number

* Jack A. Pritchard and Paul C. MacDonald give estimates ranging from 1:84 to 1:230.[215]

of other disaster stories stem from failure to verify if the woman was even pregnant.[217]

Second, bear in mind that, "Abortionists infect, doctors perforate."[218] Because of the thoroughness with which physicians learned asepsis in medical school, they seem to have been associated with relatively few infected abortions, infection being a companion of the self-induced or the husband-induced abortion.* But doctors were largely responsible for the terrible rise in uterine *perforations* in Europe from the end of the First World War to around 1930.[220] Of 120 uteri perforated during attempted abortions between 1910 and 1923 in Hamburg, for example, 78 percent were done by doctors, 4 percent by abortionists, and 18 percent by the woman herself. Of 16 uteri perforated in Rostock, between 1920 and 1930, 14 were done by doctors. In an overview of 266 other perforations in the medical literature, one scholar found that 57 percent were the work of physicians.[221]† These somber statistics suggest that "backstreet" abortionists did not often perforate their clients' uteri, because on the whole they worked competently.

New Drugs for Abortion

If new instrumental techniques alone had caused the great increase in abortion, we could stop here. But things are a little more complicated. Drugs bore a substantial share of the rise in abortion as well. In the United States perhaps one third of all abortions were still being procured with substances like ergot until the beginning of the Second World War.[223]‖ In Europe, while the percentage was lower, it was not unimportant.§ For example, although some instrumental abortions were being

---

* In twenty-two abortion sepsis cases treated in Melbourne's Women's Hospital from 1933 to 1934, the Higginson's Syringe was implicated in nine; in the others, the women mainly denied induced abortion.[219]

† Note that in absolute terms the number of perforated-abortion deaths was small. It amounted to only three or four a year in Vienna, for example, compared with around 2500 annual yearly deaths in Vienna of women aged fifteen to forty-five; many of these latter would have been abortion fatalities.[222]

‡ Of the abortions studied in one New York hospital from 1938 to 1939, 66 percent had apparently been procured with drugs, according to Virginia Clay Hamilton.[224] But Hamilton pointed out that women may overstate the frequency of drug abortion "because drug induction does not seem to carry with it the same moral odium as does mechanical interference, but also because its admission does not implicate the abortionist whom the woman, whether from fear or gratitude, feels compelled to shield."[225] The author further believed the drugs to be innocuous, and felt that women who admitted to drug abortions had probably aborted spontaneously.[226]

§ In various European studies the share of abortion with drugs ranged from 65 percent (Göttingen court cases, 1909–19) to 8 percent (Königsberg hospital, 1904–13). The data are so disparate that any statistical average would mislead.[227]

done by 1911 in York, nonetheless, according to one woman: "Most women go on taking pennyworths here and there. . . . Or they'll try as many as twenty different kinds one after the other . . . caraway seeds, salts, diachylon."[228] A scholar who analyzed one thousand two hundred replies from midwives to a 1937 questionnaire noted, "The commonest methods the midwives had observed were drugs, douching and the use of instruments and 'foreign bodies'—in that order."[229] And a British Health Ministry Committee wrote in 1939, "The most popular of all methods of attempting to bring on criminal abortion, but one successful only to a very limited extent, is the oral administration of a drug."[230] Leaving aside the question of efficacy for the moment, it is clear that drugs continued to be important in the average woman's encounter with abortion in the first half of the twentieth century. In this section I shall argue that traditional drugs for abortion like savin and ergot gave way to several new ones, and that these new drugs—lead compounds, quinine, and apiol—were, in important measure, responsible for the staggering rise in abortion after 1880.

ADULTERATED DRUGS AND "FEMALE PILLS"

Why was there any need to replace the traditional drugs? Many women, who in their personal lives had left traditional society far behind, rejected all that folklore as "superstitious," for one thing. "Today the herbs are slowly being forgotten and are little more used," wrote one scholar in 1898 of the area around Berne.[231] When in the mid-1950s Margarete Möckli asked working-class people in Zurich how much they knew about herbal remedies, only those of "peasant origin" expressed any interest.[232] Increasingly urbanized and "modernized," women were losing contact with that rustic tradition of gathering drugs in the fields and making teas of them. Some of the drugs, such as ergot, were also disappearing from the fields as the soil became more carefully cultivated. (By 1900 most ergot consumed in Western Europe came from Russia and Spain.[233])

The adulteration of traditional drugs now sold in pharmacies added further to women's mistrust. Drugs like saffron and savin, which had been heavily in demand, scarce, and complicated to prepare, offered considerable temptation to adulteration. So women would take them and get no result or become violently ill from the adulterants.[234] When in 1923 one scholar analyzed thirty-eight samples of commercial savin from five different countries, he found the English, French, and Spanish all to be phony. Only the Swiss and German were genuine, which is probably why so many of the savin references to abortion come from Central Europe.[235]

Yet even though many of the traditional teas were fading from memory, women continued to have first recourse to drugs of some kind for abortion. If in Lille, for example, women tried drugs first, it was because—according to several local doctors—of the "fear that surgical abortion inspires in healthy people. Surgery presupposes moreover a tacit confession of guilt . . . and thus is only the *ultima ratio* that women who have already had previous experience with abortion seek out." The authors continued, "How much simpler is it to go to a drugstore or a herbalist and there acquire a so-called emmenagogue for a relative or for a girl friend."[236] Indeed, it was the anonymity and simplicity of drug abortion which continued to inspire its use well into the twentieth century.

To meet this demand, manufacturers began turning out "female pills," patent medicines marketed with vague promises of "terminating obstacles" or "re-establishing your regularity." It should be clear that these proprietary pills were *not* among the new drugs for abortion. They consisted mainly of alcohol, iron salts, and laxatives and contained minimal amounts of such drugs as savin or apiol which might have been effective.[237] Yet despite numerous exposés, women would often turn first to these pills and then, when they failed, seek out instrumental abortion.[238] "You cannot afford another baby. Take this drug," friends would say to one working-class Englishwoman. "I took their strong concoctions to purge me of the little life that might be mine. They failed, as such things generally do, and the third baby came."[239] Thus, the ineffectiveness of these patent medicines helped ultimately to discredit—among both doctors and women—the whole notion of drugs as an alternative to surgery.

INORGANIC DRUGS

In the shadow of the female pills there flourished, however, several other kinds of drugs that did work. The "inorganic compounds"—drugs with bases of arsenic, phosphorus, lead, and other metals—were effective because of their dismal toxicity. Poisons, they worked by killing the fetus before the mother. Yet for a period of forty years or so these inorganic drugs figured prominently in the lives of millions of women who desperately wanted abortions.

First in vogue among them was arsenic. It enjoyed a brief history in Germany and Sweden, the latter placing controls on its sale in 1876. Of attempted abortions known to the Swedish authorities between 1851 and 1880, arsenic was responsible for one third, almost all of them fatal. In perhaps one third of those cases, the woman aborted before dying.[240] Arsenic's properties as an abortifacient in low doses are unclear.

On the heels of arsenic followed phosphorus, whose unhappy medical history begins in 1833 with the invention of striking matches.[241] Women would scrape the heads off perhaps one hundred matches, dissolve them in coffee, and drink the brew. In Sweden between 1851 and 1903 there are on record over fourteen hundred cases of phosphorous poisoning in attempted abortion, the victim surviving in only ten cases. (The big increase occurred after the banning of arsenic.) Similarly, in Germany phosphorous had a short vogue, terminated by the banning in 1907 of matches with phosphorous heads.[242] It is possible that phosphorus does produce abortion in nonlethal doses. A Swedish pathologist noted, "A number of women dying in attempted phosphorus abortions had earlier used it once or several times with success."[243] But there is no doubt that phosphorus in any dose is toxic. Its history interests us mainly as evidence of the fervor with which many women desired to terminate their pregnancies.

LEAD

Lead is a slightly different story. It was far more popular than were arsenic, phosphorus, or mercury, and there is some evidence that, in small doses, it functioned as an abortifacient without doing lasting harm to the mother. Lead plaster, called "diachylon," had been around since the ancient Greeks. Lead in flakes or powder would be mixed together with olive oil and lard to form "lead oleate," a sticky substance that could be used to hold bandages in place or to immobilize fractured ribs. Called "black stick" in England, it was sold in pharmacies in large lumps, which women would then take home, roll into small pills, and swallow for abortion.

Lead oleate has a long history in abortion. Galen thought it affected the uterus.[244] A fifteenth-century English leechbook, or herbal, gave instructions on making "diaculum" immediately following a discussion of several different oxytocic drugs.[245] In the 1860s observers in France noted how many women who worked with lead aborted spontaneously.[246] But only in the 1890s did lead oleate begin to be taken for abortion by large numbers of women, above all in England. The first cases of lead poisoning in fertile women were reported at Leicester in 1893. By 1899 the "plumbism" epidemic had reached Birmingham and Nottingham; by 1906, much of the Midlands. After delineating the exact boundaries of the poisoning cases, Dr. Arthur Hall said, "This area comprises a large number of manufacturing towns, each containing thousands of the working classes, together with a country between largely occupied by mining populations."[247] Industrial workers, not peasants, were taking lead oleate for abortion.

How does one know whether a woman has taken lead? "Look at her gums," said Dr. G. Schwarzwaeller, a gynecologist in Stettin. A blue line will appear. "She will be pale as she comes into your office, pulse regular, no fever, belly sensitive to pressure and severe abdominal pains. No other symptoms," except that she has just aborted or will do so shortly.

"It is simply astonishing how often we see this in Stettin. Among three hundred abortions I have observed since 1895, eighteen have had these symptoms."[248] Large doses, it must be pointed out, damage the central nervous system and can be fatal. Small doses doubtless poison the mother, too, but their specific mechanism for producing abortion seems to be by causing coagulation of the circulation of the placenta rather than by killing the infant outright. Rabbit experiments in which this mechanism was discovered also showed that, when given small doses, the animals were quite normal again after they had aborted.[249]* If so, perhaps these European women, in taking diachylon pills for abortion, were not acting as self-destructively as once was thought.

By the First World War, in any event, lead was widely consumed for abortion. "I found a fairly general consensus of opinion," wrote one investigator in 1914, whom the Local Government Board had sent to Lancashire, "that among the cotton operatives, a considerable proportion of the married women are desirous of avoiding pregnancy if possible, and that recently there has been a definite increase in the proportion of those who employ active means." What means? "The drug most likely to prove seriously injurious is diachylon (lead plaster), which is stocked in stick form by most of the chemists interviewed, and retailed in pennyworths, which are subsequently cut up and made into pills by the purchaser. . . . One chemist whom I interviewed admitted selling 14 pounds of diachylon last year, an amount which would cut up into about 500 pennyworths. The purchasers of this substance are almost invariably women."[251] A correspondent of the *Pharmaceutical Journal* wrote in 1906, "I refused to sell a woman a mixture of pills for that purpose [abortion] a few weeks ago; in a short time she was in the shop and told me she had been advised to take lead shot, which she obtained at the ironmonger's, and it had been effectual. From inquiries since I find it is quite a common remedy."[252] C. H. Fentiman of London advised pharmacists to refuse entirely to sell diachylon, which is used for abortion "so largely, and rarely for anything else."[253]

Only in the late 1920s did lead seem to drop off. Legislation had limited its sale in stick form (so that some women began scraping it from the backs of bandages).[254] An analyst for the Home Office thought in 1929 that lead had "completely disappeared" as an abortifacient.[255] A 1930 study of abortion in Camberwell said, "Lead seems to have lost its reputation, or else it cannot be procured easily."[256] Thus lead's history as an abortion drug lasted only about forty years. Among all the "new" drugs, it alone owed nothing to technology. Two other drugs, quinine and apiol,

---

* On the action of colloid lead aspartate, for example: "Following abortion the animals seem quite healthy."[250]

which had surfaced around 1880, now came to the fore, neatly illustrating how "medical progress" did redound to the advantage of women.

QUININE

The tale of quinine begins improbably in the mid-seventeenth century in South America with the discovery that the powdered bark of the cinchona tree reduced the fever of malaria sufferers. "Peruvian bark" or "Jesuit bark," as it was then called, won a wide reputation as an anti-fever drug among the wealthy, for only they could afford it.[257] It must have acquired some repute as a uterus-stimulating drug, too, for in 1814 we find one author recommending it for "menstrual anomalies."[258] Then in 1820 its main alkaloid, quinine, was identified, making possible the preparation of much more potent extracts. The real breakthrough, from the viewpoint of average people, came, however, in the 1870s when the first big shipments of quinine from plantations in Java—where it was being grown commercially to cash in on the huge demand—began arriving in Europe.[259] Just as it was becoming accessible, several scientific experiments suggested that quinine could initiate labor in animals, and certainly that it strengthened the tone of the uterine muscle.[260] Thus, by the 1870s quinine's obstetrical uses were becoming familiar.

Its reputation as a presumed abortifacient began to spread among the people as well. In an 1863 report on "such drugs as savin or turpentine to induce miscarriage . . . it was stated that an ague pill in use in North Witchford sometimes caused premature birth."[261] If I correctly read this elliptical text, North Witchford women were swallowing quinine for abortion. There are a few other late nineteenth century references, such as Doctor von Oefele's observation in 1897 that "quinine is widely used for abortion."[262] In 1913 a midwife ("Miss Martin") testified to the National Birth-Rate Commission that women near Birmingham took, in addition to diachylon, "quinine crystals to a very great extent; that is the present fashion."[263]

But the great take-off in quinine for abortion seems to have occurred only after the First World War, coinciding perhaps with the eclipse of lead. "It has become common especially since the Great War," wrote one pathologist in 1935.[264] Of thirty women admitted to hospital in Oslo in the 1920s for drug abortion, "most" had taken quinine.[265] Similarly, of sixty-nine drug-induced abortions treated at a Minneapolis hospital from 1930 to 1933, thirty-two had been done with quinine.[266] Working-class women in England of the 1930s commonly obtained fifty "silver-coated quinine pills" at 7s. 6d.[267] And so in 1939, a committee investigating abortion in England was able to call quinine, along with apiol and pennyroyal, a "specially favored" abortifacient.[268]

Because of the ease with which one could poison oneself, the question arose whether quinine was a genuine drug for abortion at all, or whether it merely poisoned the mother, killing the fetus in the bargain. Much comment was aroused when in 1901 an Italian doctor with quinine treated some railway laborers near Civita Vecchia for malaria; of forty-nine pregnant women among them, forty-seven failed to abort.[269] Doctors since then had observed that patients who poisoned themselves with large quinine doses would often not abort.[270] This seems to be another of those curious medical misunderstandings that have contributed to the oblivion of the abortion drugs: small doses of quinine evidently act effectively on the uterus; large doses paralyze it. Thus M. Canale, an Italian pathologist, said in 1969: "Quinine in small doses excites uterine contractions; in high ones it exercises a contrary effect."[271]*

APIOL

The third new drug for abortion was apiol, a substance found in oil of parsley. So I must pause for a moment of background. Kitchen parsley has an abortifacient tradition going back to the ancient Greeks. In the Hippocratic corpus it is recommended as a tea or tampon for abortion and for reestablishing the menses. Dioscorides mentioned it as well.[274] French peasants in Languedoc used parsley for abortion.[275] And the Germans had a saying, "Parsley helps the man onto his horse, the woman under the ground"—a reference to its supposed aphrodisiac qualities in men, its abortifacient uses in women.[276] Schoolchildren in Bremen once sang:

> Parsley, parsley, good for soup,
> Grows in mama's garden.
> Annie's gonna' be a bride.
> Better not wait much longer,
> If she wants to go to church
> Without her belly in the lurch.†

* Louis Lewin said that researchers are divided about the effect of small doses of quinine on the uterus.[272] According to one standard source, "It is now generally accepted that quinine definitely increases uterine contractions of a rhythmic character, raises the tone of the muscle, and that it may induce uterine contractions."[273]
† The *Plattdeutsch* original is more colorful than my translation:

> *Petersiljen, Soppenkruut*
> *Wasst in usem Garen,*
> *Use Antjen de is Bruut,*
> *Schall nig lang meer waren,*
> *Dat se na der Karken geit*
> *Un den Rock in Folen sleit.*[277]

Adam Lonitzer's sixteenth-century herbal mentions parsley as an emmenagogue, as does Bock's.[278] So women have long known that parsley had its female uses.

Yet if parsley did not have the same reputation for abortion as did ergot and savin, it was because nobody had yet figured out how to extract its essential ingredients. A Leipzig apothecary named Heinrich Christoph Link first discovered "parsley camphor" in 1715, observing a crystalline substance in a batch of steam-distilled parsley oil.[279]* But nobody knew what to make of this until in 1847 a couple of Parisian doctors named Joret and Homolle succeeded in cutting the malarial fever of a Breton nobleman with a decoction of parsley seeds they had boiled up. Two years later, the Paris Society of Pharmacy launched a prize contest for the best drug to replace quinine (which had become very expensive) in treating malaria. These doctors, who had continued their experiments in the meantime, submitted a formula. It involved treating parsley seeds with alcohol or ether in order to extract an oily substance they named "apiol." They started giving feverish patients the new drug. It turned out to be completely valueless against malaria, but they noticed that some of the female patients who had suffered from "amenorrhea" started getting their periods again. Thus, in 1855 Joret and Homolle announced they had discovered a powerful new "emmenagogue."[281]

Between 1860 and 1900 apiol became widely prescribed for menstrual irregularity. How it might have re-established menstruation if the woman was not pregnant is entirely unclear. But if she were pregnant, apiol apparently "re-established her regularity" by giving her an abortion. Dr. Thomas Sanctuary of Salisbury reported in the *Lancet* in 1885 that among twelve women who had missed their periods, apiol restored the "catamenia" within a week.[282] The American Roberts Bartholow exulted that, "The evidence is conclusive that apiol has decided emmenagogue power. It is a stimulant to the uterine system, and therefore . . . should not be administered [for malaria] to pregnant women."[283]

Not until around 1900, however, did apiol begin to establish itself among lay people as a drug for abortion. One Mr. Martin, "chemist, Southampton," started advertising "Apiol and Steel Pills for Ladies," the assumption being that iron was an abortifacient as well. And "Mrs. Lawrence's

* A. Fr. Walther noted the camphor in 1745, as did Carl Stange again in 1823.[280] It is to Stange that credit for the original discovery of the camphor is often incorrectly attributed. For clarity, it should be noted that *two* phenolic ethers in parsley, which are chemically very similar, myristicin and apiol, supply the active principles. Their presence varies from one region to another; German parsley, for example, is so rich in apiol that crystals of parsley camphor form at room temperature. French parsley, on the other hand, seems to contain mainly myristicin. Myristicin is also found in nutmeg, a plant that is not discussed in this book but has a long abortifacient history.

Mixture" for women who had "obstructions" turned out on analysis to contain some "yellowish green substance closely resembling apiol."[284] In 1910, Dolores G., a concierge in Oran, took thirty capsules of apiol upon finding herself pregnant. Her pregnancy continued, but she had a bad bout of poisoning from which she recovered.[285] The incident is noteworthy only as one of the few references to apiol for abortion before the First World War.

In these prewar years apiol was in all the pharmacies, sold "over the counter." The U.S. *Dispensatory* had listed it since 1868 at least.[286] The Belgian pharmacopoeia incorporated apiol in 1885.[287] In that same year William Martindale's *Extra Pharmacopoeia*, a popular English dispensing guide, listed it for malaria and "amenorrhea."[288] Apiol must have been widely sold in France by the beginning of the 1880s because complaints about adulteration were already occurring.[289] By 1913, the pharmacopoeias of Denmark and Norway were listing the drug; those of Portugal and Mexico were even giving instructions for its manufacture.[290]* A listing in these dispensing guides does not necessarily mean that bucketfuls were being sold, since their function was merely to familiarize pharmacists with the composition of various products and to establish standards of purity. Yet a link must have been forging itself in women's minds between "missing periods" and "apiol," even though doctors were supposed to be careful not to prescribe it for abortion.

Some fairly substantial drug companies were becoming involved, too, the Schimmel firm in Germany producing capsules of the crystalline apiol (parsley camphor) from around 1884.[292] The Merck Company listed all three kinds of apiol—the green oily fluid, the distilled volatile oil, and the crystalline camphor—in the first American edition of its *Merck's Index* in 1889.[293] And the Parke Davis Company of Detroit marketed apiol at least as early as 1903.[294] In the old drug indexes one encounters such "proprietary preparations" as "Apileol," made by the E. Fraquet Laboratories, 9 avenue de Villiers, Paris.[295] So somebody was taking it.

The real boom in apiol for abortion did not occur, however, until after the First World War and, above all, in Italy, France, and Central Europe. Dr. J. R. Spinner of Zurich warned in 1920 that "apiol is in the process of becoming a systematically marketed abortive, freely sold in the drugstores."[296] One German scholar argued that it was the French troops' occupation of the Rhineland in the early 1920s that "introduced apiol from the West."[297] In 1927, Dresden's Office of Chemical Analysis found apiol in many of the city's drugstores, "with veiled instructions for abortion."[298] And Halle's Professor Kochmann assured readers of the *Archiv für Toxikologie* in 1931 that apiol was used for abortion "especially

* Apiol first appeared in the French pharmaceutical *Codex* in 1908.[291]

in France, yet recently also in Germany."[299] By 1937 apiol had become, according to a Frankfurt apothecary, "by far the most often asked for . . . abortive known to the laity,"[300] despite having been made available only by prescription in 1932.

But putting it on the prescription list did not put it out of reach in Germany. One druggist kept his supply in the cellar, selling it under the counter in 1933 to four different women: two of them aborted, one didn't, and one wasn't pregnant.[301] Frau W., in her eighth month of pregnancy, got some apiol capsules in 1926 from her fiancé, who in turn had got them from a friend, who had got them from a dirty bookstore in Leipzig, which had got them from a company in Dresden, which in turn had got them from another company in Berlin that made gelatin capsules, which company had bought the actual apiol from a pharmaceutical factory in "N."[302]*

One French pharmaceutical company was by 1933 selling "several million capsules" of apiol a year all over the world.[303] Or in a city like Lille a druggist might put up his own capsules, labeling them "Three times daily for amenorrhea." When a client then appeared, he would tell her to take twelve.[304] A Marseille doctor said in 1934 that apiol had been "used as an abortive for the last ten years."[305] "We know how commonly apiol is used for abortion" wrote three Paris doctors in 1931. "Considered nontoxic by the former pharmacopoeia, this medication is sold over the counter, and there are few women who, suspecting pregnancy, do not swallow a more or less large quantity of apiol."[306]† Other Parisian doctors noted in 1941 how rare apiol poisoning was. Yet, "Everybody knows the importance which abortionists attach to this drug to provoke the reappearance of the menses."[307]

In Italy, too, apiol attained wide use after the First World War. One Roman obstetrician called it in 1928, "a product much used for the procurement of abortion. I believe it not exaggerated to say that more than half of the criminal abortions are perpetrated with this means."[308] "There are notorious pharmacies in which the sale of apiol takes place," said someone else of Rome.[309] Thus, apiol augmented a long Italian peasant tradition of abortion by decoction of parsley.

The lack of references to apiol in the literature for North America in the 1920s and 1930s could be deceiving, a sign more of the drug's lack of toxicity than of its lack of use. For in the late 1970s I placed a notice in the professional bulletin of the pharmacists of Ontario, asking to hear from those who remembered dispensing apiol in the 1930s. Many did.

---

* Note that over-the-counter sales were legal at this point.

† Apiol was dropped from the *Codex* in 1920, yet remained legal for sale. It returned to the *Codex* in 1927, to be definitively withdrawn in the 1949 edition.

In vogue in those years was "Ergoapiol," a mixture of apiol, ergot, oil of savin, and castor oil, and manufactured by the Martin H. Smith Company of New York City. "Apergol" was another apiol-based drug, distributed by the H. K. Wampole firm of Perth, Ontario. Said one man who had apprenticed in St. Thomas, Ontario, in the 1940s, "Ergoapiol was kept in a tin box for female problems. Never on display, always in a drawer. The druggist wanted to make sure it was for legitimate uses."

Oh? Which uses were those?

"Amenorrhea mainly. Ergoapiol was thought in the profession to be highly effective. The sales volume was pretty small. But Apergol, you bought it from the wholesaler by the dozen boxes. It was a pretty good seller."

Said another pharmacist who had apprenticed in London, Ontario, in the late 1920s: "I was in the——— organization. They were sales oriented. They routinely stocked apiol. We had a farm-oriented business."

The clients? "All classes. Often the man came in, for his girlfriend. If we knew them, we'd dispense it."

Another pharmacist who had apprenticed in Mt. Dennis, Ontario, responded, "If they were late in their period, they'd come in and ask 'What've you got?' We never sold ergot, by honor. But on demand we did sell Ergoapiol. We knew what they were after. But we had such low grosses that we needed the sale."

Considerable other testimony could be added to these quotes. And there is no reason to think that the United States was much different from Canada. Apiol was, after all, listed in all the drug catalogues in those years.[310]*

It is clear that apiol did produce abortions in pregnant women. But was it safe? Lead, after all, is an effective abortive but has awful side effects. My main concern in this discussion is whether technical advances had opened up to women by 1930 the prospect of abortion with *reasonable safety*. †

The question of reasonable safety ultimately did apiol in, because in the 1950s it was withdrawn from the pharmacopoeias and made a prescription drug in Britain and North America on the grounds that it was both useless and toxic. But was it either?

A now-forgotten undercurrent of medical literature maintained in the

---

* The *American Drug Index* and *Physicians Desk Reference* both listed apiol-based preparations in the 1950s and the 1960s. *PDR* was still recommending apiol as an emmenagogue in 1971![311]

† It must be emphasized that, by the standards of today's medicine, apiol has not been established as safe for abortion. This discussion is in no way to be taken as a recommendation for its use.

1930s and 1940s that apiol did, in fact, produce abortion without grave side effects. First of all, we have a number of cases in which women took apiol and aborted shortly thereafter, without serious consequences to their health. A Fribourg doctor had observed in his practice thirteen patients who aborted after taking apiol with only slight side effects. "Case 2. A thirty-eight-year-old took one package [*eine Originalpackung*] all at once. Prompt results. Only slight back pains. Expulsion of two-month old fetus two days later. No aftereffects." In three additional patients the side effects were considerable. Four other women failed to abort, though bleeding occurred in two of them.[312]* According to one specialist, eighteen documented cases of abortion without side effects were to be found by 1933 in the medical literature. He concluded that, in most cases, "Any side effects in both small and large doses were entirely absent. . . . In the last analysis the nontoxic nature of the drug is confirmed by the great number of experiences that every pharmacist has had. . . . We may thus understand the extraordinary popularity and diffusion which apiol has attained in France, Yugoslavia, and recently also in Germany."[313]

Second, the number of fatal poisonings from apiol is quite small, in view of its availability for decades and its apparent wide use by millions of women. By my count, thirteen documented deaths from apiol are on record, not counting the many "parsley decoction" deaths in Italy.[314]† Other women probably died from apiol overdoses and were wrongly diagnosed as victims of "sepsis" (because the kidney and liver damage accompanying apiol poisoning closely resembles some kinds of bacteremia). Yet in view of the many deaths from such other popular abortives as savin or phosphorus, thirteen recorded apiol deaths is few. Far more apiol users would have died in childbirth, had they completed their pregnancies.

Third, I am impressed by the number of doctors, respected figures in their time, who considered apiol nontoxic. Apropos cases of bloody urine which evidently were caused by another component of parsley called

* The doctor's intention was to warn public prosecutors of the possibility of apiol involvement in apparently spontaneous abortions, rather than to recommend its use.

† I include an apparent Ergoapiol death in 1938 in Ann Arbor, Michigan, even though it is possible the ingested substance was contaminated with "Triorthocresyl phosphate" (phosphate of creosote). At autopsy "a phosphate radical was found."[315] Excluded from this list of apiol deaths are fatalities associated with "parsley decoctions" among Italian peasants, who typically would boil a vat of parsley stems and roots for hours on end, then drink the residue for abortion. Relatively little apiol would remain after such a procedure, and the toxicity may have been associated with other plant components.[316]

In a personal communication to me, Dr. V. Mele expressed the view that the chemical composition of parsley cultivated about the Mediterranean is different from North European parsley. It would therefore, he argued, have a different toxicological effect. The reader will see that the entire question of apiol's toxicity in abortive doses awaits clarification.

"apiin," J. Chevalier wrote in 1909, "Pure apiol never produces similar phenomena and it may be used without side effects" at given doses for a number of days in a row.[317] After dismissing a number of other "female pills" as innocuous, Georg Strassmann turned his attention to "Salutol" apiol capsules: "The manufacturer admits that large doses can cause nausea. If around twenty tablets are taken at once, diarrhea and vomiting may result and presumably the contraction of the uterus as well, so that these apiol capsules represent a not entirely inefficacious drug for abortion if taken in large quantities."[318] In describing an "epidemic" of "phosphate of creosote" poisoning in the early 1930s, Amsterdam neurologist J. W. G. ter Braak remarked, "What is known is that the poison resembled in many respects the well-known abortive drug 'apiol.'. . . . Until now toxic symptoms resembling polyneuritis have never been observed in connection with apiol, either in commercial preparations or in the pure form, despite its highly frequent use."[319] The authors of a forensic medicine textbook concluded in 1940 of apiol, "In many cases abortion occurs without the mother exhibiting grave toxic symptoms. First there is uterine bleeding, followed by the expulsion of the fetus. . . . Recently numerous cases have been reported in which apiol quickly produces the desired results, especially if taken when the missing period should normally occur. . . . Despite high doses, the maternal health undergoes no serious impairment."[320] And a well-known toxicology text in current use says, "Parsley oil acts on the kidneys and the uterus, an effect which may be ascribed to apiol. . . . Pure apiol produces abortion in humans usually one or two days after internal consumption without important side effects."[321*] Thus, a number of authorities did admit (though some with disapproval) apiol's usefulness as a nontoxic drug for abortion.

How does parsley oil produce abortion? The question is unclarified to this day because research on such matters has long since ceased. It would be tedious to drag the general reader into this netherworld of pharmacology. Yet one point might be made. As with quinine, smaller doses seemed more effective for abortion than did large ones. Francesco D'Aprile, for example, found that in nine definite cases of apiol poisoning in Italy in the 1920s, the six women who had taken massive doses either died or failed to abort; the three who had taken small doses aborted and survived with relatively minor symptoms.[322] After experiments on the "isolated" uteri of guinea pigs and rabbits, Rodolfo Marri, a pharmacologist at the University of Florence, concluded in 1939 that small doses increased the tone and strength of contractions, while large doses had a

---

* Otto Gessner said that "myristicin" may also be responsible for parsley's abortive action.

depressing action on the uterus.[323] Hence the tragic paradox of women who overdosed without even achieving an abortion.*

Final question: If apiol is effective, why did it disappear? Why aren't women today resorting to it instead of having to appear before some hospital's abortion committee, claiming they'll kill themselves if they have to complete the pregnancy? There is no doubt that after the Second World War apiol went off the boards. The 1949 edition of the *British Pharmaceutical Codex* announced that it was being deleted.[325] The last edition of the *Dispensatory of the United States* to mention apiol was published in 1955.[326] The drug vanished from German pharmaceutical guides in the 1970s.† The Ontario pharmacists mentioned above recalled having sold their last Apergol or Ergoapiol in the late 1930s or early 1940s. It is not that the drug was banned for over-the-counter sale at that point, except in Germany.‡ Women simply stopped asking for it.

There are three possible explanations for its disappearance, each having some merit, and each casting some insight into women's vastly changed relationship to the medical profession.

1. A "doctor's plot" against apiol. Given the medical profession's hostility to abortion, did doctors downplay apiol for moral reasons? A bit of evidence supports this view. Dresden's Dr. H. Jagdhold, for example, was among apiol's defenders. When in 1932 the Munich *Medical Weekly* published some other doctor's erroneous statement that "apiol produces abortion only with highly toxic side effects," Jagdhold in a letter drew attention to the extensive medical literature demonstrating the contrary. The *Medical Weekly's* editorial board refused to publish his letter.[328]

It is furthermore interesting that the fiercely anti-abortionist Louis Lewin, who in his textbook on abortion drugs devoted twelve pages to phosphorus, made only a one-line reference to apiol: "In France apiol is used . . ."—along with fourteen other drugs he mentioned in the same sentence.[329] He surely knew how popular apiol had become by the time he wrote those lines in 1922. Did he want to downplay it?

If Britain's doctors were in conspiracy to deny women access to abortion drugs, the Pharmaceutical Society did not want to go along with them.

---

* The apparent paradox of little being more effective than lots may be explained as a result of the inability of placental enzymes to metabolize large doses of apiol. Instead, the liver is directly overwhelmed, without the complex interactions between enzymes and prostaglandins which would otherwise have occurred—and which might well cause the necrosis of placental tissue and thus abortion. This possible mechanism was suggested to me by Dr. Alan Seawright, Department of Veterinary Pathology of the University of Queensland.[324]

† It had vanished from *Die Rote Liste* by 1979, from *Hagers Handbuch* by 1972.

‡ Among the few restrictions of which I am aware on the sale of apiol was Canada's 1959 decree that "oil of apiol" be placed in prescription-only status. Crystal apiol, or "parsley camphor," would not have been affected by this decision.[327]

Faced with demands that some of these drugs be put on the Poisons List (and thus be made prescription-only), the *Pharmaceutical Journal* said in 1939, "The Poisons List has other uses than to serve as an ethical wastepaper basket. . . . It once more behoves pharmacy to be on its guard that any well-meaning but needless or impractical restrictions do not add one more straw to the load which the pharmacist must bear for the benefit of others than himself."[330] So if there was a conspiracy, the pharmacists were not involved.

The decision to suppress apiol from various pharmacopoeias seems to have been taken, not because apiol was an abortifacient, but because it was deemed medically useless. G. R. Brown, the secretary of the revision committee of the *British Pharmaceutical Codex*, said in 1979 that it had been necessary to "make room to describe the new synthetic drugs that were being developed at that time [1949]. There was therefore no special significance in the deletion of the monograph on apiol."[331] And Arthur Osol, chairman of the U.S. *Dispensatory*'s editorial board, said, "Since other drugs of more certain utility and less danger became available, use of the apiols diminished to a point where there was little, if any, market for them. It was because of the lack of interest in these preparations that they were eventually deleted."[332] Excising mention of apiol in druggists' guides did not, in any event, constitute banning it. It merely made pharmacists less familiar with the drug and less likely to stock it. In sum, I have seen little evidence of a transatlantic medical effort to suppress apiol in order to deny women abortions.

2. The "comedy of errors" explanation. Apiol acquired a reputation for toxicity among doctors after unscrupulous manufacturers began diluting it in 1931 with "phosphate of creosote" (triorthocresyl phosphate), which is highly poisonous. An epidemic of "peripheral polyneuritis" occurred among apiol users, similar to the outbreak of "ginger paralysis" around the same time in the United States, when manufacturers began adulterating the "extract of ginger" favored by alcoholics (in those days of Prohibition) with phosphate of creosote.[333] A number of writers began, however, to believe that this adulterant was a natural component of parsley. Thus, the *American Journal of Obstetrics* published in 1934 a note to the effect that apiol contained phosphate of creosote.[334] Frederick Taussig, in his influential book *Abortion* (1936), said that apiol should be warned against," since it contains a poison that in large doses produces nerve paralysis."[335] Thus did the myth become perpetuated.

In fact, it is astonishing how incomplete and unreliable was the discussion of apiol in reputable medical and pharmaceutical journals. Before 1934, for example, the *British Pharmaceutical Codex* confused two different kinds of apiol and proposed a chemical test for purity which turned out to be inapplicable in practice.[336] The 1947 edition of the U.S. *Dispensatory* contained no references to any research later than 1912 and ignored numerous French and Italian reports in the 1920s and 1930s about apiol's physiological effects on the uterus.[337] In 1913 the American Medical Association denounced all the volatile oils, apiol included, as general poisons with no specific effect on the uterus.[338] Thus, ten years later the A.M.A.'s Council on Pharmacy recommended the deletion of apiol from the officially sanctioned drug list *New and Nonofficial Remedies*, on the grounds that apiol and the other volatiles "inhibited the contractions of the uterus."[339] This erroneous statement was never subsequently challenged, and apiol started to be considered "useless." Wrote Torald Sollmann, the distinguished pharmacologist, in 1942, "The Apiols are administered in capsules, as emmenagogue and antipyretic. Their usefulness is doubtful."[340] I dwell at length upon this chain of misunderstandings in American medicine only because it caused the doctors, many of whom were sympathetic to their patients' desires to terminate unwanted pregnancies, to forget about apiol. It is interesting that Dr. Osol, in his letter to me explaining why apiol was dropped from the U.S. *Dispensatory*, appended a Xerox copy of the pages on apiol in the 1942 edition of Sollmann's book.

3. The major explanation, however, of the desuetude not only of apiol but of all these abortive drugs is women's own turning away from them. It is a theme of this book that a major discontinuity in "women's culture" takes place in the first half of the twentieth century, when much of the traditional body of knowledge that women had passed by word of mouth for generations stopped being transmitted. "Why did the demand for 'Ergoapiol' drop off in the early 1940s?" I asked one elderly pharmacist from a small town in Ontario. "My contemporaries knew all about it," he said, "but younger women didn't. Their mothers didn't tell them."

Ah, their mothers didn't tell them. The mothers of that whole generation of women who grew up after the Second World War did not pass on this information. And therewith it died out. The decline of abortive drugs is part of the general "medicalization" of women's health I cover in this study. For better or worse, women in the 1930s started placing responsibility for their medical fate in the hands of doctors and abandoning self-help. Able to get instrumental abortions from doctors and paramedical abortionists with relative ease (compared with one hundred years previously), women stopped using drugs. Substances like apiol had always seemed risky and uncertain. For abortion, it made much more sense to rely on the professionals. And, indeed, who can blame women for this judgment?

Let me conclude this chapter on a personal note. On the trail of apiol,

I recently asked one of the world's few remaining manufacturers of it where his markets lay.

"Here in———?" I asked, mentioning his home country.

"Oh, no," he laughed. "Women here would never touch the stuff. They get abortions in hospital. We export it to the Middle East."

It is ironical that drug abortion, once in the vanguard of women's liberation in Western society, has now passed to the Third World.

PART THREE

OTHER PHYSICAL DIFFERENCES BETWEEN MEN AND WOMEN

CHAPTER 9

Did Women Live Longer Than Men? If Not, Why Not?

IT IS WIDELY BELIEVED that women in the past outlived men. Because female life expectancy since the beginning of the twentieth century has usually been about five years longer than male life expectancy, scholars have been tempted to see in this some kind of "natural" female biological advantage.* Thus Ashley Montagu, "Life expectancy at birth is higher for women than for men all over the world . . . and this fact holds true for females as compared with males for the greater part of the animal kingdom. . . . These facts constitute further evidence that the female is constitutionally stronger than the male."[2] I cannot comment on the animal kingdom. And Montagu is correct about advanced societies in the twentieth century (though in poorer parts of the world women do not live longer[3]). But in the world we have ourselves lost—Europe, Britain, and the United States before 1900—Montagu's observation is misleading: adult women did not necessarily live longer than men.

---

*From 1900 to 1902 the life expectancy of white American women at birth was 51.1 years; of men, 48.2. In 1978 it was 77.8 for women, 70.2 for men.[1]

At What Ages Were Women More Vulnerable?

A couple of basic points about gender differences in mortality in the past:

· Male infants have always died more often than female, in nineteenth-century Europe perhaps 20 percent more frequently. For example, in Sardinia, from 1827 to 1838, 118 male babies perished in the first year for every 100 female; in Schleswig-Holstein, 128 for every 100.[4] In Europe as a whole the stillbirth rate was about 40 percent higher for males than for females.[5] Other studies have shown that male fetuses perish more often in utero than do female fetuses.*

· Older men have always been more vulnerable than older women. Excess male mortality starts around the age of forty or forty-five and continues thereafter. In England at mid-nineteenth century women outlived men by 4 percent at age forty, by 13 percent at age fifty, and by 10 percent at age sixty.

Thus, it was the advantages women had both at birth and after middle age that gave them in the past an *overall* longer life expectancy. If measured from birth, average life expectancy before 1900 for both sexes was generally about thirty-five to forty years, with women living perhaps three years longer than men.[7]

But in this book I am interested in the perceived experience of adult women, who were the bearers of the village "women's culture," women who married, had children and directed family life. Thus our "target population" is not the nine-month-old baby girl or the sixty-two-year-old grandmother. It is the twenty-seven-year-old housewife with three children. What were *her* chances of outliving her husband? That is the most meaningful question to be posed to the statistics. And the answer is, they were not very good.

Two further general observations about the world before 1900:

· Girls between the ages of five and twenty had a significantly higher mortality than boys.
· Married women in their thirties stood perhaps a 25 percent greater risk of dying than their husbands.†

These disadvanatages were usually not enough to compensate for the great female advantages at birth and at midlife, and in the past female life expectancy on the whole ended up slightly higher than male. But if we ask, What were the chances that a nine-year-old girl would die

---

*In a study of United States' vital statistics from 1922 to 1972, Marilyn M. McMillen finds a primary sex ratio in fetal deaths of around 120 males for every 100 females.[6]

† The actual percent varied: "25 percent" is from Norway, from 1871 to 1880, where at ages thirty to thirty-four, 69 married men died per 10,000 males; 85 married women, per 10,000. Thus, female mortality at that age was 23.2 percent higher than male.[8]

before her male playmates, or a woman of thirty-eight before her husband, the "natural biological advantage" that women are thought to have disappears.

In the very distant past adult men outlived women at almost all ages. In seven out of eight series for prehistoric populations between the Neolithic and the Early Iron ages, males had a higher expected age of death. In the Neanderthal series, for example, men at age twenty had an estimated life expectancy 40 percent longer than that of women. (Statistics on child deaths were not available.)[9] G. Acsádi and J. Nemeskéri, who have recently summarized this research, conclude that in prehistoric times "expectation of life for males was longer by about 20 percent."*

A whole series of village studies, done by historical demographers, demonstrates an excess female mortality, sometimes during a woman's fertile years alone, sometimes across her entire life. For example, Keith Wrightson and David Levine, in a study of the English village of Terling from 1550–1724, found that at age twenty-five, the average man would live 6.6 years longer than the average woman. Even at age fifty-five he would still outlive her by 1.7 years.[11] In eighteenth-century Mittelberg, peasant husbands would outlive their wives by six years on the average; between 1840 and 1849, by 12 years! Only women married in Mittelberg after 1890 would finally start surviving their husbands.[12] The statistics in other places are not so extreme, yet most point to a substantial male advantage.[13]†

By the middle of the nineteenth century we have the reliable statistics assembled by national record offices. They show the pattern of women dying more often than men at *younger* ages and outliving men at older ages. In 1850, for example, American men outlived women from ages ten to thirty-five.[15] In the Duchy of Oldenburg, between 1831 and 1850, females had an 8 percent greater probability than males of dying between the ages of five and twenty, a 25 percent greater probability at ages between thirty and forty.[16] Then after forty in Oldenburg women would live longer. In Prussia and Schleswig-Holstein at mid-century young girls and married women in their prime were all more at risk than males of comparable ages.[17] In Norway and Belgium at mid-century it was mainly adolescent girls whose mortality rates were significantly higher than boys'.[18]

Only in the last quarter of the nineteenth century did females begin to outlive males at all ages (table 9.1). If an identical death rate for men and women is considered 100, numbers in table 9.1 greater than 100 mean excess male mortality, less than 100 excess female mortality. Note that only in 1896–1900, for example, does the excess mortality of

---

* These authors also demonstrate a surplus female mortality for the Roman era and for medieval Hungary.[10]

† Only the Swedish data, in the series of which I am aware, show higher female life expectancy at all ages during the "traditional" period.[14]

TABLE 9.1

Male Death Rates as a Percentage
of Female Death Rates, According
to Age (England, France, and Italy,
in the Nineteenth Century)

Age	Percentage
France (1850–52)	
1– 4	103
5–14	92 (overcome* in 1925–27)
15–24	100
25–34	96 (overcome in 1880–82)
35–44	96 (overcome in 1865–67)
45–54	113
55–64	109
England and Wales (1851–55)	
0	122
1	102
5	102
10	96 (overcome in 1866–70)
15	97 (overcome in 1896–1900)
20	98 (overcome in 1861–65)
25	98 (overcome in 1861–65)
30	98 (overcome in 1856–60)
35	100
40	105
45	113
50	115
55	112
60	111
Italy (1901–11)	
0	110
10	79 (overcome by 1950–53)
20	95 (overcome by 1921–22)
30	88 (overcome by 1950–53)
40	100
50	125
60	114
70	101

NOTE: Over 100 = females live longer; less
than 100 = males live longer.
  * Year after which male mortality higher
than female (i.e., greater than 100).
SOURCES: See notes to tables, page 384.

English girls in their late teens dissolve. The surplus of deaths among
French girls ages five to fourteen ceases only in 1925. And the greater
mortality of Italian women in their thirties comes to an end only in
the 1950s.

All these nineteenth-century females had, at birth, a longer life expectancy than men. But in view of women's higher death rates than men at many particular ages, it is difficult to see any natural biological advantage working in their favor. Of course, one could argue that at age thirty women were exposed to exceptional risks as a result of childbearing or whatever, and that these excessive hazards momentarily neutralized their natural genetic protection. But, similarly, one could argue that males at birth were exposed to exceptional hazards, as a result of having larger heads, or that at age sixty they were exceptionally at risk as a result of having spent lives at grinding field labor. In sum, the record of the past suggests that neither sex had any kind of inborn, genetic protection against the vicissitudes of fate. Mortality differences at any age were probably a result of the particular hazards that men or women faced at that age.

Diseases Especially Affecting Women

The diseases discussed in this chapter, which affected women in vulnerable age groups, are not "women's diseases" but ailments that more often claimed the lives of women than of men. By far the best cause-of-death statistics for the nineteenth century come from England. So let me try first to pin things down for that country.[19]

The higher death rates for girls are, at first glance, no big mystery. In the middle of the nineteenth century (1848–72) they died of infectious diseases. One quarter of deaths among girls of the ages of five to fourteen came from scarlet fever, a streptococcal infection of the blood. Fourteen percent of them died of typhus and typhoid fever (the two had not yet been differentiated). And slightly more than one in ten died of pulmonary tuberculosis. For each of these diseases girls had a higher death *rate* than boys and, thus, a special predilection for that particular disease.

For teen-age English girls the story is also clear: half of the deaths among fifteen to twenty-four-year-olds were from pulmonary tuberculosis; a further 11 percent, from typhus and typhoid fever. At this age, too, females are more disposed than males to die from these causes, having a 22 percent higher death rate from TB, for example.

For women in childbearing years, respiratory TB was again the number one killer, causing 40 percent of all deaths among twenty-five to forty-four-year-olds. Heart disease carried away a further 6 percent, and childbearing yet a further 6 percent. The special predisposition of women to TB continued—at least in England—into this age group. But death rates from heart disease for men in their thirties and forties were slightly higher than women's.

TABLE 9.2

*Male Death Rates as a Percent-
age of Female Death Rates for
Selected Diseases (England and
Wales, 1848–72)**

Ages 5–14	
Typhus-typhoid fever	54
Scarlet fever	96
Respiratory tuberculosis	69
Diseases of nervous system	83
Heart disease	88
Bronchitis	91
Ages 15–24	
Typhus-typhoid fever	96
Scarlet fever	91
Respiratory tuberculosis	83
Cancer	88
Heart disease	90
Diseases of digestive system	86
Ages 25–44	
Scarlet fever	82
Respiratory tuberculosis	96
Cancer	33
Diseases of digestive system	89

NOTE: Over 100 = males have higher mortality; less than 100 = females have higher mortality.

* When all causes of death are considered, females in England in this period had higher death rates than males only at 15 to 24 (97 male deaths per every 100 females'). The data in this table, however, suggest the particular diseases that may have been involved in those places where, at given ages, women did in fact die more often than men.

SOURCES: See notes to tables, page 384.

Thus at first inspection the picture is straightforward. When women lived less long than men, it was mainly because they got TB more often— and also were slightly more affected by the diseases of filth and insanitation.

There are, however, other diseases to which women in these vulnerable age groups were subject (table 9.2). Numerically they may not have carried the same weight as TB, but it is intriguing to note them anyway.

Young girls in England were, for instance, quite subject to heart disease, probably as a result of rheumatic fever (another streptococcal infection, like scarlet fever). At ages five to fourteen their death rates were 13 percent higher than boys'; at ages fifteen to twenty-four, the same.

In teen-age years the enormous excess female mortality from cancer begins to appear (see page 242 ff.). And females aged fifteen to forty-four died considerably more often than males of afflictions of the digestive system.

The digestive system? Each of these findings is more surprising than the last, for today males perish more often than females from all of the previously mentioned diseases; although some, like scarlet fever, have virtually ceased to be fatal.* It is impossible to understand women's greater vulnerability in the early years of life—which flip-flops only toward age forty as men become more vulnerable—without looking more closely at some of these maladies.

TUBERCULOSIS

When the tubercle bacillus settles elsewhere in the body (scrofula), the disease has no particular gender pattern; but when it settles in the lungs (pulmonary tuberculosis), it has in the past been, for unclear reasons, a disease of girls and young women. Latvian male peasants in the pre-Christian era said, for example:

> I'd rather marry a fart-box
> Than take on a barker;
> A fart-box scampers 'cross the field,
> A barker lacks the stamina. [21]

A "barker" meant probably a young woman with tuberculosis, a brutal reference to her hacking cough. In 1842, Doctor Rame wrote of Lodève, "Pulmonary phthisis [tuberculosis] is the principal endemic malady raging among adolescents and adults. . . . It strikes more women than men, and among the former, especially young girls are the main victims. It afflicts above all those who live most secludedly, and whose life is divided between exercises of devotion and the duties that their calling imposes on them"—an apparent, though baffling, reference to young nuns.[22] The pallor and bloody cough of the tuberculosis victim certainly became a Victorian symbol for the martyrdom of delicate young women.[23]†

---

* English women in 1977 died slightly more often than men of digestive diseases, but this represents an exception to the international pattern.[20]

† England appears, however, exceptional in its excess of female TB deaths. Elsewhere any special female susceptibility to TB ceased with adolescence. In Danish towns, for example, males older than fifteen had from 1876 to 1885 a higher TB death rate than females. The same is true for Norway from 1871 to 1875 and for Stockholm from 1891 to 1900.[24] Men's sickness rates from TB in Leipzig, from 1887 to 1905, were 7 percent higher than women's at the ages of fifteen to thirty-four, 25 percent higher from thirty-five to fifty-four.[25] In Geneva during the 1730s men aged twenty to forty-four had a TB death rate of 7 per 10,000 population; women, only 5—a finding computed from Elizabeth Wicht-Candolfi's data on *phthisie*.[26]

HEART DISEASE

Historically, women of all ages seem to have been more afflicted with heart problems than have men. (England is an exception, where excess female heart deaths stopped at age twenty-four.) In Danish towns, between 1876 and 1885, there were 71 male heart deaths for every 100 female deaths at ages five to fifteen; 79 at ages twenty-five to forty-five.[27] Whereas 5.9 young men per 1,000 were off work in Leipzig because of heart problems, 7.0 younger women were; among the middle-aged there were almost twice as many women as men.[28] In the twentieth century, this female excess would reverse itself as rheumatic fever, the main cause of heart disease in women, became less virulent and less frequent.

"GASTROINTESTINAL" DISEASE

One fascinating finding is how many more women than men died from ailments of the gut tube and the abdominal organs (in reality a diverse group of diseases, but early "nosologists" lumped them together on the basis of common symptoms). Consider table 9.3. A clear excess of female deaths (ratios lower than 100) appears for late adolescence in England and Denmark, and for women in their fertile years in England, Denmark, and Norway. Women's death rate from "intestinal" disorders was almost double that of men in Geneva during the 1730s.[29] Whereas 95 men died in Breslau, between 1687 and 1691, from "tumors and internal ulcers," 161 women did so.[30] The number of female deaths attributed to "peritonitis" in Berlin from 1877 to 1896 was in some years more than double that of males. In the age group thirty to thirty-five the disproportion was breathtaking: 1 male peritonitis death in 1883; 28 female.[31] Forty-seven percent more young female workers than male took time off because of "disorders of the digestive organs" in Leipzig at the end of the nineteenth century.[32] And whereas women represented only 40 percent of all admissions to the Mantes hospital around 1900, they had 56 percent of the appendectomies.[33]

What was going on? Why all this abdominal disorder for women? Several factors were involved:

· Much of this "peritonitis," "enteritis" and "appendicitis" was clearly infected abortion and the sequelae of childbed fever. This point has been made in previous chapters. The reader is reminded that many maternal deaths were concealed under other diagnoses—a fact that helps account for women's excess mortality in the fertile years. There is simply no other explanation, for example, for the wild disproportion between the sexes in peritonitis in Berlin. Yet seventeen-year-old deaths from gastroenteritis were probably not obstetrical in nature, so something more must be involved.

TABLE 9.3
Male Death Rates as a Percentage of Female Death Rates for Gastrointestinal Disease (England, Denmark, and Norway, in the Nineteenth Century)

Age	Percentage
England and Wales (1848–72)	
1–4	101
5–14	104
15–24	86
25–44	89
45–64	102
+65	107
Denmark, towns (1876–85)	
5–15	80
15–25	81
25–45	70
45–65	91
+65	122
Norway (1899–1902)	
15–19	78
20–29	108
30–39	86
40–49	107
50–59	120

NOTE: Over 100 = males have higher mortality; less than 100 = females have higher mortality.
SOURCES: See notes to tables, page 384.

· Some digestive disorders genuinely are more frequent in women. In the United States in the 1930s women had six times more gallbladder disease than men, for reasons that are still uncertain. (Today gallstones are found in three times more women than men.[34*]) We have, from this historical evidence, no way of determining the exact nature of the affliction, and I note only that women probably *were* sabotaged by their gut tubes more often than were men.

· Young women once were particularly victimized by peptic ulcers (from the stomach's digestive acid) and died considerably more often from perforations of these ulcers than did men. One nineteenth-century British surgeon saw six times more perforations in women in their twenties than in men.[36] After the First World War this pattern was to reverse

* According to Leslie Schoenfield, gallstones are found at autopsy today in 20 percent of women and 8 percent of men.[35]

itself, as perforations tended to become a disease of middle-aged men.[37] Perforated ulcers, for our purpose, are extremely interesting as the diagnosis is usually simple to establish: "sudden agonizing pain, boardlike rigidity of the abdominal wall, and in most cases collapse and death within twenty-four to forty-eight hours."[38] Thus the observation that these ulcers tended to afflict primarily young women is probably true.

· Women in their fertile years were considerably more subject to fatal pelvic infections than were men. In a later chapter I discuss this in detail but note here that burst tubal abscesses—associated, for example, with gonorrhea—might easily have been misdiagnosed as colitis. According to Hermann Fehling, "acute pelveoperitonitis" was not even recognized before the nineteenth century.[39] Thus, when we encounter these mysterious excess female deaths from things like peritonitis—of which six female patients of the Edinburgh New Town Dispensary died in the 1820s, and only two men—the cause could well be ruptured abscesses of various kinds, gynecologic in origin.[40]

Or it could be anything. The point is not to establish retrospectively exact diagnoses, but to note how much more vulnerable were teen-age girls and fertile women than men to fatal diseases of their abdominal organs.

Note that "men's diseases" did exist. Men were especially subject to diabetes before the First World War, and had, for example, in Denmark a death rate 75 percent higher than women's.[41] (Today that pattern has practically reversed itself, as women die more often of diabetes than do men.[42*]) Men died then, as now, substantially more often from alcoholism: in Denmark in the 1880s, 53 male deaths annually per 100,000 population, 6 female. But, above all, men died more often from violence, accidents, and suicide. Thirty-seven men perished in Breslau from accidents in the late 1680s; 8 women. In Norway at the end of the last century, 133 young men but only 8 women per 100,000 died of "accidents and suicide."[44] In fact, if one deducts deaths from violence, females aged five to forty-four in England had a higher death rate on the whole than did men.[45] Most of those deaths were from infectious diseases. I harp on this subject because today in medicine the view is widespread that women have greater "biological" protection from infectious disease than do men (being more subject instead to "auto-immune disorders").[46] On the basis of the historical record, that view is simply incorrect. A natural female immunity to infection greater than the male's does not seem to exist.

---

* Women in the United States in 1977 also had a higher morbidity from diabetes, registering at all ages more office visits per 1,000 population than did men.[43]

The Sources of Women's Higher Death Rates

RURAL LIFE

Nothing in women's genetic makeup predisposed them to die more often at age thirty-three of tuberculosis or typhoid than men did. It was the harsh world in which they found themselves. Women were more liable than men to die at certain ages because their lives at those ages were much harder than men's, and their resistance to infection was lower. Two circumstances in particular emerge: the grinding routine of field work in rural areas, and the rigors of married life. Separating the two is difficult because most women before 1900 were likely both to live in the countryside and to be the mothers of families. Yet we have some aids.

Table 9.4 shows how much greater in rural areas was the tendency for women to die before men. In the Grand Duchy of Oldenburg, for example, rural women in their thirties had a 30-percent greater mortality than men; urban women only a 10-percent greater mortality. Whereas Danish men in their thirties had a 19-percent *lower* mortality than women in the countryside, men in the cities had a 13-percent *higher* mortality than urban women. At almost all ages when women were generally vulnerable, rural women were considerably more vulnerable than urban women to dying before their men died.

The thinness of the historical sources makes it difficult to play "Mirror, mirror on the wall, who had the worst health of all?" be it peasant or proletarian women. Each by modern standards had ghastly existences. Yet to set by every horror story from the Industrial Revolution there are similarly dismal tales from the lives of women in the countryside. Keep in mind, for example, how much *more* subject rural women were likely to have been to physical injury. Here is an entry from 1698 in the daybook of Dr. Frizzun, who practiced in a Swiss village: "On May 24 I began treating Frau Neisa because an ox had stepped on her hand. The hand was much swollen and had a large cut on the lateral margin which ached greatly. I treated her once daily until the 27th, and left behind medicine for four days."[47] There are many such entries in the journals of the old country doctors.

Peasant women were described as aging prematurely in terms I have rarely seen used for urban women. Thus Franz Mezler on the countryside around Sigmaringen: "The young girls are already wilting at an age when elsewhere one finds many fresh young beauties. Most of them devote themselves to farmwork and to the truly heavy tasks involved with it; the others are occupied with spinning, sewing, and knitting, rarely keeping

TABLE 9.4

Male Death Rates as a Percentage of Female Death Rates, Rural versus Urban (Oldenburg, Denmark, and Norway, in the Nineteenth Century)

Ages	Rural	Urban
	Oldenburg (1855–64)	
0–5	108	104
5–10	96	109
10–20	95	86
20–30	110	117
30–40	77	91
40–50	99	115
50–60	103	121
	Denmark (1840–44)	
20	111	143
30	81	113
40	90	163
50	124	169
	Norway (1899–1902)	
Deaths from tuberculosis		
15–19	78	89
20–29	122	140
30–39	83	98
Deaths from other diseases		
15–19	108	114
20–29	95	113
30–39	75	114

NOTE: Over 100 = males have higher mortality; less than 100 = females have higher mortality.
SOURCES: See notes to tables, pages 384–85.

their health and often losing their periods." From age ten on, Mezler continued, "women die increasingly more often than men, in the country-side especially because of misery, and lack of care when they are sick. It is not unusual to see women going about with skin infections [*Rothlauf*], open sores on their feet, hernias and prolapses which plague them unto the grave."[48] Dr. Goldschmidt wrote of another part of Germany, "The beauty and freshness of the young poor people is unfortunately rather short-lived; it usually lasts little beyond childhood. . . . Often I have mistaken a mother, showing me her child, for the grandmother."[49]

Do you have varicose veins?, Gertrud Dyhrenfurth asked peasant women around 1900 in a Silesian village. Ten out of seventeen said Yes.[50] Of the thirty-one women whom two midwives interviewed on behalf of another scholar in a Baden village, five were described as "worn out" [*verbraucht*]. Of those five, one had born seventeen children; one, thirteen children; and three, twelve children.[51] It is thus not surprising that when Dr. Mezler totted up the deaths in Sigmaringen between 1776 and 1804, he found that fifty women as opposed to twenty men had died of "hydrops" (fluid-filled abdomen); thirty-four men and forty-seven women were dead of chronic lung disease, mainly TB. He said, "We should also consider the many rheumatic and convulsive afflictions, the heart ailments, the stomach cramps and liver problems with which people around here drag themselves about for years."[52] Who knows what these diseases really were. But in Sigmaringen they struck after women who were ground down by years of hard work.

Chronic exhaustion appears again and again in descriptions of rural women's life. The peasant women whom one female anthropologist interviewed toward the First World War in Württemberg spoke of their weariness from *die Eile* ("being rushed"). "She is so rushed that the peasant wife scarcely makes it to the table. She is the last to sit down and often the first to get up again. During the dinner she hurries to and fro, bringing in new dishes. In addition she looks after feeding the small children."[53] Thus, these women's lives were jammed with fixing meals, trimming grape vines, and pitchforking manure. "It is laborious work," said Frau B. Walkmeister-Dambach in 1928, "to haul the fertilizer out to the fields and spread it. In most places this has to be done on steep slopes. Another hard job is turning over the soil, which is still done with spades. Later comes getting ready the seedling potatoes and planting them. Cultivating the potato field is left entirely to the woman, as is weeding the grain field, which the woman often does kneeling, for days on end."[54] Which job do you think is hardest?, Dyhrenfurth asked the Silesian women (actually paid agricultural laborers). One said "Threshing with the flail and spreading manure." Another replied, "Digging ditches while I'm pregnant." Said another, "Carrying around grain sacks and spading."[55]

In the last quarter of the twentieth century some of these tasks might strike us as good exercise. But when combined with ceaseless childbearing and poor diets, field work probably had the effect of reducing the ability of rural women to withstand infection. Wrote Elisabeth Baldauf in 1932, "Overexertion poses even greater problems for rural women in that they get no rest at the time of menstruation, of pregnancy, or while breastfeeding. Abdominal complaints are often the result."[56] After commenting on the excess female mortality in the less developed areas of Europe like Galicia, Friedrich Prinzing said, "Even for old women there is no relief. The propertied peasant's wife has to work just as hard as the aging female laborer, whether her husband helps alongside or just watches and commands, or indeed passes his time in the tavern, as not infrequently happens." Prinzing went on to reflect how all this might harm one's health.[57]

In the 1920s and 1930s these terrible conditions started to end, or at least the excess female mortality in the countryside began to disappear. But not until the 1930s did rural Norwegian women, between the ages of thirty and thirty-nine, begin to outlive their husbands. (Urban women of that age in Norway had outlived men ever since appropriate tabulations began in 1889).[58] Irish rural women in the 1930s still had death rates higher than had men of comparable ages. This was much less true in the cities. But not until the 1950s in Ireland would women begin outliving men at every age.[59] Thus rusticity helped make for greater mortality among women than among men, as the former were growing up and in their prime years.

FAMILY LIFE

In most series of statistics, married women in their fertile years had higher mortality than single women and higher mortality than their husbands. In the 1850s unmarried Dutch women would expect to end up living 3.7 years longer than men; but married Dutch women would live 1.5 years *less* than their husbands. Not until the 1930s, in fact, would their life expectancy at the age of twenty outdistance their husbands'.[60] Nor was Holland singular. While single Norwegian men, aged twenty to twenty-four, had in the 1890s a mortality rate 67 percent higher than single women, married men had a rate 32 percent *lower* than their wives.[61] In France during the 1850s, 7.1 married men in their thirties would die annually per 1,000; 9.1 married women. Only after childbearing was over, in the forty to fifty age group, did married French men start to have a higher mortality than women.[62] In Prussia single women in their twenties and thirties easily outlived single men; not so for married women, who had a mortality of 6.4 per 1,000; married men only 5.8. Only after age forty would married women in Prussia outlive their husbands.[63] These figures are an indictment of the impact of traditional marriage upon the lives of women.

Contemporaries were not blind to how family life hurt women's health. "The rural mother has to suffer unimaginably in giving birth," wrote a Rotenburg doctor in 1784, in reference to the wretched midwifery of the time. "After the first or second birth her health is lost."[64] Wilhelm Brenner-Schaeffer sounded the theme—which I just noted—of how quickly young women lose their beauty, but this time in connection with childbirth. "The blossoming young woman remains pretty only in the beginning; then her features start looking coarser and more massive. After a few deliveries she has the appearance of a matron."[65] Here is Joseph Wolfsteiner, from the same area, on how women's appearance changed as domestic life went on. "When they are in their twenties, and more strikingly in their thirties, their walk loses in liveliness and suppleness and becomes awkward; the body forms lose their roundness and become squarish; the back takes on a slight hump; the shoulders become hunched over; their facial features become slacker and eyes and expression take on a slight shadow. Women who have given birth several times appear matronly and much older than they really are."[66] Of course, one might well say the same of men as they grow older. Yet these women died more often. That is the point.

Was childbearing the "married women's disease"? After earlier chapters in this book, the reader will be tempted to explain married women's higher mortality in obstetrical terms. That judgment would be hasty. Repeated deliveries probably did deteriorate the health of married women—even after discounting direct obstetrical mortality—by making them highly anemic and thus less resistant to infection (see pages 247–54).

But even after we remove obstetrical deaths, married women still died more often than their husbands. In a study of 1869 first marriages in four different nineteenth-century communities, Arthur Imhof found that after the 94 maternal deaths were deducted, women still had a higher mortality than their husbands: 374 non-obstetric deaths among the women, only 334 among the men.[67] Even if childbed represented the second or third leading cause of death among fertile women, in absolute terms its contribution to women's overall mortality was not overpowering: 6 percent of all deaths between the ages of twenty-five to forty-four in mid-nineteenth century England, 10 percent in Denmark, 5 percent in Ravensberg County, and so forth.[68] In a study of 2,614 American women born from around 1700 to 1824, Bettie Freeman found no real correlation between the number of children a woman had (the average for the group born before 1750 was 7) and the number of years she lived after the age of forty-five (about twenty-nine more years on the average).[69]

So things are more complicated. It was the general routine of overwork and undernutrition that endangered married women, not the specific risks of dying in birth. Only in the first quarter of the twentieth century would married women become less vulnerable than their husbands to these general hazards of family life.*

---

* The surplus mortality of married Norwegian women, however, vanished only at some point between 1929–32 and 1949–52.[70]

Cancer as a Woman's Disease

Cancer is not, in fact, a women's disease. In the United States in the mid-1970s, the incidence of new cases was 21 percent higher among men than among women. And in that period men had a 56-percent higher mortality rate from cancer than had women.[71] The real incidence of cancer has probably changed little over the ages—so little that some writers refer to the disease as "species-specific," meaning that the species *Homo sapiens* has probably always had about the same likelihood of getting cancer.[72] Quite reliable data for Berlin, Hamburg, and Switzerland, going back to about 1900, show little change in cancer mortality, once the aging of the population has been taken into account (because cancer strikes more often among older people).[73]

But whatever the real rate of cancer, the argument of this section is that before 1870 or so, people *thought* that cancer was mainly a women's disease, because the only cases they were able easily to diagnose were the "external" cancers that afflicted especially women: breast, cervix, and to some extent the upper two thirds, or "body," of the uterus. (Tongue cancer was the other important "external" neoplasm, but it affects men more than women; its overall incidence, in any event, is not high.) Today these gynecologic cancers bulk fairly large in women's lives. American women, for example, had from 1969 to 1971 an 8-percent lifetime chance of getting breast cancer, a 4-percent chance of cancer of the uterus, a 1-percent chance of ovarian cancer. The most common nongynecologic cancer in women, by contrast, is cancer of the colon and rectum (a 5-percent chance).[74] No other site approaches these in frequency.

In the past cancer was diagnosed in women far more often than in men. In Verona from 1760 to 1839 doctors saw cancer in 142 men, 994 women.[75] Whereas 17 percent of all deaths in women were attributed to cancer in the town of Einbeck from 1700 to 1750, only 7 percent of male deaths had that diagnosis.[76] In Landau in the Palatinate, 1 man died of cancer from 1826 to 1829; 10 women.[77] "Scirrhus" (an old-fashioned word for a hard cancer) was assigned as the cause of death to 40 women in Dresden between 1828 and 1837, to only 10 men.[78] And even these statistics—inadequate as they are because the vast majority of cancers in both sexes were undoubtedly attributed to such causes as "old age" or "consumption"—are dominated by the gynecologic cancers: in Prague of 121 cancers diagnosed in *both* sexes over the years 1814 to 1823, 77 were breast and uterine cancer.[79]

The diagnosis of cancer improved considerably during the nineteenth century as autopsies were done more often and the microscope came into use (1902 for the first time in Middlesex Hospital, which had a large cancer ward).[80] Yet even so, official statistics reflect a disproportion of female cancers that must have been out of line with the real balance. The following table shows the male death rate from cancer as a percentage of the female, for ages twenty-five to forty-four:

England–Wales, 1848–72	33
Denmark, towns, 1876–85	53
Norway, 1899–1902	71
United States, 1976	83[81]

If the American statistics from 1976 reflect anything like the real situation, men at midlife tend to die of cancer 17 percent less often than women. Thus, the English statistics for the mid-nineteenth century, which show the female death rate three times higher than the male, must reflect the greater ease of diagnosing the more common female cancers—to wit, breast and uterine cancer. The people of the time, however, probably believed the statistics and imagined cancer for people in the prime of life to be primarily a women's disease.

If past ages did think of cancer as being "women's lot," what particular implications did that assumption have for women's attitudes to their bodies? This fascinating question cannot be answered directly because I have seen almost no evidence on what women in village life thought about cancer generally or about their neighbors who became afflicted with it. Several features of breast and uterine cancer loomed, however, prominently for its victims.

BREAST CANCER

The ulceration of breast cancer was one. Around 1780 an English gentlewoman found "a lump in her breast" about the size of a pea. It grew a bit, and Dr. Hamilton removed it. "In about three years afterwards this lady was alarmed by the appearance of another glandular knot, similar to the former, at the upper margin of the scar." Dr. Hamilton removed this one as well, "but in a little more than a year after it healed the mamma itself became greatly diseased, and adhered to the parts beneath it. . . . The breast, now become a cancer, ulcerated and discharged a corrosive ichor. The ulceration spread." The woman ultimately died from a cancer that had spread throughout her body, but for a long time she had to live with this ulcerating breast.[82]

A cancer itself has no smell, nor particular effluvium; but as it advances, the necrotic tissue around it becomes infected and produces an odorous discharge. This (in addition to pain) was one of the distinctive problems of breast cancer. Of 356 women admitted with breast cancer to Middlesex Hospital between 1805 and 1933, 68 percent had ulceration.[83] It was about a year after her menses ceased that Mrs. G. of Glasgow noticed "a number of small, hard colourless tumors on the surface of the left breast." When Dr. John Macfarlane first saw her, "she was confined in a semi-recumbent position, and was much emaciated. Her countenance was anxious, and of a dark leaden colour; respiration rapid and laborious. . . . The integuments on the front part of the chest . . . but especially those over the mammae, were studded with scirrhous tubercles, some of which were superficially ulcerated, had a livid appearance, and discharged a thin bloody fluid."[84] Mrs. G.'s cancer had clearly caused many problems, but in her last days she and her attendants would also have to cope with these discharges on her chest.

Is there evidence that women were more concerned about breast cancer than about any other disease? That the fear of cancer imprinted women's culture any more than, let us say, the fear of cholera? There are hints. The local doctor in St. Pölten said in 1813, "We often observe scirrhus on the breasts of women here." (He meant lumps.) "How much is the risk feared that this disease might transform itself into cancer. Then the scirrhus becomes painful, breaks open, and transforms itself into an open, malignant sore."[85] Presumably he was referring to his patients' anxiety as well as to his own. One of the puzzles of Europe's demographic history is the systematic refusal of women in some regions to breast-feed their children. Dr. Johann Ebel, of Appenzell Canton, suggested in 1798 that a folkloric belief that lactation caused breast cancer may have been responsible. His own theory was equally off the mark: "Bloodletting during pregnancy, and a modest diet after giving birth should have the desired effect against tumors of the breast and thus free the mothers of Appenzell from the terrible fear, which drives them to deny their infants the healthiest and most precious nourishment"—meaning breast milk.[86] Because failure to breast-feed was associated with a high infant mortality, we must assume that Appenzell women were fearful about their own chances of getting breast cancer.

Medicine could give little relief to victims of breast cancer before the nineteenth century. Opium "hardly afforded a small truce to her sufferings," said Dr. Hamilton of the woman I have just described.[87] Morphine, the major alkaloid of opium, was not isolated until 1806, and not available in pharmacies until the 1820s.[88] With anesthetics the terminal agony of cancer patients could be managed, but only for short periods.[89]

Traditional surgery had been equally futile. Since the ancient Greeks, surgeons had attempted to cut off cancerous breasts, seizing them with great pincers and then performing mammectomy.[90] But a medium-term solution to the "local difficulties" of breast cancer would not come until in 1882 the Baltimore surgeon William S. Halsted began to remove not only the breast but the underlying muscles and lymph nodes as well ("radical mastectomy"). Previous surgeons had been plagued with the recurrence of cancer in the chest and upper limb because they had left behind small bits of tumor which would then proliferate. Halsted removed most of the "pectoralis major" and "minor" muscles. (Press your arm against your side; the chest muscle that bulges forth is "pec major.") This operation would leave the patient with a physical deficit but provided remarkable guarantees against a recurrence of the cancer in that area.[91] Whereas other nineteenth-century surgeons who did only mastectomies or "lumpectomies" had a local recurrence rate of 51 percent to 82 percent, Halsted's patients had a local recurrence of only 6 percent.[92]

Halsted's operation would have been unthinkable without asepsis and anesthesia, and so—along with many other new procedures—it was a child of the 1880s. (He reported it in 1891.) By the First World War it was being widely done, and for the first time in history, breast cancer victims had some practical relief. Alas, not a long-term cure, for they would almost as surely die of their cancers as would untreated patients. Most "treated" patients with "grade 3" (quite advanced) breast cancers would be dead after fifteen years. But grade 3 *untreated* patients were dead after three years.[93]* Women thus had by 1900 some relief from a particularly unpleasant aspect of breast cancer.

CANCER OF THE UTERUS

Cancer of the uterus has many awful features, but I wish to emphasize its insidiousness for older women. Some uterine cancers may be quickly spotted. If the bottom third of the uterus, or cervix, becomes cancerous, pathological changes will be visible in a vaginal examination. But if the top two thirds, or body (also called "corpus"), of the uterus becomes cancerous, the first evidence may be nothing more than unusual uterine bleeding. It is for that reason that post-menopausal women who find themselves "menstruating again" become alarmed. Whereas *cervical* cancer tends to be a disease of women in their forties and early fifties, the age distribution of *corpus uteri* cancer clusters in the late fifties and early sixties. In fact the peak incidence rate of corpus uteri cancer is age seventy.[94] Uterine bleeding may have other causes, but the whole question of "getting one's period again" filled older women with apprehension.

Premodern medicine did little to alleviate the uncertainty. Put some

---

* The mean survival of grade 3 untreated cases (1902–33) was twenty-two months; of treated cases (1936–40), forty months.

of the discharge on a tampon impregnated with gallnut, greater celandine, and saffron, said an ancient authority. If the tampon changes color, it's cancer.[95] A forty-seven-year-old Parisian woman, menopausal for two years, "was surprised all of a sudden by [uterine] bleeding," which then continued for two years "with the discharge of a very fetid purulent matter." François Mauriceau saw her on 21 September 1669, two weeks before she died of a "carcinomatous ulcer of the uterus . . . as I had foreseen from the deplorable state in which I found her." Mauriceau observed, "All these hemorrhages that come to older women, after their menses have ceased for a number of years, are always fatal if they continue more than a month or two."[96]

Mauriceau was a distinguished surgeon, and his observations quite sensible. But consider the total confusion in which the less luminous found themselves. Here we have London surgeon Robert Semple, writing on "Menstruation at Advanced Periods of Life": "I have always considered menstruation as a very important function in the female economy." He went on to present cases. "In the year 1833 Mary Owen, aged 77, a pauper patient in the workhouse of the Liberty of the Rolls, was placed under my care with an abundant menorrhagic [excessive uterine bleeding] discharge. She was in much pain. She had not been in such a state, she said, for these last thirty years. In a few days, however, she died." He presented several similar cases, with equal puzzlement. Nowhere does he mention the possibility of cancer.[97] One can imagine the bewilderment and apprehension of his patients.

Among the diseases discussed in this book, uterine cancer aroused the most foreboding even in doctors. "Of all the calamities to which a sex that seems destined to support the largest share of human misery is subject, the cancerous uterus is heaviest," wrote a London surgeon in 1795.[98] It could not be reliably diagnosed, for as John Leake said, "The signs of a cancerous womb are very uncertain and obscure, being often confounded with those of conception, dropsy, or other affections." And Leake deemed it incurable when the cancer had advanced to the point where it could be diagnosed.[99] Unlike such diseases as uremia (kidney failure), to which males were probably more subject because of prostate disorders, uterine cancer had generally a grim course. Thus Leake: "a slow fever attended with nightsweats, a habitual diarrhea, pain and want of rest alternately consume the patient's strength. Clots of corrupted blood are discharged with excessive pain and forcing down, and sometimes fluid blood in large quantities escapes from the vessels corroded and eaten away by the extreme sharpness of the cancerous humor."[100] "Death from uterine cancer is usually horribly protracted," wrote Lawson Tait a century later.[101]

It is difficult to know to what extent this sense of medical helplessness and horror was shared in the women's culture. German women had special terms for the clotted discharges of the disease: *eine Versammlung* ("the clumps") or *der Brand* ("the blight").[102] Swiss peasants in the Simmenthal appear to have devised a special poultice for uterine cancer: "Take goat dung and mix it with honey and put it on top so the cancer and fistula will die."[103] Willughby tells stories—all too depressing to relate here—of women who came to him for relief from various genital cancers. They may have sought advice from other women before seeing doctors. But after he himself had proven powerless to relieve their sufferings, they continued to seek out quacks and other doctors until they died. Thus at the point when they saw him, cancer victims had left the resources of other women behind.[104] Possibly the women's culture simply resigned itself to helplessness in the face of the awesomeness of the disease. How to wrestle with the terminal symptoms of uterine cancer may have been such an intimate issue that it has no folklore.

The first real progress in lightening this historic burden came with abdominal surgery in the 1890s: the disease could be managed, if not cured, by removing the cancerous uterus ("Wertheim's Operation").* A second major weapon was added in 1903, when clinical radiation therapy began.† The change in the lives of the victims was revolutionary. Whereas between 1900 and 1910 only 20 percent of the corpus uteri cancer patients treated in the University of Pennsylvania hospital survived for five years, by 1926 to 1930—with the combined use of radium and hysterectomy—51 percent were surviving.[107] By the 1960s almost 80 percent of women with corpus uteri cancer survived at least five years, and over 60 percent were surviving fifteen years and longer.[108] Uterine cancer death rates are now declining dramatically.[109] Thus, I am happy to see my general argument—that the first quarter of the twentieth century saw a great amelioration of women's vulnerability—confirmed with the resistance to this disease.

Blood and Iron

Iron-poor blood, or anemia, interests us because its main impact upon women is to make them feel tired and be less resistant to infection.[110] That is its main impact upon men, too, but anemia was far more common in women historically. For example, in Leipzig at the end of the nineteenth century, 77 women per 1,000 members of the Sick Fund made claims for anemia; 4 men per 1,000.[111] The "Peckham Experiment," a survey

---

* Ernst Wertheim first performed his operation in 1898.[105]
† By 1918 radium therapy for cervical cancer had "become usual" in Dublin's Rotunda Hospital.[106]

of 2,000 London families from 1935 to 1939, found one third of the men and 57 percent of the women anemic; between the ages of sixteen and twenty one quarter of the men were anemic and 70 percent of the women.[112] While one has to be quite anemic before symptoms show up, 45 percent of the 1,250 working-class wives surveyed in various English communities in the mid-1930s thought they had those symptoms.[113] So among poorer groups of women in the past we may assume the incidence of anemia, as defined either by blood tests or by the presence of symptoms, to have been high indeed.

You become anemic when (1) you get less iron in your diet; (2) your body's demands for iron increase; or (3) you lose blood.

1. Virtually no one today becomes anemic from a sudden decrease in dietary iron, although it is conceivable that in the past the sudden falling away of something like eggs, or the annual pig that families raised, would knock out much of their iron intake and leave them with a negative iron balance. Yet they would have gotten iron from the soil admixed with their food (an iron source today in Third World countries[114]), from iron pots and pans, and from the garden vegetables that most rural families grew themselves. So it is difficult to see decreases in dietary iron as responsible historically for anemia.

That generality has one important exception. One could ingest sufficient iron, yet it might be blocked from absorption in the intestine. One is a chronic laxative-taker, and the food tends to rush through the gut tube with little chance of absorption; one is deficient in vitamin C, which plays a role in iron absorption. Such problems were all far more pronounced in the pre-1900 world than today. Then the entire population constantly dosed themselves with purgatives; then scurvy (a disease involving a deficiency in vitamin C) was common; and then dietary iron would come more in vegetable form—more difficult for the digestive system to extract—than in the form of meat.

2. Women's demands for iron particularly increase during pregnancy as their blood volume expands. If the argument of chapter 4 is correct that historically women did not supplement their diets during pregnancy, they probably incurred significant iron deficits in childbearing—deficits that worsened with each additional pregnancy. The women we have just witnessed so hollowed out and exhausted by age thirty-five were probably, among other things, severely anemic.

3. The most important factor in anemia was probably blood loss. It began with menstruation. As we will see, a particular variety of iron deficit struck girls around the time of menarche and continued through young adulthood, probably tied to blood loss through the menses. Bleeding from hemorrhoids (a common traditional complaint), from peptic ulcers,

from hookworm, and from the gynecologic damage I describe in the next chapter—all were greater sources of blood loss for traditional people than they are today.

A capital source of blood loss was therapeutic bloodletting, so beloved of both folkloric and academic medicine. I noted in chapter 4 how often "prophylactic" bloodletting was done during pregnancy. Men and women alike had their annual spring "bleed" to "clear out their systems." One Swedish doctor said, toward the middle of the nineteenth century, that it was "rare for anemic women from the countryside to seek medical attention before already having bled themselves two or three times from a foot vein and having been cupped at several other points, which makes such cases difficult to heal."[115] They would be indeed.

Thus valid *a priori* reasons exist for believing the incidence of anemia higher in the past. But how severe? Up to a certain point, anemia that can be detected in the laboratory is clinically invisible. Symptoms begin to appear only when the negative iron balance is such that, having used up the iron stored in the bone marrow and the tissues, the body starts stripping iron from the red blood cells in the plasma. Under the microscope the cells are small ("microcytic") and have an enlarged pale space in the middle ("hypochromic"), meaning they have less hemoglobin. (The iron is carried in the hemoglobin.) Hence the current term "hypochromic microcytic anemia" for the chronic iron-deficiency anemia of the past. Only when the bone marrow starts turning out these peculiar red blood cells do most of the symptoms of anemia begin to appear: in women, losing one's period, feeling "not 100 percent"; in severe cases, having spoonlike depressions in one's fingernails, cracks at the corner of one's mouth, headaches, and so on. Severe iron depletion of this kind is rare today. A study of South Wales found that only six women in every thousand were severely anemic.[116] But by laboratory standards, many additional women are somewhat anemic. According to William Crosby, the incidence of "mild anemia" in the United States is something less than 10 percent of all menstruating women[117] (the fertile years are always emphasized in these studies as the period of greatest blood loss for women). And complaints of tiredness, though not "spoon nails," may well emerge at these lesser degrees of depletion.

In the absence of blood tests—which hospitals didn't use regularly before the 1890s—the traditional medical criteria for anemia in women were sweeping: pallor, tiredness, constipation, heartburn, gastrointestinal upset, heart palpitations, breathlessness, and so on. But a hundred different disorders could have produced these symptoms. Mr. Foote reported the case of Charlotte ————, unmarried, thirty-six, a history of irregular periods, and pallid complexion ("chlorotic aspect"): "Her present symptoms are palpitation, dyspnea [difficulty of breathing], cough, pain in the chest and loins and between the shoulders. Her legs are edematous [swollen]; she has no appetite; her pulse is 80, and soft; tongue clean; bowels confined."[118] In fact, Charlotte could have had anything imaginable, including iron-deficiency anemia. Heart disease or early tuberculosis spring immediately to mind. Her symptoms went away in ten weeks, after (despite) Foote's treatment of her with iron and purgatives.

Most anemia in men and women has historically been hidden in the fog of imprecise diagnoses and absent laboratory findings. Our knowledge focuses basically upon one small group: young women who were thought to have chlorosis. Chlorosis, named after the Greek *chloros* for "green," means essentially iron-deficiency anemia. It was believed to be a disease of girls between puberty and marriage, in whom observers thought they saw a greenish tinge—hence, such designations as "the green sickness." Physiologically, people may take on a greenish hue, as in a kind of leukemia called "the green cancer," or in certain pathological conditions associated with "biliverdin jaundice." But it is most unlikely that any anemia victims actually assumed this greenish caste: the straw yellow of jaundice and the pallor of the tubercular were more likely to have been the colors of chlorosis.

In the days before blood tests, when doctors said a young woman was "chlorotic," they meant that she was pale, weak, and menstruating irregularly or not at all. It is striking how often these combinations of symptoms have recurred across the ages. The ancient Greeks believed, "Such women as cannot conceive . . . appear green, without fever, and the viscera are not in fault; these will say that the head is pained and that the menstrual discharge is vitiated and scanty. . . . Those who have green color, without decided jaundice" also, the account went on to say, eat clay and soil—an allusion to a form of "pica" (earth eating) which sometimes occurs with mineral-deficiency diseases like anemia.[119]

The first comprehensive description of young women's anemia, however, came in 1554 from Johannes Lange, who called it "the virgin's disease." "You rightly ask with what kind of disease is she afflicted: since her face, which in the past year was distinguished by rosiness of cheeks and redness of lips, is somehow as if exsanguinated, sadly paled, the heart trembles with every movement of her body; the arteries of her temples pulsate and she is seized with dyspnea in dancing."[120] Many accounts of such vague symptoms, bundled together as "chlorosis," followed over the next three centuries. Gotha's Johann Storch wrote, "I had to treat a number of girls for chlorosis, or anemia, in spring of 1721, among them a sixteen-year-old of delicate constitution . . . and two older sisters, because they were in this age, had been ill for over a year and had very pale complexions." He went on to present the usual list of symptoms for chlorosis: "the transformation of the skin of the whole body but especially the face from a pink to a pale green," listlessness in "otherwise industrious girls," headache and toothache, fainting, shortness of breath, and so on.[121]

Interest in chlorosis was not confined to academic medicine. A traditional Swiss remedy for "anemia in women" said, "Get up early before sunrise and dig a sod of grass from the garden or meadow. Urinate in the hole. Turn the sod upside down and press it back into the ground." In theory the anemia should be drawn out through the urine into the grass to wither as the grass withers.[122] Peasants in Württemberg distinguished between two kinds of chlorosis: "florid anemia," which was associated with young women just starting to menstruate; and "growing-pains anemia," associated with "weak blood" in adolescent development. The florid variety was thought to be more dangerous because the "blood climbed into your head."[123]

This distinction between the two kinds of anemia was elaborated in academic medicine as well. Anemia could be diagnosed in anyone once Johann Duncan discovered in 1867 pale (hypochromic) red blood cells under the microscope.[124] It is significant for my purpose that doctors continued to insist on the *two* varieties of anemia, because only young women were at risk of one of them: chlorosis. In Compiègne around 1881, for example, Doctor Douvillé counted twelve deaths from "anemia," fifteen deaths from "chlorosis."[125] Leslie Witts recalled, "When I was a medical student immediately after the First World War my teachers used to speak of going to the outpatient department in the old days, seeing the benches crowded with greenish or pasty-faced girls and young women, and murmuring sadly to themselves, 'Nothing but chlorosis.' "[126] An older Danish practitioner said in 1931, "Only young clinicians, who have never seen chlorosis with their own eyes, could doubt the identity of this disease."[127] In 1955, Dr. H. St. H. Vertue of Guy's Hospital was still making the same distinction between the two kinds of anemia that Vienna's Bartholomäus von Battisti had made in 1784:

Vertue: In chlorosis the menses are "scanty," rather than overabundant as in anemia.[128]

Battisti: "There is, however, another kind of anemia . . . which we especially encounter in the countryside. It happens to sturdy women when they find their periods suppressed."[129]

Thus for the doctors of a not too bygone era, chlorosis existed. Whether it was a medical figment, a real disease now defunct, or a kind of cultural behavior in women somehow induced by "nineteenth-century Victorian capitalism" has never been resolved.

Several scholars have argued that chlorosis increased during the nineteenth century, although the abundance of earlier references makes that argument unlikely.[130] But the feature of chlorosis most relevant for my purposes is its astonishing *disappearance* in the first two decades of the twentieth century. Whereas a Hamburg general hospital admitted 201 chlorosis cases in 1901, only 3 were diagnosed in 1923.[131] In 1898–1900 chlorosis represented 18 percent of admissions in combined statistics on several large British hospitals; by 1913–15, only 8 percent.[132] Nor was this decline simply an artifact of changing diagnoses. Thirty-four of the women admitted for chlorosis in Guy's Hospital from 1907 to 1909 had hemoglobin "scores" of less than 60 (out of 100), meaning severely anemic; there were only eleven from 1913 to 1915.[133] When chlorosis declined from twenty-three cases in 1898 to two in 1906 at the Massachusetts General Hospital, Richard Cabot commented, "The most remarkable fact about chlorosis today seems to the writer to be the very convincing evidence that it is disappearing."[134] One French lung clinic had not seen a single case since 1911, said someone in 1924.[135] In Kolding, Denmark, by the 1920s chlorosis was seen "extremely seldom."[136] And H. Sellheim said in 1926 that, while in Germany "the intractable forms of anemia (pernicious anemia) seem to have increased, iron-deficiency anemia [*Bleichsucht*] has as much as disappeared."[137]

What caused this remarkable decline of anemia in women generally and of "chlorosis" in young women in particular? Several explanations have been advanced:

· Better medical diagnoses, so that anemia was no longer confused with tuberculosis and other diseases that produce pallor and weakness. It will be obvious that some cases of "chlorosis" were missed diagnoses of other diseases, as when we find chlorosis "turning into" TB.[138]* Yet one study of 378 chlorotics found that only 5 later died of TB.[140] Indeed, as J. M. H. Campbell pointed out, it is precisely because most cases ended "favorably" that we are entitled to conclude other diseases were not lurking under the label of chlorosis.[141]

· The abandonment of corsets and of Victorian "modesty" generally. Several writers have tried to link chlorosis to tight lacing, on the grounds that corsets might have compressed the vagus nerve, thus slowing gastric secretions and causing dyspepsia. Other equally farfetched physiological theories have been proposed in an effort to associate chlorosis with a "middle-class" life style.[142]†

The overriding piece of evidence against this interpretation is the ubi-

* Dr. Ashwell said, " . . . If the disease terminates fatally, it will frequently, if not generally, be in phthisis."[139]

† Robert P. Hudson argues that corsets might have compressed the common bile duct.[143]

quity of chlorosis among working-class and peasant women, women who demonstrably did not wear corsets nor lounge about feebly all day. Dr. Boëns-Boissau, for example, found it widespread among the teen-age girls who went down in the Belgian coal mines to work (their chlorosis later appears in Emile Zola's *Germinal*).[144] Numerous small-town Swedish doctors, who in the 1850s answered a questionnaire about the health of the population, commented on how widespread chlorosis was in the countryside. They believed it a recent phenomenon but did not mention tight lacing, and it is inconceivable that all this anemia could have been caused by the rustics strapping themselves into corsets.[145] When one finds chlorosis widespread in rural Unterfranken and in the industrial city of Lodève, one might really wonder whether tight lacing was at fault.[146] Campbell reported chlorosis "especially common among domestic servants" in London. And among chlorosis sufferers in the Boston area, "relatively few cases occur among the well-to-do"; domestics far exceeded any other occupation.[147] My own feeling is that those scholars who have linked chlorosis to some particularly "confined" condition among "middle-class Victorian women" have placed too much credence in a few doctors who happened to have middle-class practices and whose patients practiced tight lacing.* But the majority of chlorotic women were working-class, and the disease seems to have been just as frequent in the countryside as in the city.

· Better iron therapy. On the face of it, this explanation appears unlikely because iron had been recommended for anemia ever since the Seville physician Nicolas Monardes wrote on the subject in 1565.[150] The English doctor Thomas Sydenham popularized iron therapy in 1685 when he recommended "iron filings . . . washed down with wine of wormwood." He said, "Thus are cured hysterical complaints. Thus also the so-called female obstructions, especially chlorosis, or green-sickness."[151] It was, however, only in 1831, when Pierre Blaud advocated the use of ferrous sulphate mixed together with potassium carbonate, that it became possible to take large amounts of iron in easily absorbable quantities. The ferrous sulphate was an "iron salt," which has remained until now the basis of iron therapy.† Blaud's nephew, a chemist, marketed the pills all over the world as "the veritable pills of Doctor Blaud."

All other things being equal, chlorosis would probably have come to

---

* Sarah Stage discusses chlorosis in the context of how doctors "preferred weak women"; according to her, we find physicians "sentimentalizing illness . . . until the wan and wasted woman became a perverse ideal of feminine beauty."[148] The empirical basis—such as it is—for statements of this nature would be in the observations of doctors like Vincent Harris that almost all the outpatients treated for anemia at Victoria Park Hospital had no occupation and lived at home. According to Harris, "Chlorosis is a condition observed among the well-to-do classes."[149]

† The ferrous carbonate in his pills, by contrast, was relatively unabsorbable.[152]

an end at this point, as the new therapy of iron salts in massive doses became generalized. Unfortunately, iron therapy fell into disuse when in 1885 the German chemist G. von Bunge cast doubt upon the absorbability of iron in this "inorganic" form. Iron became rehabilitated only in the 1920s, just as chlorosis went into its final tailspin.[153] Whether a relationship exists between the vicissitudes of physiological theories about iron and its actual use remains to be seen. Yet of the major explanations offered for the abrupt diminution of anemia in the female population, this one strikes me as the most likely.

In any event, my purpose is not to trace the history of anemia but to demonstrate its role in the relative ill-health of women vis-à-vis men. There is a close coincidence among the prevalence of tuberculosis, the high incidence of peptic ulcer (a bleeding disorder), and the tendency to anemia—all among girls and young women. These health problems doubtless stood in reciprocal relationship: the ulcers exacerbating the anemia, the anemia increasing the susceptibility of young women to infectious disease. Clearly the important question is, Why did this tangle of pathology exist among young women historically, suddenly to be obliterated in the first two decades of the twentieth century? It is a disappointment to me that I do not have a new theory to place instead of all the old theories about "capitalist oppression" and the Victorian "woman on a pedestal." But at least we are able to see the inadequacy of the old theories. By the first quarter of our own century, for inexplicable reasons, the greater vulnerability of women than men in certain age groups to disease had come to an end.

CHAPTER 10

Diseases of Sexual Significance

WOMEN are subject to many more kinds of pelvic disease than are men. To list them all would have about the same interest for the general reader as a gynecology textbook. Instead this chapter will argue that two sorts in particular were "sexually significant" for women in the past: (1) those acquired from men in intercourse, and (2) those that would make a woman feel sensitive about her body in sexual situations. This special "sexual" vulnerability constituted a major source of victimization for women. They would fare worse than men in dealing with sexually acquired diseases, and the vicissitudes of pelvic disease would expose them in their own eyes to humiliation in front of men.

The History of Vaginal Discharge

Perhaps one woman in every four who goes to a gynecologist today does so because she has a discharge.[1] These discharges come from the uterus and vagina, range in color from clear white to yellow-green, sometimes smell offensive, and may make intercourse painful. Most today are easily treatable and—when they do not come from conditions like uterine cancer—go away quickly. But in the past they were not so easily treatable and represented a terrible affliction for women, who would go about for years with these fluids oozing from their vaginas. Aside from the odd case of gonorrhea which turned into peritonitis, these discharges rarely represented life-threatening diseases. But they were a constant reminder of the special sexual burden of womanhood.

The history of these discharges reaches far back in time. A fifteenth-century English leechbook recommended for "the superfluities of the mother [uterus]" that people "seethe calamint in water, and therewith wash [the woman] from beneath."[2] Cold water, said an Urnerland doctor in 1811, is a "time-tested means of combating the nauseating odor that not infrequently manages to lurk beneath the loveliest dress. . . . It is especially useful in summer, when the emanations collect in the lips of the vagina, become acrid, and make the flesh sore, causing the white flowers."[3] "The whites," "white flowers," or "fluor albus" were the classic medical labels for any viscid vaginal or uterine discharge. "Leukorrhea" is the modern term. These discharges were once thought a separate disease, rather than just a symptom of different underlying diseases. And because women found them so annoying, they were among the few gynecologic conditions for which medical help was sought. As a result we know more about the history of vaginal discharge than about most other aspects of women's health.

When women today have these discharges, one of the following is probably at work:

· A vaginal infection from a "protozoan" micro-organism called *Trichomonas vaginalis*. Although one adult woman in every five harbors some of these "trichomonads" in her vagina, far fewer women have symptoms. Lots of men, too, carry "trich" in their penises. But whereas men seldom have symptoms, women with clinical infections notice a fetid odor coming from their vaginas, a bubbly yellow-green discharge, and a fierce itching.[4]* *T. vaginalis* was first observed in 1836.[6] But not until the 1930s did doctors begin routinely identifying it in office examinations.

· A vaginal infection from a yeastlike organism called *Candida albicans* (formerly "monilia"). Again, maybe one woman in five has candida growing naturally in her vagina,[7] but only a few notice symptoms. Yet when these "yeast infections" strike, they are highly vexing: a discharge like cottage cheese runs from the vagina, accompanied by intense itching and painful sex.

· Gonorrhea. On this I shall have more to say (pages 263–67) but note here that theoretically the greenish discharge of the gonococcus

---

* Trichomonal infections in men occasionally cause symptoms in the urethra, but they account for relatively little of overall male nongonococcal urethritis. "NGU" itself is not frequent in men, occurring annually in only about 4 men per 1,000 population. Thus, symptomatic trichomonal infections are far more common in women.[5]

has always been differentiated from the "whites." William Smellie wrote in 1752 that, unlike normal "fluor albus," gonorrhea produced "inflammation or ulcers within the labia." "Gonorrhea is likewise distinguished from the Fluor Albus by its continuing all the time of the menstrual discharge."[8] Yet many past observers in practice did not bother to distinguish between them, and we may be sure that among some of the young women "made infertile by the whites" were gonorrhea victims.[9]

· A whole range of bacterial infections of the vagina, either a rodlike bacterium named *Hemophilus vaginalis* or members of the streptococcus and staphylococcus families. Their symptoms are not "characteristic," and we know little about them historically.

· Various bugs infecting the cervix. "Acute cervicitis" is usually the result of gonorrhea, but chronic infections of the cervix associated with damage from childbearing are likely to have been more common in the past. They produce a thick, yellow, pus-filled discharge.

So the "flowers" historically could have meant all of the preceding infections. One additional source of leukorrhea in the past, however, which rarely occurs today, is the whole dismal array of post-delivery infections. Once the connective tissue of the pelvis, the uterus, or the tubes was infected, pus could trickle out literally for years. "A weaver's wife at Wossall, in Staffordshire, about the year 1654, came unto me, complaining of much pain in her back, and heat about the outward parts of her body," related Percivall Willughby. "She said that this happened after a hard labour, and that many skins, and lumps of flesh came from her body, after her delivery." She had many other symptoms, but what interests us is that "she had a whitish, sordid matter, which continually issued from her. And it did much inflame and moisten those parts [the vulva]. And the humour had a raw, faintish savour. . . . What became of her, after I went to London in 1656, I know not."[10]

Whatever the cause, these vaginal discharges were once extremely frequent. Vienna's Friederich Colland complained in 1800 how difficult it was to find a proper wetnurse because these women were so deceitful. "When they present themselves for their interview, they usually wash and clean their private parts, then stick in a small sponge (which they remove before entering the house), and finally put on a white dress so that the malignant nature of their leukorrhea will not be recognized."[11] This passage suggests both that their prospective employers inspected their genitals, and that the "whites" were normal in the class of women from whom these nurses were recruited. Within a six-year period in the late eighteenth century, 446 women appeared at the Aldersgate Dispensary in London for "fluor albus" (by contrast, 270 for heavy periods).[12] Was this a lot of women? Keep in mind that, given the modesty of the day, women rarely sought the help of a male doctor for vaginal discharge unless they were absolutely in extremis. As a Danzig doctor explained, "Women think of leukorrhea as such a common complaint that for it alone they consult a doctor only in the most severe cases."[13] When, in 1877, Syracuse gynecologist Ely van de Warker examined 34 women in John Humphrey Noyes's famous "Oneida Community," he found that 11 had "large" amounts of leukorrhea.[14] Even in the 1920s in London, when Marie Stopes was counseling mothers in her birth control clinic, many clients had discharges and could not be fitted with cervical caps. Said Dr. Maude Kerslake, who worked in the clinic: "Only a few of these women had previously sought medical advice. . . . Often they said they had been told [a discharge] was natural and they must put up with it."[15]

Much evidence exists, in other words, on the ubiquity of copious vaginal discharge in past times. To avoid overwhelming the reader with the scores of obscure doctors in remote villages who have commented on it, I shall just make several specific points.

Leukorrhea was not solely a "middle class" disease associated somehow with "invalid" women in polite society. Many voices cry out from the hinterland:

· Doctor J.-B. Denis Bucquet, writing in 1808 from Laval: "Leukorrhea is almost universal. The women of every age and every class are equally subject, and frequently the disease is carried to the extreme"[16]—meaning, presumably, that it was among the terminal symptoms of uterine cancer or pelvic peritonitis.

· Doctor Rame on Lodève in 1841: "Uterine catarrh is so common that few of the fair sex are exempt from it."[17]

· Dr. F. J. Werfer on Gmünd in 1813: "Among the female sex, single and married, the white flowers are very frequent, and even in the country-side it is now appearing more often than before. This is doubtless the result of a more coddled upbringing."[18]

· Dr. Johann Rambach on Hamburg in 1801: "The whites are very widespread, and indeed more so among the women of the people than among the well-to-do. Few women succeed in avoiding it, at least under most circumstances."[19]

And so on. Dozens of these "medical topographies" were published in the first half of the nineteenth century, and for many of the writers leukorrhea was—perhaps alongside anemia—the most salient aspect of the medical care of women.

A second special circumstance is the prevalence of the whites among women working in industry. A Viennese pediatrician noted how often young girls in the spinning industry had it "as a result of continual sitting."[20] Around Wangen in Württemberg, a Dr. Zengerle noted that "one of the most frequent morbid phenomena among our female population is the so-called white flowers. In our fatherland there are few regions where so many female individuals afflicted with this ailment are to be found." The doctor droned on, concluding that "as a cause of the high frequency of this disease must be regarded the life of sitting which occupies peasant women for half the year. From October until April women are occupied from early morning until late at night almost continually with spinning, sewing, and knitting [on an industrial scale]."[21] In Glarus Canton, F. Schuler thought leukorrhea was generally "occasioned by factory work." Women cotton printers had vaginal discharges more often than women weavers, he noted in 1872, and he believed the "warm humid air" of the printing works to be at fault.[22] A doctor in the French textile town of Elbeuf was struck by the leukorrhea of "women and young girls" in the various cloth workshops, "where they used braisers to warm their feet from the dampness."[23]

These doctors' theories about the causes of this exceptional "industrial" leukorrhea were all silly. Nonetheless we might ask what aspect of industrial work made women more susceptible to vaginal and uterine infections. In view of the fact that both married and unmarried were at risk, it was probably not some particular circumstance in their domestic lives, such as a husband's tendency to drag home a trichomonal or gonorrheal infection from prostitutes. These "white flower" epidemics among industrial workers resemble strikingly the epidemics of "vulvovaginitis" among prepubescent camp girls of our own time—transmitted by infected towels or uncleanliness within populations of women living close together.[24] The women of Wangen, clustering together in the same farmhouse for industrial "outwork," would have been exposed to vaginitis epidemics as well.

What about the possibility that all these reports of women's vaginas smelling bad stem more from male fantasies than from reality? In the medical imaginations of the past danced sometimes fantastical sexual images.[25] Why not here as well? Several kinds of evidence suggest that copious vaginal discharge really did alarm the women who had it, as opposed to merely their middle-class medical attendants.

For one thing, a number of folkloric remedies for leukorrhea existed, handed down from generation to generation. Popular medical advice from the sixteenth century insisted that "for the white disease you take the roots of white roses, put them in a wine decoction and drink down the wine for a few days."[26] "If the mother [the uterus] is cooking only slime," said Bavarian peasants, a woman can take rosemary, sauerkraut water, plantain, or twenty other different botanical brews.[27] For the "whites"

Swiss peasants swallowed "white sausage and white lilies that have been boiled in water."[28] Even in the 1970s rustic women in the Moselle department would give themselves vaginal injections made from walnut leaves for leukorrhea.[29] In view of this extensive tradition of folk medicine, it is unlikely that "the whites" were mainly the product of overworked male medical imaginations.

There are less direct hints, too, that vaginal discharge upset the women who had it, as well as their doctors. Working-class women in Britain referred to leukorrhea as "inward weakness" or "waste."[30] In Finnish communities "a woman with the whites is seen as unchaste. The whites are generally thought of as a grave disease, which considerably weakens a woman, finally making her infertile"—an apparent reference to gonorrheal discharge.[31] Mrs. S., a thirty-three-year-old Londoner, had had an "uninterrupted yellowish discharge, in large quantity, and of a very offensive character," for about three years. "On some occasions" this discharge was said to have "produced sores on the fingers of her laundress."[32] Now, it is most unlikely that her laundress did in fact get dermatitis from Mrs. S.'s dirty linen. The point is that the laundress and Mrs. S. both thought she had (and Dr. Francis Ramsbotham agreed on being told about it), thus showing that they all imputed extreme virulence to these discharges.

Vaginal discharge is relevant also insofar as it affected relations between men and women, reinforcing traditional women's sense of themselves as hobbled by nature. What evidence exists that men were sensitive to leukorrhea, or women embarrased by it? Here the sources are largely quiet, for these attitudes are buried in the historical silence that envelops the body's other secret functions. The Latvians, in the pre-Christian era, had, to be sure, a song about it:

> *The pecker goes a ploughing*
> *With a red hat on.*
> *The pussy comes with lunch*
> *Wiping her tears away.*

In the view of the editor of this folksong collection, the pecker's "red hat" means the glans penis, and the pussy's "tears" are possibly a discharge.[33] If so, this is one of the few cultural representations of the private drama of leukorrhea and is interesting especially because these folksongs were usually devised and transmitted by males.

Behind vaginal discharge lay the striking insalubrity of common people in former times. They lived in filth, did not wash themselves, and were afflicted with lifelong infections and infestations of the skin, the ears, the eyes, and the hair. But it is the genitalia that interest us here. After noting the extraordinary frequency of uterine infections in the Rhön district, Dr. K. H. Lübben went on to talk about how dirty the inhabitants were: "Most get their first and last bath from the midwife."[34] One third of the midwives who, toward 1900, responded to a hygiene questionnaire in Hungary, reported that women in their district never bathed, "unless they fall accidentally into the water," as one put it. Bathing was "not customary," "not the fashion here," "unknown." One midwife said that women bathe for the last time just before they are married. Another said that "women get bathed for the first time when they are born, for the second time after they die."[35] Maria Bidlingmaier, the young German doctoral student who lived among the peasants of two Württemberg villages, reported that the only parts of their bodies that women ever washed were face, hands, and feet. "How fortunate that the rough clothes and the constant activity rub clean the rest of the body" (this meant ironically).[36] The medical officer of health in Roding reported in 1860, "The women wash themselves only on Sundays and holidays, stopping after face, neck, arms, and feet. They consider the washing or cleansing of their private parts to be sinful and improper."[37]

Women's premodern sense of cleanliness shows itself most vividly in the area of menstrual hygiene. What did peasant women use when they menstruated? The answer seems to be basically that women from the popular classes menstruated onto their clothes. Someone in Frankfurt lodged in 1457 a complaint against the leprosy inspectors, on the grounds that they insisted in completely disrobing a dead woman suspected of leprosy, despite the fact that she had just menstruated before she died. The inspectors might have noted that *by the state of her clothing*, the complainants said.[38] Even early in the twentieth century Finnish country-folk believed it positively harmful to wear pads during menstruation, "because women are cleansed of evil and dirt during their monthlies; so that the cleaning will be unimpeded, the genitals must not be stopped up with a cloth or pad." The clothes onto which the woman had bled, moreover, "must be washed in secret and only in a bit of water."[39] Even in more advanced areas of Europe like Switzerland, the custom of letting the menses flow unhampered persisted until quite recently. A Swiss woman recalled her girlhood in the 1890s: "At most, underpants were worn only in the coldest winter. People called them unhealthy, and said the body has to get air. Nobody even thought about washing there. . . . Only when I started getting my period was I permitted to wear panties, and then only because my godmother insisted."[40]

I am not saying there is anything nasty about menstruating onto one's clothing. The point is that all this dried blood would have been an excellent growth medium for micro-organisms, caked either on the clothes or in the woman's skin folds. Similarly, the argument in regard to "dirt" is not that women smelled bad because they did not wash themselves. Indeed, we know today that douching the healthy vagina is unnecessary and hurtful. Rather, the dried sweat, dead skin cells, and dirt that accumulated about the folds of the thighs and the labia offered a perfect nesting ground for pathogenic organisms. For people who lived before the 1850s it was probably such organisms—the streptococcus, coliform bacteria from the bowel, and the staphylococcus—that caused most leukorrhea. Trichomonal infections women could easily get from their husbands. Yeast organisms were omnipresent—given people's casual ways with fecal matter; and we know that they played a significant role in vaginal infections because of the "epidemics" of infant "thrush" that occurred from time to time. (Thrush is a candidal infection of the mouth and is acquired by babies at birth from the yeast infections in their mothers' vaginas.)[41] Gonorrhea before 1850 was probably not an important cause of leukorrhea. But no more favorable atmosphere for the other vaginal infections could be imagined than dirty people living together in close contact.

When were women finally relieved of chronic vaginal infections? I have seen no evidence linking the dissemination of cheap cotton underwear after 1850 to a lessening of complaints about "chronic leukorrhea." Yet there probably was a connection. If my argument about insalubrity is correct, the across-the-board advance of personal hygiene in the second half of the nineteenth century must have reduced vaginitis in the same way that it seems to have cut back pediculosis, scabies, septic dermatitis, and the other diseases of insanitation.

Medical care probably made little difference until the 1930s. Which is not to say that "traditional" medicines—either academic or folkloric—were entirely inefficacious. The most common source of vaginitis—trichomonads—may be combated by increasing the acidity of the vagina or by killing the organisms. Johann Osiander, for example, recommended in 1838 douches with oak bark (acidic) and injections with a decoction of sage leaves (a volatile oil in sage appears to destroy trichomonads).[42] Douches with boric acid and tannic acid for leukorrhea have a long history in both medicine and folklore.[43] It is possible that douching with bicarbonate of soda might have palliated the acid discharges of *Candida albicans* (yeast infection), although that method is not recommended today.* None of the traditional remedies would have been effective against the gonococcus or the streptococcus.

The problem with these traditional approaches was that, alongside the drugs that probably did work, the sources would mention twenty or so

---

* The fifth edition of the *Merck Manual* recommends bicarbonate of soda for an "acid discharge"[44] but see Robert W. Kistner's *Gynecology.*[45]

others that probably did not work. For example, the first edition of the *Merck Manual*, a standard reference guide which began to appear in 1899, lists for leukorrhea no fewer than sixty-four different drugs (plus "spinal ice bag" and "cold sponging"), including "lead salts" and "iron sulphate."[46] The patience of the victim would have been exhausted long before she reached the few remedies that offered some relief. The 1923 edition of the *Merck Manual* is similarly filled with useless remedies.[47] So inadequate was understanding of the basic causes of vaginitis in those years that gynecologist Arthur Curtis would write about yeast, "Whether these organisms are incidentally present or are the essential cause . . . remains problematical."[48]

Then things began to look up. In the late 1920s a highly effective organic compound named "gentian violet" began to be used for candidiasis.[49] After 1936 the sulfa drugs would sweep away bacterial sources of cervicitis and vaginitis. And in 1955 the drug metronidazole ("Flagyl") was discovered, replacing the dangerous arsenical "Stovarsol" in the treatment of trichomonal infections.[50*]

So if we ask, When were women liberated from the fear of smelling bad in front of men? the chronology is not as precise as for, let us say, the conquest of post-delivery infection. Indeed one might argue that a change in their own sense of autonomy has been as important as any pharmaceutical or medical advance. Yet certainly by the Second World War chronic vaginal discharges of whatever color had been vastly reduced.

Venereal Disease

Venereal disease, or V.D.—defined as syphilis and gonorrhea— is not terribly important for our purposes because most women who lived before 1850 never had it. A long, slow increase, however, in the frequency of both syphilis and gonorrhea began late in the eighteenth century and continued until the middle of the twentieth. By 1911 almost half of all working-class men in a city like Graz had contracted gonorrhea sometime in their lives, and many communicated it to their wives. Coming into contact with the gonococcus does not necessarily mean that one will have symptoms. Yet 16 percent of those married men in Graz who admitted an infection said that their wives had "abdominal troubles"—together with leukorrhea. Those women, and many others, probably had advanced gonorrhea. Thus, to understand more recent developments in women's lives we must pause for a moment at V.D.[51]

How many women had V.D.? Hard to say. We must keep in mind that about a third of those infected with syphilis recover spontaneously.[52]

* Stovarsol had been in use since 1923.

Perhaps four fifths of the women exposed to gonorrhea never show any symptoms of the infection and become "asymptomatic" carriers.[53] So we have no real way of knowing how many men and women in the past may have been exposed or have had only brief bouts.

The historical record of V.D. begins in the sixteenth century. From then until around 1850 gonorrhea and syphilis remained at the margins of the population: a disease of soldiers, students, and prostitutes. Even when normal women became infected, it was not necessarily through intercourse, since one may contract gonorrhea simply through the exposure of a fresh drop of pus to a mucous membrane or a sore. The same is true for syphilis. Kissing, close living together, or suckling an infected infant will suffice to spread it. Thus, a syphilis epidemic in Lausanne in 1683 was largely nonvenereal in nature: Daniel Montandon, who had come from Neuchâtel, infected his new bride: "She infected her sister; the two sisters infected the infants whom they had taken as nurslings; these infants infected their mothers and other nurses; the scourge spread."[54] A syphilis epidemic around 1837 in Cologne was spread by one of the "suck-out women" (women paid to suck the milk from the breasts of new mothers who didn't want to breast-feed) who had syphilitic sores in her mouth.[55] In fact, in late-nineteenth-century Sweden, of 4,176 cases of syphilis whose origin was known, fully one third did not come from coitus. Two hundred and eleven cases were owing to mothers and nurses premasticating the baby's food; and over 1,200 resulted from "living in close proximity."[56]

Yet the average woman with V.D. would have been infected because her husband brought it home from a trip. The medical literature is filled with these sad little stories. A horseman's wife near Gotha, who had born four children, was infected by her husband after he returned from a voyage. He underwent a "salivation" cure, meaning that he was treated with mercury. She, however, began to have irregular periods and did not again become pregnant, although she noticed at that time no other symptoms. But several years later began a series of attacks of what sounds like acute pelvic inflammation. After one she finally felt something "burst in her side," and died shortly thereafter, probably of a ruptured fallopian tube filled with pus (for which her initial bout with gonorrhea would have paved the way).[57]

A Norman gentlewoman, having been "greatly indisposed" for eight days by the "white flowers," summoned Guillaume de la Motte to attend her. She had a leaden sensation in her lower abdomen with some pain and much itching. De la Motte, "knowing that the conduct of her husband had not been aboveboard," immediately diagnosed a "genuine dose of clap" (*vraie chaudepisse*); and indeed, the husband confessed several days later that he had "made a present of it to Madame his wife."[58] Thus, accidents happened.

Until the nineteenth century my impression is that these accidents remained more or less isolated. Then a dramatic increase in V.D. began, starting probably first among the lower classes but spreading by 1900, via the channel of their husbands visiting prostitutes, to middle-class women. V.D. cases admitted to Paris's civil hospitals increased from 2,200 in 1804 to 5,300 in 1837, considerably outdistancing the city's population increase.[59] Patients with V.D. in Finland's hospitals climbed from around 1,000 in 1831 to 2,600 in 1848, to 8,600 in 1870.[60]* These statistics have limited value, because not until 1838 did Philippe Ricord publish his empirical test for differentiating gonorrhea from syphillis. And not until 1852 was chancroid—the third of the major venereal diseases— clearly diagnosed for the first time.[61] As is well known, the discovery of the gonococcus itself would await Alfred Neisser's work in 1879. So until the twentieth century we have only hints that V.D. was on the rise. Yet considerable evidence supports this impression and I have no doubt that V.D. did become more prevalent during the 19th century.[62] A whole revolution in extramarital sexual behavior, which I have described elsewhere, was causing in Europe and America a huge increase in all venereally transmitted infections.[63]

Then around the First World War a sudden jump in V.D. occurred. Gonorrhea in Swedish women was reported only 537 times in 1911, 5,400 times in 1919—and the level remained high thereafter.[64] One experienced German midwife had never seen a case of gonorrhea until 1914.[65] Although national statistics on syphilis in the United States do not begin until 1919, 113 cases per 100,000 population were reported in that year. The peak was reached in 1943 with 447 cases per 100,000. Gonorrhea increased as well, though less drastically, in the years between the two world wars.[66]†

If we ask what were women's and men's relative chances of getting V.D. in those years, the risks, though divergent, in no way meant that the average woman would be "spared." Among members of the Sick Fund in Leipzig between 1887 and 1905, 5.7 males between the ages of fifteen and thirty-four per 1,000 were ill with V.D.; 4.2 females.[67] In 1900, Berlin doctors treated 14 males per 1,000 adult population for V.D. and 4 females per 1,000.[68]‡ A nationwide U.S. survey in 1928 found the prevalence of V.D. as follows, in cases per 1,000 white population:

* The latter figure is for syphilis only, which was, however, probably somewhat overdiagnosed.

† Some part of this fourfold increase in syphilis comes from better reliability in diagnosing it.

‡ In small towns and villages, .8 males and .3 females per 1,000 population.

	Male	Female
Gonorrhea	5.7	2.1
Syphilis	5.1	2.8[69]*

By these years V.D. had long ceased to be a disease of the down-and-out. In Berlin in the 1890s, 25 percent of the students were being treated for V.D., 16 percent of the salesmen, 13 percent of the waitresses, but only 9 percent of the factory workers.[70] Many of the patients whom Emil Noeggerath saw in his New York practice were infertile women whose middle-class husbands had infected them just after marriage: "Mrs. S. from Williamsburgh, the second wife of a merchant whose first wife died after an abdominal infection, was married two years ago as a healthy young woman; she began suffering immediately after the wedding, namely from leukorrhea and profuse menstruation, in addition to abdominal pain. Six months after the wedding the pain was so severe that she had to take to her bed, acutely ill with the symptoms of pelvic peritonitis."[71] In other words, Mrs. S.'s husband had communicated to her a gonococcal infection which he carried without symptoms in his urethra; his first wife had probably died of a ruptured tubal abscess, for the gonococcus speeds across the uterus and into the tubes, where it paves the way for deadlier, more invasive pathogens which create so much pus that the abscess bursts. Now Mrs. S. herself had such an abscess; it had ruptured, giving her a powerful abdominal infection.

Two points may now be made:

1. Gonorrhea, once it climbed into the tubes, created a significant amount of abdominal pain for women through "pelvic inflammatory disease" ("PID") as it is now called. One woman in every seven who contracted gonorrhea would, in the pre-antibiotic era, end up with a tubal infection.[72] Indeed, the vast majority of all tubal infections were probably touched off by gonorrhea. The gonococcus was found for the first time in tubal pus in 1886,[73] and therewith the understanding began that many women who complained of deep pelvic pain for which no apparent cause could otherwise be found, may have been suffering from the advanced stages of venereal disease.†

2. Gonorrhea made a large number of women infertile before they

---

* Because V.D. is often underdiagnosed in women, the real rate for them was probably higher.

† The gonococcus was cultivated in more than 70 percent of all tubal infections in Chicago about 1920.[74] Howard C. Taylor believed that much former "perimetritis" was probably salpingitis.[75]

wished to be. Readers of this book will probably be startled to see infertility suddenly identified as a cause of problems in the lives of women historically, because I have occupied myself mainly with women who bore far too many children. Yet beginning in the last quarter of the nineteenth century, and continuing until perhaps the Second World War, there was a significant rise in the percentage of women who were entirely infertile, or who became so after bearing only one child.[76] Most of this new infertility probably stemmed from gonorrhea, nesting in the tubes and sealing them off so that the ovum could not be fertilized by the sperm. A German midwife spoke of the "typical one-child gonorrhea marriage":[77] The husband infects the newly married wife, but she has time to conceive just one child before gonorrhea blocks her tubes, making her infertile. According to Noeggerath's statistics from New York, of eighty-one women who married already-infected men, thirty-one became pregnant. Of these thirty-one, eight failed to carry to term. Of the twenty-three who did, twelve bore only one child.[78] (Syphilis, by contrast, reduces fertility mainly by killing the fetus late in pregnancy or by causing badly debilitated infants to be born who die soon afterward.[79]) These venereal infections may have had a role in decreasing the birth rate at the end of the nineteenth century. It is interesting that Italy's Liguria region, where in the 1930s more than one woman in ten had been childless all her life, also had one of the highest reported V.D. rates for a period fifty years earlier. The same is true for the regions of Lazio, Umbria, and Campania.[80]

So here is a pattern of vulnerability that does not fit the general plan: things got *worse* for women, rather than better, in the last quarter of the nineteenth century and thereafter. To be sure, Paul Ehrlich's discovery of "Salvarsan," which he announced in 1910,* gave some relief to syphilis victims.[81] But no specific treatment for gonorrhea was available until the marketing of the "sulfa" drugs began in 1936. Penicillin, which provided the final victory over syphilis, started to be used for that disease only in 1943.[82] Even today one couple in ten is unable to have children, and in 30 percent of those couples the fault lies in the woman's tubal disease, perhaps one half of these cases gonorrheal in origin.† While the other "diseases of sexual significance" had greatly receded by the 1930s, V.D. has until today continued to remind women of an unequal "natural" vulnerability to sex.

* The patent was taken out in 1909.
† Richard H. Schwarz estimated that 60 percent of acute PID is caused by gonorrhea.[83] Of 563 cases of acute salpingitis—in which there was a bacteriological finding—at Lund University Hospital from 1960 to 1967, the gonococcus was cultured in 40 percent. Gonococci, which were likely to have been the origin of an unknown additional number of cases, would have been displaced by other pathogens by the time the tests were made.[84]

Long-term Damage from Childbirth

Injuries sustained in birth might remain throughout life. And once a woman has been mutilated in giving birth, her sex life will certainly be altered. Note that in a brutal or long drawn-out delivery, a number of structures in the pelvis might be damaged. In the 1890s, Dr. W. J. Sinclair was called to a young woman who had just given birth: "When I first examined her, the uterus was found to be completely prolapsed, and it was so lacerated that the anterior and posterior halves of the cervix, projecting from between the nates [buttocks] looked like two separate organs, and the perineum was torn completely through into the anus."[85] A woman who had suffered this way in childbirth would find her life entirely transformed: simple bowel functions, walking, the fear of yet another pregnancy. . . . To women thus damaged, the notion of "the joy of sex" would be meaningless.

Such pelvic injuries were not uncommon. I discuss three of them in this section: "fistulas," or openings betweeen the vagina and neighboring organs; tears of the perineum which might extend back to the anus; and the tendency of the uterus itself after several difficult labors to slide down the birth canal, even hanging out between the woman's legs. These terrible conditions were very much bound up with a woman's whole notion of "femininity" or "womanhood" in previous times, and if we wish to understand those women we must grapple with their injuries.

FISTULAS

Most starkly awful, but least common, of the various gynecologic sequelae of childbirth were fistulas. A bladder-vaginal, or "vesicovaginal," fistula occurred when the infant's head was jammed for long periods in the vagina, cutting off the circulation to the thin septum of tissue separating vagina from bladder, so that a hole would form in the septum. Sometimes the hole would actually be torn during the delivery, as forceps or a perforation hook were introduced to end the labor; or it might appear on its own a week later.*

"Rectovaginal" fistulas were less common but equally feared. The tissue between rectum and vagina might be split under similar circumstances, creating an opening that would let feces and gas pass directly from the rectum into the vagina. Willughby told of a London midwife, who through manual manipulations caused a long tear in the posterior wall of the mother's vagina. "With this affliction the woman was much disquieted. For ever afterward her excrements came forth by the birth place."[87] After

---

* Of the vesicovaginal fistulas that Thomas A. Emmet repaired at the New York Women's Hospital (probably during the 1870s), thirty had appeared during the delivery, forty-three after the delivery—an average of ten days later [86]

her second delivery, a baker's wife in Negreville suffered a rectovaginal fistula, "from which fecal matter escaped without her feeling it and obliged her always to wear pads to receive it." De la Motte, who reported this story, examined her and was able to pass his thumb through the rectum into her vagina.[88] One can imagine how distressing this condition might have been to the woman. Mrs. D. of Hull got a rectovaginal fistula after a hard instrumental delivery in March of 1833 and found, five days later, that "she had lost all power of retention, and the feculent matters passed from her involuntarily as she lay in bed." George Fielding attempted to repair the hole, "so as to enable her to have some command over the feces, a matter of great importance to one who appeared scrupulously neat and cleanly in her personal habits."[89]

Far more common, however, were fistulas between vagina and bladder. The first one on record occurred to the young princess Hehenit of the eleventh dynasty in Egypt around the year 2000 B.C. Her mummy "shows a vesicovaginal fistula, probably caused by a protracted delivery, as a result of her abnormally narrow pelvis. This delivery also caused her death."[90] Because they were virtually incurable, these fistulas have always fascinated medical writers. The Arab doctor Avicenna, who flourished in the eleventh century A.D., remarked that "the bulk of the fetus may cause a tear in the bladder which results in incontinence of urine." And Luiz de Mercado, a physician in Valladolid, declared in 1597, "What an empty and tragic life is led by the affected victims and how great are their embarrassments . . . uncontrolled urine runs from the fistula with ease."[91]

In truth, the lives of the victims were miserable. The German surgeon J. F. Dieffenbach wrote in 1836, "A sadder situation can hardly exist than that of a woman afflicted with a vesicovaginal fistula. A source of disgust, even to herself, the woman beloved by her husband becomes, in this condition, the object of bodily revulsion to him; and filled with repugnance, everyone else likewise turns his back, repulsed by the intolerable foul urinous odor. . . . The labia, perineum, lower part of the buttocks and inner aspect of the thighs and calves are continually wet, to the very feet. The skin assumes a fiery red color and is covered in places with a pustular eruption. Intolerable burning and itching torment the patients, who are driven to frequent scratching to the point of bleeding. In desperation many tear the hair, which is coated at times with a calcareous urinary precipitate, from the mons pubis. The refreshment of a change of clothing provides no relief, because the clean undergarment, after being quickly saturated, slaps against the patients, flopping against their wet thighs as they walk, sloshing in their wet shoes as though they were wading through a swamp."[92] Mrs. Dröhnen, who appeared in 1786 at the Göttingen Clinical Institute to be treated for "a fistula of the urinary bladder and the rectum," had endured hers for fourteen years.[93] An elderly woman living in a large Canadian city recently recalled how, as a young wife in Nova Scotia, she had been left with a fistula by a midwife. "All my passages ran together," she said. She expressed great embarrassment, she told an interviewer, "at having to live this way with her husband, since she had to wear a diaper constantly, was often soiling her clothes, and was irritated and chafed regularly. . . . Because she could not bring herself to discuss her experiences with other women, she lived silently with this burden for many years. . . . She said she was always terrified of being pregnant again."[94] One can imagine so.

How common were these fistulas? Because they tend to happen in primitive obstetrics—brutal hauling at the mother combined with highly protracted labor—few statistics have been kept on them. In almost two thousand deliveries supervised by the Westminster General Dispensary in the 1770s, only one fistula occurred.[95] But under less enlightened regimes the frequency was probably higher. Paul Portal, writing in 1685, sounded as though he saw them often. In one delivery "I was careful not to injure the mother, for in a number of similar cases I have seen tears in the vagina and even in the urethra and the rectum, from which women suffer great hardship for the rest of their lives, uncontrollably defecating and urinating via the vagina."[96] In a five-year period toward 1900, the gynecology outpatient clinic in Tübingen treated thirty vaginal fistulas, which represented about 1 percent of all patients seen.[97] Is thirty a lot or a few? It depends on how many women in the region gave birth; yet the accident was obviously not extraordinary. Fleetwood Churchill called it in his textbook "not very rare."[98] In a follow-up study in the 1920s of ninety-eight women who had endured "failed forceps outside" deliveries, the Edinburgh Royal Maternity Hospital found three of them fistulous.[99] My reading of this fragmentary evidence is that fistulous women would not have been unfamiliar to the average villager—and it would take only one or two to create a collective sense in the women's culture of how singular was the sexual burden that women had to carry.

Fistulas were the archetypal accidents of "granny deliveries"; and once trained midwives and doctors began to take over, they happened less and less. Horribly protracted labors, where the child's head would be stuck in the vagina for three days, were now terminated by forceps. By the late nineteenth century several authorities agreed that vesicovaginal fistulas in particular—"the one great injury of parturition of former generations"—were now on the decline.[100]

Also during the nineteenth century an operation was devised to correct these fistulas. They had stymied traditional surgeons, who could not figure out how to visualize the relatively inaccessible anterior vaginal wall, and who had trouble keeping the sutures from tearing free. Some successful repairs had been done, the first in the United States being John P. Mettauer's in 1838.[101] But nobody had been able reliably, time after time, to close up fistulas. Then in one of the famous stories of medical history, James Marion Sims, a surgeon in Montgomery, Alabama, was called in 1845 within the space of a month to see three young fistulous black women. Fistulas were a source of considerable alarm to the owners of slaves, for such women were unusable for work and sometimes committed suicide rather than living on "year after year in misery and ostracism." In any event, Sims took these three women into his little cottage hospital, paid their upkeep, and for the next four years tried to discover a cure, finally making himself world-famous by doing so.[102] Ironically, Sims has been much vilified by recent historians for this accomplishment on account of his having "used black slaves for his experiments."* But whatever the ethics of doing gynecology in the antebellum South, Sims's operation became widely done, and the lifelong suffering brought by these incurable fistulas was over.

LACERATIONS

If fistulas declined over the years, a second kind of gynecologic damage probably increased during the nineteenth and early twentieth centuries: tears of the perineum. As the reader will recall, the seam that extends from the base of the vagina to the anus is called the "perineal body," and in a difficult forceps delivery—or if the child's head is too large or the mother's soft parts too rigid—that space will tear apart. If the tear extends to the external anal sphincter muscle, the woman will lose voluntary control over defecation (she may also get a rectovaginal fistula). Thus, given any looseness in her bowel movements, she will soil her clothes and contaminate her vagina. Owing to the greater use of forceps in the nineteenth century, the frequency of this injury probably increased.[104] But as perineal tears may be easily sutured, the epoch at which these tears had greatest significance in women's lives was before 1900, when such tears were commonly not repaired. Then the woman would suffer fecal incontinence for the rest of her life if the tear involved the anus; and even if the tear involved only the perineum, her vagina would hang open from the bottom.

* Thus the account of Sims's life in one popular "women's studies" text: "The pioneering work in gynecological surgery had been performed by Marion Sims on black female slaves he kept for the sole purpose of surgical experimentation. He operated on one of them thirty times in four years, being foiled over and over by post-operative infections. After moving to New York Sims continued his experimentation on indigent Irish women in the wards of the New York Women's Hospital."[103] Fistula is not even mentioned.

In the experience of one eighteenth-century French surgeon, tears involving the anus occurred perhaps once in every thousand deliveries.[105] On 8 September 1704, de la Motte was called to see a young woman about a month after she had given birth. A perineal tear had destroyed her control over her bowel movements, and "she was compelled to defecate without being able to control it for a single instant, which was very incommodious for her, not only on account of her friends, but because she dared not expose herself in public or in going to church, unless at a time when no one was there."[106]

Less drastic perineal tears were far commoner, as I pointed out in chapter 7 (page 171). They also mattered a good deal to the woman concerned. One working-class English mother, just before the First World War, described her first birth: "The time came. I was in labour thirty-six hours, and after all that suffering had to be delivered by instruments, and was ruptured too badly to have anything done to help me. I am suffering from the ill-effects today. This is thirty-one years ago."[107] Thus one sees what women endured before the repairing of such tears became routine.

While the skilled urban midwives I described in chapter 3 did, in fact, repair tears,[108] other traditional birth attendants did not. Jacques Mesnard, a surgeon in Rouen, explained in 1753 that he repaired only tears involving the muscles of the anus; for lesser ones he recommended "anodyne cataplasms."[109] A Frankfurt doctor said in 1884 that local midwives paid no attention to tears of the perineum: "You cannot expect that the midwife is going to summon her archenemy [the doctor] to insert a couple of sutures, and thereby confess to her clients that she has reached the limits of her ability."[110] Marie Stopes, who knew the lives of working-class London women through her clinic, wrote in 1925, "Doctors come away after however serious and painful a delivery and leave the mother with a lacerated cervix, often with a torn perineum, with not only no attempt at an operation to right these things, but without even examining to discover whether they have arisen or not." One woman had "a very badly torn perineum and prolapse."

Stopes asked her, "Don't you suffer a good deal from back-ache?"

"Tears came into her eyes when she replied that her back ached nearly every day, so much so that several times a day she had to lie down with racking pain and was unable to do her house work."[111]

I hesitate to mention this, in view of the calamities not relating to intercourse which these injuries created for women. But, in part, women were sensitive to tears of the perineum because they feared their vaginas would become too big to satisfy their husbands. We know about women's anxiety regarding vaginal size only because of the popularity of various creams that promised to make the vagina return to normal. Midwives sold them. De la Motte fumed against some "myrtle water" that midwives and nurses were selling to this end, and called it an aid to "brutal passions" and, moreover, "illusory."[112]

If the perineal body was torn, a fair chance existed that some of the surrounding muscles of the pelvic floor would be torn as well. Without dwelling on anatomical detail, let me just mention that lacerations of the "urogenital" and the "pelvic" diaphragms weaken the ability of the vagina to resist the intrusion of other abdominal organs. Thus, after a difficult delivery the bladder, the urethra, the intestines, and the rectum may all tend to press in upon the vagina. A woman whose rectum is prolapsing into her vagina, for example, will have to place a finger in the vagina and push the wall of the rectum back as she defecates.[113]

PROLAPSE OF THE UTERUS

The organ, however, that far more than any others would try to press into the vagina after difficult childbearing, was the uterus. When the uterus begins to slide down the birth canal, the condition is called "prolapse," or "falling of the womb." And when the body of the uterus actually hangs outside of the vaginal introitus, dragging an inverted vagina behind it, the condition is called "procidentia." The woman looks as though she has an elephant's trunk between her legs. Procidentia today is very rare. But given the brutal and prolonged labors of yesteryear, it happened often.

First of all, how frequent was prolapse of any kind? Of twenty women laborers whom Gertrud Dyhrenfurth interviewed in the early 1900s in a Silesian village, five had some degree of prolapse.[114] A French midwife, Mme. Rondet, said in 1836 that she had encountered in her practice "a great number of women afflicted for a long time with falling of the womb" and of other pelvic organs. "I sigh when I see these unfortunate creatures condemned to spend all their lives in pain" because they were "too modest to see a doctor." (Mme. Rondet, it must be said, was advertising a pessary she had invented.)[115]

Many of these uteri were fully procident. A Boston hospital, for example, treated 683 of them between 1875 and 1928.[116] A doctor in Port Hudson, Louisiana, expressed astonishment in 1859 at how common it was in slave women. He had seen cases among the field hands in which "the uterus protruded nearly as large as a coconut," and attributed it to the "ignorance and obtrusive interference of our plantation accoucheurs and 'nigger midwives.' "[117] Indeed, in Ilza Veith's view, "it was the observation of uterine prolapse" that suggested to classical medical writers—

who believed that the peregrinations of the womb inside the body were the cause of hysteria—"the possibility of a migratory organ."[118] Hence, in the past the organ often protruded from the vagina.

In women's own perceptions, prolapse, and especially procidentia, must have been like the clap of doom upon their femininity. According to Mme. Rondet, in moderate prolapse "the woman feels the sensation of a foreign body in her vagina and an uncomfortable weight upon her rectum. Walking and long standing make it worse. The least exercise tires her out, and she is at ease only in bed or when sitting." When the uterus actually falls out, Mme. Rondet continued, "it may become inflamed or tumefy, and become so large that it no longer pops back in at night. I have even seen them eaten away by gangrene." (She might have added only that continuous urinary tract infections also accompany advanced prolapse.) In 1834 she saw one patient whose procidentia went back ten years. For the previous eighteen months the woman had not left the house. "I found her with her uterus between the thighs, about the size of the head of a two-year-old child."[119]

Thus one might understand that the village women's culture had devised remedies for this malady. In the household book of one Bourbonnais farmer there were two prayers against uterine prolapse plus one home remedy: "In the name of the Father, the Son and the Holy Spirit you make the sign of the cross with a baby's left shoe; then you take the shoe and push back in the part that is hanging out, saying, 'Saint Blaise, put it back that we may see it no longer.' "[120] A popular English women's health guide from the fifteenth century said, in Beryl Rowland's modern translation, "Sometimes women have such difficulty in bearing a child that the skin between the two privy members [the vagina and the anus] breaks apart and is just a hole, and so the uterus falls out there and grows hard. To help women in this trouble, first boil butter and wine together for half an hour; and when the liquid is all warm put it in the uterus."[121] Many other remedies are to be found in other sources.[122]

One might stress how far prolapse was a disease of lower-class rather than of middle-class women—one reason that our historians of women have taken little note of it. The women of the people were much more likely to have traumatic deliveries, to lurch from bed soon after, and to spend their lives in standing—all predisposing factors (or at least deemed to be by the doctors of the time).[123] Thus Dublin's Thomas Madden in 1872: "The after-effects of lacerations of the perineum are even more distressing with patients of the working class than is the case with women of a higher social condition." His own experience with the "wretched denizens of the crowded tenements of the lanes and back streets of the

capital of the poorest country in Europe has confirmed the observation—
the wives of our artisans and laboring-men undergo far more hardship
and privation, and at the same time perform as much labor as their husbands. The whole of the domestic duties of women of this class . . .
act as powerful predisposing causes of prolapse of the womb." And if
the perineum was destroyed, he continued, *they could not even wear a
pessary to correct it.* [124]

Thus these injuries fit together in a circle of misery: if a woman's
perineal body were not stitched back together, she would be doomed to
live with her prolapsing uterus forever. And even if she could tolerate
a pessary, those available before the vulcanization of rubber were unap-
pealing. Mme. Rondet described the traditional ones available to her working-class clientele: "They become coated with a fairly thick calcareous
incrustation and give off a fetid odor. Thus festering, they become a
permanent cause of irritation . . . of the uterus and vagina, which turn
into sites of ulceration and of abundant purulent discharges." [125]

The effects of these pelvic injuries upon the woman's sexuality can
be imagined. One German doctor saw "a considerable number of women
whose uteri were so greatly sunken that their husbands found it difficult
to insert their penis." [126] According to Dr. Munaret, women seemed to
feel that procidentia made them "disgusting in the eyes of their
husbands." [127]* Members of families afflicted by prolapse did not tend
to leave memoirs about the state of their feelings, so perhaps we shall
never know their true sentiments. Nonetheless, one Los Angeles woman
who suffered from some kind of prolapse and had to wear a pessary,
sought divorce in 1886 because her husband refused to "control his lust-
ful desires" and "unnatural excesses." She was "frequently for weeks
at a time obliged to wear mechanical appliances to keep her parts in
place, but even while wearing such appliances he would force her to
submit." [129]

The story of how prolapse came to be correctible surgically is quite
technical, and I shall not go into it. The essence is that between 1908
and 1921 two surgeons in Manchester, England—Archibald Donald and
William E. Fothergill—worked out the technique of what was called for
a while "the Manchester operation"—appropriately because so many
women in that industrial city suffered from prolapse. [130] The operation
put an end to a lot of useless earlier surgical meddling and erased yet
another source of inequality between the sexes.

---

* Bernard Christian Faust said in 1784 that husbands regarded prolapse as so "disagreeable"
that they would become unfaithful. [128]

The Average Woman and "Women's Diseases"

Today the average woman goes to the doctor 3.5 times a year. Only one tenth of these visits are primarily for "gynecologic" reasons, so whatever may have been true of the past, "women's diseases" today do not dominate the health care of women.[131] Moreover, whether she goes to the doctor or not, the average woman today will have an "acute genito-urinary disorder" only once every ten years. In 1977–78 there were ten such disorders for every one hundred females in the population.[132] Typically today the average woman is laid up with pelvic problems less than one day a year and suffers five times as much time lost from flu.[133*]

How about the past? How prominently did pelvic disorders loom in women's lives? It is partly a matter of whom one listens to. Recalled Paris midwife Louise Bourgeois in 1626, "I used to be astonished to see the village women, up until the day they gave birth, carrying about sheaves of grain on their heads without hurting themselves. The reason for remaining well was that since youth they have been accustomed to this exericise, which relaxes the ligaments." She clearly considered them in blossoming health.[134]

Against her assessment may be balanced Catharine Beecher's informal survey of the health of American women toward the middle of the nineteenth century. In the towns where she stopped on lecture tour, "I requested each lady first to write the initials of ten of the married ladies with whom she was best acquainted in her place of residence. Then she was requested to write at each name, her impressions as to the health of each lady. In this way, during the past year, I obtained statistics from about two hundred different places in almost all the Free States."

A typical entry from this survey:

"Batavia, Illinois. Mrs. H. an invalid. Mrs. G. scrofula. Mrs. W. liver complaint. Mrs. K. pelvic disorders. Mrs. S. pelvic diseases. Mrs. B. pelvic diseases very badly. Mrs. B. not healthy. Mrs. T. very feeble. Mrs. G. cancer. Mrs. N. liver complaint. Do not know one healthy woman in the place."

Beecher then presented evidence from her own family: "I have nine married sisters and sisters-in-law, all of them either delicate or invalids, except two. I have fourteen married female cousins, and not one of them but is either delicate, often ailing, or an invalid. . . . In Boston I cannot remember but one married female friend who is perfectly healthy." Beecher ultimately taxes our credulity, but concluded that "a terrible decay of female health all over the land" had taken place.[135]

Bourgeois versus Beecher. The whole thrust of this book is that Beecher's

---

* Restricted activity: 48.8 days a year per 100 persons, excluding childbirth.

judgment is the more accurate. We saw in the last chapter how women's mortality rates were higher than men's in the time of life when women were most exposed to these diseases. I shall examine in the next chapter a kind of "subculture of suffering" which women erected to shelter themselves against these maladies. At this point an overview of the major women's diseases might be welcome.

To our aid comes a statistic that Dr. Paul Mundé compiled on admissions to the gynecology ward of New York's Mt. Sinai Hospital between 1883 and 1894: "The gynecological patients of Mount Sinai Hospital enjoy all the privileges which can reasonably be expected by patients from the lower classes who pay nothing for either board or medical attendance."[136] So we are talking not about middle-class women who sat around and played the piano all day, but about a heavily immigrant population, desperately poor, whose health was still thoroughly "traditional."

A striking finding of table 10.1 is how few women's diseases were the kind of psychogenic complaints associated with the "Victorian woman." Mt. Sinai was not treating women for "the vapors," "hystero-epilepsy," "ovarian madness," or any of the other mental conditions that a whole generation of historians has now identified with the condition of women in the nineteenth century. The twenty-two "hysteria" patients and the single "nymphomaniac" represent a tiny minority.

Half of the gynecology patients at Mt. Sinai had serious infections: the kinds of pelvic inflammation I have just described, "ovaries filled with pus," infections of the uterus. Unlike the "women on the pedestal" about whom we have heard so much, these were desperately sick people.

A further quarter of the women suffered from long-term sequelae of traumatic labor: lacerated cervixes, perineums split in two, the contents of the pelvis tumbling into the vagina, and eighteen fistulas.

Nine percent were admitted for large tumors and cysts, the smallest portion being for cancer. In general, more than one woman in ten in those years had "fibroid" tumors of the uterus, and some of them would turn up at Mt. Sinai.[137]* But ovarian cysts in particular were the bane of women before the rise of abdominal surgery. The cysts would swell up with fluid to monstrous proportions and have to be tapped periodically through the abdominal wall. Nine hundred and seventy-eight pints of fluid were removed over a period of time from the cyst of one English woman.[139] Nonmalignant uterine tumors could also grow to huge dimensions. So Mt. Sinai was doing surgery to remove such diseased ovaries and uteri. (It must be pointed out that in the shadows of this mainline surgery grew an ominous procedure, called "Battey's Operation," to remove *healthy* ovaries for vague "mental indications." Yet the great major-

---

* James N. West argued that only a small portion of them needed to be removed.[138]

TABLE 10.1

Diagnoses of 3,687 Patients Admitted to the
Gynecologic Service of Mt. Sinai Hospital,
New York (1883–94)

Gynecologic sequelae of childbirth:
  518 cervical lacerations
  184 lacerations of perineum
  65 rectum prolapse (rectocele)
  37 bladder prolapse (cystocele)
  40 uterine prolapse
  13 vesicovaginal fistulas
  __5 rectovaginal fistulas
  862 (23% of all patients admitted)

Pelvic infections:
  691 infections of tubes and ovaries
  626 peritonitis
  297 infections of lining of uterus (endometritis)
  103 pelvic abscesses
  79 infections of pelvic connective tissue (cellulitis)
  28 bladder infections (cystitis)
  __20 vaginitis
  1,844 (50%)

Tumors—cysts:
  10 cysts of broad ligament
  130 uterine "fibroid" tumors
  128 ovarian cysts
  __60 cancer (including 5 breast cancer)
  328 (9%)

Other:
  213 uterine malpositions
  90 overly narrow cervixes ("stenosis")
  31 amenorrhea
  22 hysteria
  1 nymphomania
  296 miscellaneous
  653 (18%)

NOTE: The numbers refer to diagnoses, not to patients, since
a few patients had more than one diagnosis. Obstetrical cases are
excluded from the total.
SOURCE: See notes to tables, page 385.

ity of "oöphorectomies," or removal of ovaries, were done for physical disease.[140]*

The table is silent about "endometriosis," a disease that is common

---

* Lawrence D. Longo finds "inflated about tenfold" Ely van de Warker's often-quoted estimate that 150,000 women had undergone Battey's operation.[141] In 281 operations on the ovaries and tubes between 1883 and 1894, the Mt. Sinai Hospital did only 5 for such "psychic" indications as "reflex neurosis."[142]

among women today and was first diagnosed only in 1921. In endometriosis the kind of tissue that lines the uterus spreads to other organs in the pelvis, causing painful little cysts.*

About one patient in ten, finally, fell into a rather murky grabbag. The 296 "miscellaneous" diagnoses were mainly for infrequent conditions like polyps on the labia and abscesses about the anus. Of interest is the remainder of the "other" category: women admitted for uterine malpositions, overly narrow cervixes, and the like, because it is not clear that these women were really sick. The nineteenth-century medical imagination had its share of fantasies, one of them being that a uterus that tips either too far forward or backward ("anteverted" or "retroverted") was a source of problems and should be treated. Many thousands of useless "uterine suspension" operations were done in order to correct these anomalies, which are largely harmless (save for the backward-tilting uterus which painfully drags down the ovaries or becomes "incarcerated" in the hollow of the sacrum during a pregnancy).[144] Today perhaps 20 percent to 30 percent of the female population has a backward tilting uterus; the vast majority of these uteri cause no symptoms of any kind.[145] In those days, however, surgeons intervened perniciously and needlessly, themselves victims of inadequate medical knowledge. (There are less charitable explanations as well of these many unnecessary operations.) Yet the victims of meddling were remarkably few, compared with those women whom nature, childbirth and their husbands all had victimized by giving them huge cysts, unwanted pregnancies, and "bucketfuls of pus" in their pelvises. If we insist on seeing the nineteenth century as "the age of the womb"—in the sneering phrase of one historian[146]—then it is because these late-nineteenth-century doctors had finally identified ways of surgically relieving women of age-old miseries, and not because a "male medical establishment" had somehow begun "preying" upon previously healthy females.

Indeed, one of the most poignant notes in this whole story is the inability of many outside observers then or now to understand the pain that women were undergoing. It is perhaps to us a surprising point that most women who lived in the past accepted pain as a normal part of their lives. Dr. Jane L. Hawthorne, who practiced at Marie Stopes's London clinic, said, "I had not been attending the Mothers' Clinic more than a few weeks when I began to realize that among the many women coming to the Clinic a large percentage were suffering from disease of the pelvic organs as well as from malformation of the pelvis and pelvic viscera. In the majority of cases the individual was quite unaware of the fact that

---

* John A. Sampson first reported in 1921 endometriosis ("endometriomata") in "perforating hemorrhagic (chocolate) cysts of the ovary."[143]

there was anything wrong." Dr. Maude Kerslake, who also worked in the clinic, added, "One general fact that stands out is the large number of women more or less injured after confinement who seem to consider it is a woman's lot in life always to suffer from various aches and pains and never to expect really good health."[147]

Contrasted with the women's resignation to their suffering, we have the indifference of the outsiders:

· Many of the doctors of the time. A health survey of England in the interwar years found one "woman of 43 who has ten children and three miscarriages (four children have died), has had bad hemorrhage for nine years; this has resulted in a weak heart. Her doctor puts it down to a 'certain age,' and tells her to rest in bed!"[148] Hunter Robb, a Baltimore surgeon, cautioned his colleagues in 1892 about women seeking morphine for "ill-defined pelvic pains." He bridled at the notion of prescribing for patients with "minor pelvic lesions," because "they will seem to demand immediate relief at all hazards. . . . Nervous symptoms predominate in these cases as a rule."[149] Interesting here is Dr. Robb's failure to make any insightful, imaginative leap into the lives of his patients. Were these women actually in pain? And what could be done to alleviate pain? were questions he never asked.

· The *traditional* husbands. I emphasize "traditional" because with modern family life, many husbands became quite sympathetic indeed. The traditional husband, however, usually trivialized or ignored a wife's physical complaints. "If your dog limps or your wife cries, it's not going to be a big surprise," said French peasants. "Women's troubles, like the dawn, both by midday they are gone."[150] In 1889 the twenty-four-year-old wife of a soldier near Odessa appeared at the local hospital. About six weeks before, she had started bleeding from the vagina, had abdominal pain and painful urination. "From that time on, the genital bleeding had continued steadily. Nonetheless, despite her intolerable pain, her husband was unable to abstain from intercourse with her."[151] (In fact, he had ruptured her vagina.) If what I have suggested elsewhere about the empathy of the modern couple is correct, this kind of husbandly indifference would be unusual in the twentieth century.[152] It was, however, normal in all previous centuries, and expected by women.

· Most spectacular, however, has been the failure of some current historians to understand the suffering of women who lived in the past. One study concluded that women who took to their beds because every step was painful, or who complained of deep pelvic pain for which their medical attendants could find no obvious cause, did so because "male chauvinism encouraged women to become invalids."[153] Doctors, in this analysis, wished women to become "weak, dependent, and diseased." And the women went along by adopting the "role of patient." According to another historian, operations on the ovaries were done only to "women too rebellious to be tolerated."[154] Still another historian felt that "largely psychogenic, feminine illness represented a symptom of internal conflicts." There were advantages to invalidism, she says: "Sickness generally meant repeated visits to various doctors and specialists." If women showed symptoms of distress, it was because they were "writhing under the decrees of the era that fettered their activities."[155] In none of this literature is the possibility admitted that women in the past might actually have been sick with vaginal infections or suffered from cystitis or endometriosis. To assert that their maladies were all in their heads ("psychogenic") is to trivialize the experience of these women in exactly the same way as the men of the day trivialized it.

Postscript: The Average Man and "Men's Diseases"

Did men never suffer from diseases of the genitals? Were women the only ones to get sick?

Men did, in fact, suffer from several quintessentially male problems. Yet I shall argue that they were unlikely to have much affected a man's sexual self-image because: (1) these conditions were not frequent, and (2) they occurred very early or very late in life, but rarely in between. At some level, however, these male genito-urinary disorders did become noticed, and mocked, in the village culture. For the Latvian women sang:

> *You ladies have some fun.*
> *I have lost my yearning.*
> *The nut bag of my husband*
> *Cracked open in the middle.*[156]

It is unlikely that many men's scrotums "cracked open in the middle"— an apparent allusion to a testicular abscess. Yet two diseases in particular did afflict males.

EXCESSIVE GROWTH AND INFLAMMATION OF THE PROSTATE GLAND

The prostate sits just beneath the bladder, surrounding the male urethra. While an *inflamed* prostate ("prostatitis") makes ejaculation and urination very painful, an *enlarged* prostate ("benign prostatic hypertrophy") closes off the urethra, making it hard to pass water. Rarely before age forty do men's prostate glands start to enlarge, but when they do, the condition rivals in dreadfulness any of the women's disorders I have described. "The most distressing accompaniment of an enlarged prostate," explained James Hingeston, is that the rectum bulges out at the anus, "presents itself red and excessively tender, with a copious drainage of mucus." The prolapsed anus and the accompanying hemorrhoids "result from the powerful muscular efforts which the patient makes to expel his urine. In the act of micturition [urinating], he straddles his legs, bends his body forward, and grows red in the face; the anus descends, and the feces sometimes escape at the same moment into the old man's clothes, while the urine drips out along the urethra, drop by drop, hot as melted lead [the man probably had an infection, too]. . . . Life becomes a loathsome burden to himself, and an offence to all who are concerned about him." And so forth, until the penis, buttocks, and thighs become benumbed, "and the patient only suffers from the sense of a large ball lodged in the rectum, and this ball he is always straining to expel."[157] Finally the urine backs up to the kidneys, and he dies of uremia, if he is lucky, for that is a relatively gentle death. If not, he will die of blood poisoning as some portion of his urinary tract ruptures or becomes infected. "He died in the greatest pain," said Thomas Shapter of one of his Devonshire patients. "On this occasion I witnessed the paroxysms of pain expressed by loud and bitter laughter."[158]

So older men would not escape a sense that nature had designed for them special trials, just as uterine cancer was the "angel of death" of the women's world. Yet not many men died of things like "retention of urine" (which we may assume to be caused mainly by an overgrown prostate). In Geneva from 1730 to 1739 only 16 did so, out of 1,550 adult male deaths.[159] Although the men's death rate from "nonvenereal diseases of the genito-urinary system" in England between 1848 and 1872 was almost three times as high as the women's, such deaths were nonetheless only 1.4 percent of all male deaths. By contrast, in England women's cancer death rates were more than twice as high as men's, to say nothing of women's mortality from childbed, ovarian diseases, and so forth. Moreover, in the prime of life—let us say ages twenty-five to forty-four when women were most exposed to childbed deaths—very few English men died of genito-urinary causes.[160]*

STONE

Traditional men were far more subject than were women to stones of the urinary tract—hard little pebbles of uric acid which, when caught in the kidney or ureter, cause agonizing spasms of pain, and which in the bladder can block the outflow of urine, in addition to being wildly painful. France's Emperor Louis Napoleon III died of bladder stone in 1873.[161] So did fifteen Breslau men in the years 1687 to 1691; only ten

* At ages twenty-five to forty-four the obstetric death rate was three times as high as the male genito-urinary death rate.

women.[162] In general fifteen to twenty men fell ill with bladder stone for every woman.[163] As a "male disease," bladder stone has a history stretching back to Hippocrates (kidney and ureter stones being generally undiagnosable before the invention of the X-ray). Hippocrates, however, recommended that physicians not involve themselves with the removal of stones, and over the centuries a special corps of "lithotomists" outside the medical profession devoted themselves to making an incision in the bladder by going via the rectum, and then jerking out the stone with a hook or with forceps.

The operations of these "town-square" lithotomists (who pursued their profession in public, in the town square) are among the most grizzly in all the accounts of traditional medicine. Relatively ignorant of the complex anatomy of the region, these stone-cutters would slice through major arteries, causing great pain and much loss of blood. In an operation in 1831 in Gloucester, England, the surgeon, after several failed efforts to extract the stone, approached the patient with an air of "dreadful determination to succeed. His right foot was placed . . . against a chair, which was supported by a pupil; the scene became animated, though horrible. The straining and creaking of the forceps, as they occasionally lifted the suffering wretch from the table (they twice pulled him off it)—his wild, agonizing shrieks, and entreaties for forbearance, after continuing for nearly two hours, gradually became more faint. . . . When the stone was shown to him it was doubtful whether he saw it. . . . He expired a few minutes after being carried to his bed."[164] But so exquisite was the pain of bladder stone that men were willing to submit. The Marechal de Lorges at the court of Louis XIV watched a master lithotomist, the famous "Frère Jacques" of the children's song, operate successfully upon twenty-two poor patients, all of whom survived, before undergoing it himself, and succumbing.[165]

Yet in statistical terms bladder stone does not seem to have been common, in either sex. In 1834, Dr. John Forbes of Landsend in Cornwall thought it rare; he had noted only three in the Dispensary register in seventeen years, and had not seen one personally. He wrote, "Dr. Montgomery, who has resided in this district many years, informs me that he has only met with one case of stone in the bladder, and had been informed of two others."[166] Thomas Shapter, writing of Exeter in 1842, said that stone of the bladder is "comparatively rare here," and that urinary disorders generally were "not very frequent," except late in life.[167] Thus, although stone, as a surgical challenge, has attracted attention in the history of medicine, it is unlikely to have figured greatly in the lives of ordinary men.

Over the last century bladder stone has greatly decreased. It seems likely that as societies become increasingly industrialized, the location of stone moves up the urinary tract.[168] Thus, bladder stone in East Anglia declined from 187 cases admitted to a hospital in the 1870s, to 27 in the 1940s. Stones in the kidney or ureter, on the other hand, have now become frequent; and because of them, each year 1 man in every 100 will seek out a doctor.[169]

Prostate disorders have become an even greater threat in men's lives. A forty-year-old man today has a one in ten chance of facing surgery for benign prostate enlargement if he lives to be eighty.[170] And prostatic cancer among older men is now the third most common cancer, after lung and colon-rectum. It is found at autopsy in up to 46 percent of all men.[171]* Perhaps if all those traditional men had lived to be eighty, they would have faced these problems as well. But they did not; and at age thirty-seven in 1800 prostate disorders did not loom prominently.

Ironically, urinary disorders have shifted from being men's to women's diseases. In 1977–78 in the United States, 8 percent of all women visited a doctor for a urinary condition (mainly bladder infections), and only 3 percent of all men did so (the most important single complaint being infections of the urethra not caused by V.D.). Genital disorders, despite the upsurge of prostate complaints, remain today heavily female. While 4 percent of all men sought out a doctor in 1977–78 for genital complaints (of which prostate infections were most important), 17 percent of all women did so.[172]

So how does the fact that genito-urinary disorders have now become a female rather than a male problem help "liberate" women, in view of my contention that women have become freed of the physical complaints that were the anchor of their sexual submission in past times? The answer is that toward 1900 genito-urinary problems started to become easily correctible for both sexes, with the exception of infections, for which relief would appear only in the late 1930s. At the same time as hysterectomy for fibroids was introduced for women, safer bladder-stone operations, which involved making an incision above the pubic bone rather than in the rectum, were coming in for men. In the 1920s, as abdominal surgery for ovarian problems was becoming relatively risk-free, surgeons devised new techniques for treating the prostate gland in men (by inserting a tool in the penis rather than continuing to poke about in the perineum).[173]† Thus these dreadful genital and urinary conditions were ameliorated for both sexes at once, resulting in a sexual "advantage" for neither.

* In men older than fifty. Only one third of the cases found at autopsy are "manifest clinically."

† Suprapubic prostatectomy, also an important procedure, was first described in 1887; yet transurethral resection was to become the more common.

CHAPTER 11

Changing Alliances and the End of Victimization

THIS BOOK BEGAN in an effort to find the origins of modern feminism. One reason has now become fairly clear for the fact that women in the seventeenth century were not demanding the vote or insisting on being admitted to a university: they had an overwhelming physical disadvantage in relation to men. Before 1900, women were saddled with large numbers of unwanted children; they were less well fed than men, were dragged down by anemia, enervated by all kinds of diseases for which there is no male counterpart, and in every way imaginable denied the platform of physical equality which is the ultimate launching pad of personal autonomy.

But there is a second reason. I remarked in the preface on the striking fact that in past times, not only were women objectively at a disadvantage, but that subjectively they accepted their disadvantaged status as part of the natural order. They concurred in society's judgment that they were poisonous, diseased, and inferior. And as long as they believed this about themselves, feminism—which presupposes a basic equality between men and women—would have been unthinkable.

In this final chapter I attempt to do two things: to show how women acquiesced to the male view that femininity was corrupt and dangerous; and to suggest that at the roots of modern feminism lay a fundamental switching of alliances, once women began to cast off this view of themselves. As the various kinds of victimization I have described in this book began around 1900 to dissolve, women were in the process of turning from other women to men as their main source of emotional support. The village women's culture assumed that a woman's best friends were other women, that only women could give solace for the sufferings that life had in store. When women began to see femininity as a basically positive rather than a negative force, they left the women's culture behind and sought out men as their major emotional allies. Men have changed, in other words, from being women's enemies to being their best friends.

Traditional Male Fears of Women's Bodies

It is probable that male fear of demonic "feminine" qualities had existed since the dawn of time. The high culture of Western civilization is drenched in this theme from the Greek tragedies on. Through popular culture as well rode a visceral male fear of women's "magical" powers. According to Martine Segalen, the French proverbs "that compare the woman to a devil are doing more than evoking metaphoric allusions. We see from these rituals that she has the power to evoke the devil, that she is the devil herself." Thus, according to one body of proverbs, "a husband who beats his wife will undergo her magical vengeance, notably in the form of her sexual domination."[1]

This male fear of women's sexual power strikes the keynote: something about the uterus, and the sexual and reproductive functions associated with it, represents a magical threat to men. Because the culture of traditional Europe was dominated by male visions, these fears of women's physical qualities were to become incorporated in the culture as a whole, and to end up being believed by both men and women.

Of all male fears of women, most wrenching was the fear of the uterus. Ever since Hippocrates, academic medicine had assigned to the uterus bizarre qualities, such as the ability to wander about the abdomen or to send the woman into hysterical fits.[2] But these attributes, amplified fearfully many times, turn up as well in popular culture, among people who had never read a medical textbook nor had any notion of "academic" medical teachings. This folklore also survives long past the demise of academic theories about uterine influences.

In much of Europe's popular culture, the uterus was thought to be alive—not just part of a living body, but a separate animate creature housed inside a woman. And an elaborate body of folklore existed for feeding or appeasing this animal once it became aroused, causing "colic" or "macica." Some people thought of the uterus as a frog "with many legs that is supposed to stay in the body, because you have to die when the colic [or frog] creeps out to your throat."[3] According to one account from the Tirol, a woman became ill on a pilgrimage and lay down on the grass. "Scarcely was she asleep when the uterus, and the attaching ligaments crept out of her mouth into a brook, swam around and crawled back inside. When she awakened, she was healed."[4] Imagining the uterus as a live animal presupposed an enormous peasant ignorance of anatomy, the more so because, according to one Tirolean woodcutter, a man could have a uterus too, which would creep from *his* mouth as well.[5] Yet certain it was in peasant folklore, that uteri were mainly the property of women.

Even among peasants who did not animalize the uterus, the view prevailed that it could migrate about the human body. "Globus hystericus," or inability to swallow, was ascribed in these regions to the uterus rising in the throat. And to get it back down, a woman needed merely repeat, "Womb high, womb low, get back to the old place that God has sent you. In the name of God the Father, the Son, . . ." et cetera. The victim would thereupon make the sign of the cross three times.[6]

To persuade the demonic uterus to behave, women in Saxony would conjure it, "Womb you rascal, get the hell back to your own house."[7] Whereupon presumably the aches of uterine cancer, or whatever "woman's disease" was being cured, would subside. The point is that any organ to which such life-threatening, life-saving qualities were assigned could not help but take on a fearsome aspect in the eyes of men. If the demonic bodies of women had to be controlled, it was first because of the uterus inside them.

One fearful thing to emerge from the uterus was menstrual blood. Male phobias about the menses are as old as time and known in virtually every society on record.[8] Albertus Magnus, a thirteenth-century medical scholar, said that a priest had asked him to write his book about the "Secrets of Women" because "menstruating women carried with them a poison that could kill an infant in its cradle."[9] Guillaume de la Motte described how a menstruating servant woman had turned his white wine into vinegar by touching the bottle: "It was so sour that no one could drink it."[10] Thus the traditional medical mind.

Menstrual taboos lingered far longer in the peasant mind. Even in our own century, menstruating women in Provence had to keep themselves "strictly away" from the wine cellars while vinification was taking place.[11]

And these taboos stretched from wine to virtually everything else on the table. In the Sologne district a menstruating woman could not touch the salted pork or approach the newly killed pig. She would cause the salad dressing to spoil, the mayonnaise to curdle, the very flowers in the fields to lose their aroma.[12] In Hungary the menstruating woman was barred from making preserves, sauerkraut, pickles, or "paradise apples" or from baking bread. And if her husband had sex with her, he would be "unclean for seven days."[13]

One might argue that women themselves have always rejected these raging male fantasies, confident in the knowledge of their untruth. But, no. Women in Europe's traditional culture seem to have agreed about the toxicity of their own menses. In the late 1960s a couple of ethnographers interviewed women in a French village about whether salt pork would go bad if a menstruating woman touched it. Although there was some divergence of opinion, one woman did say, "Oh boy! Once I caused the entire barrel to go bad. It's true. I wasn't thinking at all. I just went in there. And when I went back later for some more bacon, it was all green."[14] One could cite the ritual purification of orthodox Jewish women after menstruation, or Hildegard of Bingen's view of the menses as punishment for sin, as further evidence that women in the past internalized the assumption that their own discharges were polluted.[15]

Even more ghastly, however, were the emanations of the *pregnant* uterus. Later pronatalism on the part of officials has covered the tracks of traditional male unease about the uncleanliness of pregnancy. European lords and officials who wanted for populationist reasons to see the number of bodies on their lands increase, made certain that pregnant women received special favors, rather than suffer discrimination.[16] Yet beneath the officialdom, traditional European society harbored profound suspiciousness about the pregnant woman's power to contaminate the world about her. In Finland, according to Pelkonen, she "was not permitted to attend church or to show herself in public places; and she was requested not to attend baptismal feasts." In Finland's Swedish-speaking coastal areas it was explicitly written that she is "not worth any more than a sow. She should keep as much as possible at home and not mix among others, and all this not just because people think she is more susceptible to evil spirits, but because she would contaminate others with her uncleanliness."[17] In one part of Hungary it was believed that not only the mother was unclean but *all the women who had come in contact with her during birth* as well (my italics). None of these women were permitted to cook, make dough, or do the laundry during this period.[18]

A religious practice called "churching" provided the most consistent evidence of a male disposition to believe women's bodies dangerous to society. Churching is a religious decontamination of the new mother four to six weeks after delivery and gives her permission to re-enter society. The custom was found among the rites of all the Christian churches, east and west, before the Protestant Reformation and, even though rejected by the Puritans, continued to be practiced in the Anglican and Catholic churches until the twentieth century. According to Leviticus 12: 2–8, a woman shall be unclean for seven days after the birth of a boy, and for fourteen days after the birth of a girl. For a further thirty-three days in the case of a boy, and sixty-six days for a girl, she shall not enter the sanctuary. Finally she shall make offerings to the priest at the door of the tabernacle, when she shall be "cleansed from the issue of her blood."

These biblical utterances continued to resonate powerfully in European society two thousand years later. Here's what happened if a woman left her own property before she was churched: "In Liebau people believe that if a new mother goes into a strange house before she's had the religious ceremony, it will burn down. Hirschberg people ward her off with a broom if they see her coming. In Jauer she is not permitted to fetch water from the well before churching, or else it will become contaminated or dry up."[19] In Heveser County in Hungary the new mother would be churched and her infant baptised after two weeks; thereupon "there's a big cleanup. The house is freshly whitewashed, thoroughly polished up and sprinkled with holy water."[20]

The mechanics of the ceremony drove home even more forcefully the point that a woman was *contaminated* in the act of giving birth. In the Münsterland the new mother remains standing at the door of the Protestant church until the pastor fetches her, "his surplice in one hand. The mother grips the surplice with her left hand, holding a consecrated candle in the right. The pastor begins to pray, and thus do both advance to the altar. Here the pastor reads from the beginning of the Book of John, after which he lets the mother kiss the appropriate page of the Bible."[21] Similarly, among French Catholics in Alsace, the mother awaited the priest at the door of the church after Mass. "She is sprinkled with holy water, and handed a lighted candle. After giving thanks to the Virgin, the mother kisses the hem of the priest's robe, and lets herself be led to the altar, where she deposits an offering."[22] The message to the mother is clear: You're contaminated.

What is striking is the extent to which women themselves, and their female neighbors, insisted on churching, rather than just going along reluctantly with the dictates of male society. Women in late-medieval Flanders would no more do without churching than without baptism, according to one scholar: "Every woman, married or not, feverishly rushes toward this rite of 'purification.' " People said that a mother who died before her churching did not have the right to be buried in a cemetery.[23]* There were "parts of England where the neighbours will not allow a woman who has recently been confined to enter their houses until she has been churched."[24]

If a mother died in giving birth or perished of an infection before churching, traditional peasants mobilized a final set of defenses to protect themselves from her. Death, for Europe's peasants, was always enveloped in ominousness, and a rich folklore surrounded the odors of a disease like cancer, a "burning sensation on the fingers" being ascribed to a discharge from the cancerous uterus. But most foreboding of all was the death of a mother in childbed because she was in a position to do magical harm to the community. Given how common death in childbirth was, traditional Europe had frequently to confront the question.

The dying mother's very appearance spelled gloom. "Dwarves are responsible for the death of many a new mother," they said in the Weichsel-land. "You can see that her face has been scratched up by the beards of the fellows."[25] In Toulon they went through the paces of churching anyway, even if the mother had died, to ward off the baleful consequences of her soul remaining on earth. "People gathered in the victim's room; her clothes and her jewelry were laid out on the bed. The godmother brought over new shoes. The infant was dressed, and then when the church bell sounded, the godmother cried out to the dead mother, 'Missus, Mass is going to start. Let's get going.' Then the cortège left the bedroom, and if they heard the creaking of planks on the floor or the stairs, they said, 'It's the soul of the mother in her new shoes who's going to the churching mass.' "[26]

Some of the justifications for outfitting the dead mother with new shoes sound benign. "If a woman dies in childbed," they said in Alsace, "she leaves behind her a living infant. Before burying her, it's necessary to give her a pair of well-made and solidly nailed shoes, for the road to eternity is long, and she'll have to take it back each night for four weeks in order to nurse her child."[27]† But villagers had to face a more alarming possibility: that the mother's soul might return to haunt them if she were not properly disposed of. The superstitious of Provence believe that, unless churched properly, the mother's dead soul would come back and *insist* on it. So goes a story that a shopkeeper whose wife had died in childbed omitted the churching and, instead, quickly remarried one of his employees. The new bride was haunted by tapping sounds when she was alone, and only after she had laid out the former wife's clothes on

---

* The Church, however, resisted this view of burial.

† G. Lammert said in 1869 that people put slippers under the bed of the dead mother for six weeks because during this time she returns each night to look for her child.[28]

the bed and conformed to the other details of the "retroactive churching" did the soul depart in peace.[29] To make sure that the mother's soul departed, peasants in North Friesland would throw a needle, thread, some linen cloth, and a pair of scissors into the open grave, "so that she'd be able to get along," and not return as a specter.[30]

Around the year 1000 peasants in Saxony had more radical means to ensure that undelivered mothers who had died in birth would not return to haunt them: they drove a stake through her and her unborn child in the grave. (The village women would also drive a stake through an infant who had died before baptism, in order to make sure that it would not arise from its grave and do damage.) Fears of this kind persisted in Saxony until at least the sixteenth century.[31]

To protect the community, corpses of women who had died in childbirth were often buried off in a corner of the cemetery, next to the murderers and suicides, or indeed buried outside the cemetery wall entirely. Despite Martin Luther having thundered in 1525 against the practice of putting dead mothers "behind the cemetery wall," we find in 1528 the Breslau City Council insisting that new mothers not be buried "along the walkway, where people go by or have business to do, but away in a corner or next to the wall where there is little activity."[32] In 1713 the Breslau Protestant Consistory reviewed the question: "It was earlier the custom here to surround new mothers' graves with fences in order not to infect other people with the contagious matter with which their bodies were full. But the supposed uncleanliness of these poor women does not exist," wrote one of their legal experts. Nonetheless the Breslau City Council decided to continue burying dead mothers outside the cemetery, and within protective gates, to preserve passers-by from their "corrupt emanations."[33]

Make no mistake. It was to protect the community from the dead mother, and not vice versa, that these measures were taken. The village of Niebusch stipulated in 1790 that women who had died in childbirth were to be buried apart because "all women between fifteen and forty-nine would pay dearly if they happened to walk over her grave accidentally at a certain time of month."[34] Further protection was assured the Silesians by tying a linen string around four stakes marking the edges of the new mother's grave, in the belief that "maidens and young wives would die in their own childbed if they were to cross such a grave."[35] In a village near Essen a white handkerchief was secured atop the grave with four posts, because, unlike the other deceased, mothers would ascend into heaven only after the cloth had moldered away.[36]

These mothers were, then, contaminated; and if you wanted to punish your boy friend for his faithlessness, you had, in Bohemia, only to throw some dirt from such a grave into his face.[37] What could better be calculated to drive home the message: Women's bodies are dangerous.

Female Bonding as a Defense against Male Fears

In the other chapters in this book I have argued that the women's culture was a culture of "solace," a place where the bodily misery of womanhood would find understanding. But the women's culture functioned also to defend women from the malignant aggression of men.

How did traditional women respond to the terrible insults to their sexuality we have just seen? To some extent, of course, they accepted male views, internalizing the belief that their menstrual blood was sullied, their lochia dangerous to society. Otherwise, they would have refused their subordination. Even today it is other women, and not men, who in parts of Africa perform the mutilating "female circumcision" rites, showing to what extent women are capable of internalizing male myths about themselves.[38] Similarly, in traditional Europe midwives helped internalize the view of childbed as a time of contamination by taking the infant to church for baptism, so that the "unchurched" mother could remain at home.[39]

Yet there slumbered underground a current of female resistance to these male fears, and it represents the main form of female "bonding" in traditional society. I shall argue that this female solidarity crystallized around childbirth and the lying-in period, the time when women were considered most dangerous to the external world.

Of course, other occasions for bonding among women existed as well. One thinks of the work bees that occupied several evenings a week each winter: many were women-and-girls-only affairs, though so often were men included that it is hard to see the custom as a quintessentially female experience.[40] Martine Segalen has shown how exclusively feminine was the periodic household laundry: "No man would dare approach the laundry, so feared is this group of women, whose power is increased by their number."[41] Village women were willing to intervene in wife beating much sooner than were village men, as Roderick Phillips has pointed out for Rouen.[42] Preparing for the pre-Lenten Carnival, for the annual harvest home, and for the other ceremonies that dotted the village calendar gave married women many occasions to be together.[43] But on none of these occasions did men deem them to be contaminated, *nor did they deem themselves to be vulnerable.* Only in childbed did this whole mesh of fear and vulnerability between the sexes become visible.

Accordingly we observe much female bonding, some of it explicitly against males, in the period of delivery and lying-in. When, as we saw in chapter 4, the neighbor women clustered about the bed of the birthing mother, they were offering support. But something else was going on as well. "A new mother should never be alone," said the villagers. And when the other women were present, they performed various rites around her bed—as, for example, in Austria removing their aprons and tying them crosswise as a binder about her abdomen. This kind of ceremony helped ward off "all that brings evil and harm."[44]

After the birth some kind of "women's feast" would take place. It might be at the time of baptism (remember that the mother was not actually at the baptism) or simply in celebration of a successfully negotiated birth. Reinhard Worschech stresses the specifically female character of these baptismal fetes: "For the female community, baptism is the most important event in a person's life."[45] One local count forbade in 1619 these parties "because until now many of them have drawn a great number of women; after the baptism they are offered not just a meal with all its unnecessary costs, but also much singing, screaming, laughing, and commotion which takes place in the new mother's presence."[46] The midwives of Speyer were admonished in 1775 to prevent these celebrations, "because in the countryside it is custom that new mothers overeat and drink too much at these baptismal parties. . . . All commotion must be kept away from the new mothers."[47] In the Hunsrück region all the neighbor women customarily visited a new mother. And they came with their own children, who brought presents for the baby. By the nineteenth century, an ethnographer tells us, "such visits were not conceivable without the Hunsrück 'national drink,' brandy; nor were they conceivable without much yelling and screaming. Thus it was ordered in Sponheim County that before and after a delivery not more than four women should be present with the new mother, and that an appropriate stew should be served."[48] These postpartum fêtes were said to last in some areas "for days."[49] They are found in France as well and everywhere formed an intimate part of the life of traditional peasant women.[50] Note that these were women's festivals, no men invited. It is significant that the one big women's fête in village life took place at the time when women were thought to be most contaminated: childbirth.

Bonds of female solidarity tightened finally when the new mother lay dying. In the Allgäu it was the neighbor women who did the death watch if another woman had died (pregnant or not).[51] A church order of 1521 in Franconia specified that the corpse of a new mother should be borne to the funeral service by other women: "In front of the church the corpse is sprinkled with holy water by the priest; then the women bear the body into the church."[52] Although it was unusual for neighbor women to serve as pallbearers, in both Germany and France they nonetheless constituted themselves as a separate group in the church service and in the funeral cortège.[53]

Why do we not know more about these key rituals in a woman's life? Why are the details to be garnered only in obscure ethnographies? It is because this aspect of women's culture was regarded with massive uneasiness by men, because recovery celebrations after childbirth and funeral arrangements for dead mothers inspired the deepest male fears of the magical powers in women's bodies. In other words, what the women suffer should remain their own business. As they said in Alsace: "Women's problems at dawn are gone like the morning dew."[54] The message is: We men don't want to know about it.

The Demystification of Women's Bodies

In the long haul from traditional society to the rational bourgeois culture of the early twentieth century, men's fears of women's bodies largely vanish. Accordingly, a mainstay of female bonding has been cut away, and an entirely new gender pattern of political affiliation has emerged. Women have begun to see other men, especially their husbands (and to a lesser extent their doctors)—instead of other women—as their main allies. Female bonding, if my argument is right, has thus been vanquished both by improvements in health and by the companionate marriage.[55]

In this interpretation I oppose a considerable corpus of recent scholarship that argues that in the nineteenth and early twentieth centuries women found themselves in *opposition* to the "snare of family sentiment."[56] It seems to me more likely that the romanticizing of male-female relations that occurred in the nineteenth-century companionate marriage *liberated* women from this terrible burden of traditional male fear. As new ties of sentiment snaked out to enmesh the couple, men's previous anxieties about the malefic powers of women's bodies were put to rest or, at least, pushed deep down into the psyche.

What evidence exists for my interpretation? For one thing, it is clear that traditional forms of female bonding did expire. One doesn't see thirty neighbor women standing around the delivery suite of a modern hospital. In rural France in the twentieth century women still clustered about the delivery scene, but increasingly mothers were saying, "I never liked all that. I told my mother-in-law, please leave. You can't believe the fuss that caused." Who was asked to remain behind? "I told my husband, you stay."[57] Some scholars have argued tha' ie woman's emotional isolation in modern marriage created new forms of bonding among women.[58]

Yet by the mid-nineteenth century the modern couple's insistence upon family intimacy and privacy had clearly weakened the strength of the emotional associations women were able to sustain with each other outside the nuclear family. One scholar has shown, for example, that starting around 1830 American husbands began to replace neighbor women in participating in a wife's childbirth.[59]

For another thing, there are hints of a transition period in which the death of a new mother is still seen as a distinctive kind of death, but the special burial rites now protect *her* from the baleful influences of the surrounding world, rather than the community from her. An ethnographer writing just before the First World War explained the Württemberg custom of putting four posts and a rope around a new mother's grave as an effort to "preserve her peace."[60] In some Württemberg counties "new mothers are so highly esteemed that if they die, people believe they become blessed."[61] It was true that, in the Swiss Vorderprättigau, people accorded the corpse of a new mother special attention, letting her lie longer on the bier than other deceased—but only to make sure that they did not risk burying someone alive.[62]

Not too much should be made of these isolated examples of apparent sentimentality in the singling out of new mothers for special treatment among the dead. Yet the contrast between them and the Saxon practice of driving a stake through her body is nonetheless striking. The sentimental mode of family life had doubtless imposed itself by the time these newer practices were recorded. So perhaps we have in these reformed rites a litmus test for male fears. In any event, after the 1920s full-term maternal deaths became so rare that any apparatus of custom surrounding them fell inevitably into desuetude, and death in childbed ceased to be a focus for female bonding.

But that is a technical explanation for the decline of this complex interaction of male fear and female response. It is similarly technical to argue that male fears of women began to evaporate because medicine was able to demonstrate that women did not have live frogs in their bellies, and that the horrible odors of puerperal infection were caused by bacterial rather than by demonic action.

Behind these technical changes, however, lies a vast drama of cultural change as well, in which the old women's culture was dissolving, making way for the romantically involved couple of the modern world. The dissolution of this culture occurred in two stages. First, new styles of family sentiment burst on the scene around 1800, making men more receptive to tenderness. This new style of family life—middle-class in origin—also encouraged women to spend more time with their husbands and families than with other women. All this happened late in the eighteenth or early in the nineteenth century (except among the peasantry), and was not in the slightest initiated by the changes in health discussed in this book, which generally occurred about a hundred years later. But the "modern family" gravely undermined the women's culture.

The death knell of the women's culture was not, however, sounded until women ceased to need a "culture of solace." Only then—after the suffering that had provided the initial impetus for women to hang together, had come to an end—would female bonding cease or, at least, cease to be a major rival of the family. By the 1920s the classical pattern of women's suffering had ended. The physical problems that had driven women into each other's arms for comfort since time out of mind had been alleviated by modern medicine, by relatively safe and accessible abortion, by a shift in mortality patterns to the disadvantage of men, and by the many other changes we have seen in this book. As a result, no physical reason remained either for fearing men's contempt or for seeking sisterly solace; and the shift in allegiance from the women's culture to the family was completed.

The first quarter of the twentieth century has often appeared as the decisive period for these health changes. That is also the time of the first of the two great surges of feminism in the twentieth century. The evidence is, thus far, purely circumstantial, but it suggests to me that this first great wave of feminist enthusiasm was made possible by the securing of good health for women. If I am right about this conjunction of health, feminism, and modern family life, the first surge of feminism would turn out to have taken place in alliance with men rather than in the context of traditional women's culture. The men were "new men," remolded by the modern family into affectionate husbands, and quite unlike the contemptuous, brutal males we have seen in most of this book. This strikes me as a nice irony and reminds us how short is the historical pedigree of the *second* great wave of feminism in our century, that occurring between 1965 and 1980, which would take place in alliance against men.

APPENDIX

Sources for the "200-Year Survey" of Maternal Sepsis Deaths*

The survey rests on a sampling of the enormous literature on puerperal fever. I tried to find accounts of individual cases that gave the date of parturition, the date of onset, and, where fatal, the date of death.

INFECTED AT HOME

Percivall Willughby, *Observations in Midwifery* (East Ardsley: SRP, 1972), reprint of a 17th-century manuscript, pp. 79–80, 105–06, 127–29, 171–72. Four cases in and near Derby, 1638–69.

Paul Portal, *La Pratique des accouchemens* (Paris, 1685), pp. 183–86, 291–94. Two cases in Paris, 1671 and 1679.

François Mauriceau, *Observations sur la grossesse et l'accouchement des femmes* (Paris, 1694), pp. 45–46. One case in Paris, 1672.

Phillippe Peu, *La Pratique des accouchemens* (Paris, 1694), pp. 231–34. One case in Paris, date unknown.

Guillaume Mauquest de la Motte, *Traité complet des accouchemens*, rev. ed. (Leiden, 1729), pp. 228–29, 454, 578, 580–81, 584, 623–28, 631–34, 722. Thirteen cases in and around Valognes (Normandy), 1683–1721.

Johann Storch, *Weiberkranckheiten*, 8 vols. (Gotha, 1746–53), VI, 171, 201. Two cases, probably in Gotha, 1722.

Frederick Hoffmann, *Opera Omnia physico-medica*, 2nd ed., 6 vols. (Geneva, 1740), II, 73. August Hirsch states that Hoffmann's three cases occurred as part of a 1725 epidemic in Frankfurt. *Handbuch der historisch-geographischen Pathologie*, 2nd ed., 3 vols. (Stuttgart, 1881–86), III, 292.

Georg Wilhelm Christoph Consbruch, *Medicinische Ephemeriden nebst einer medicinischen Topographie der Grafschaft Ravensberg* (Chemnitz, 1793), p. 139. One case, date not given.

William Butter, *An Account of Puerperal Fevers as They Appear in Derbyshire* (London, 1775), pp. 34–48. The case I selected occurred in 1765.

Ernest Gray, ed., *Man Midwife: The Further Experiences of John Knyveton, M.D. . . . During the Years 1763–1809* (London: Robert Hale, 1946), pp. 22–23, 27. Two cases in London, 1765–66.

Charles White, *A Treatise on the Management of Pregnant and Lying-In Women* (London, 1772), pp. 246–51, 254–57, 283–85, 290–95, 300–02. Seven cases in Manchester, 1770–72; one elsewhere.

Friedrich Osiander, *Beobachtungen . . . Krankheiten der Frauenzimmer* (Tübingen, 1787), pp. 3–12. One case in Kassel, 1781.

* Listed in chronological order by date of publication or by date of a particular case taken from a publication. For abbreviations used in references, see page 318.

Alexander Gordon, *A Treatise on the Epidemic Puerperal Fever of Aberdeen* (London, 1795). Reprinted in Charles Meigs, ed., *History, Pathology and Treatment of Puerperal Fever* (Philadelphia, 1842). I took only seven of the seventy-seven cases he describes, 1788–91, pp. 36–46 of the Meigs edition.

Kenneth Cameron, ed., *Shelley and His Circle, 1773–1822* (Cambridge, Mass.: Harvard University Press, 1961), I, 186–95. The death of Mary Wollstonecroft, London, 1797.

William Hey, *A Treatise on the Puerperal Fever . . . in Leeds and its Vicinity 1809–1812* (London, 1813). I took the first three of twenty-six cases, 1809–10. Reprinted in Meigs, *Puerperal Fever*, pp. 88–101.

John Armstrong, *Facts and Observations Relative to the Fever Commonly Called Puerperal* (1814). Reprinted in Meigs. I took three cases, Sunderland, 1813, pp. 204–14 in the Meigs edition.

Thomas West, "Observations on some Diseases, particularly Puerperal Fever, which occurred in Abingdon . . . 1813 and 1814," *London Medical Repository*, 3 (1815), 103–05. General account.

Augustus B. Granville, *A Report of the Practice of Midwifery at the Westminster General Dispensary during 1818* (London, 1819), pp. 161–78. Eight cases.

Case book of Gideon A. Mantell, a doctor in Lewes. Three cases from 1820; the document is currently in the possession of the Alexander Turnbull Library in Wellington, New Zealand.

William Campbell, "Observations on the Disease usually termed Puerperal Fever," *Edinburgh Medical and Surgical Journal*, 18 (1822), 195–225. I took two of fifteen cases in this epidemic, Edinburgh, 1821.

Robert Lee, "Cases of Severe Affections of the Joints after Parturition," *LMG*, 3 (1829), 663–66. Case in London, 1828.

John Roberton, "Is Puerperal Fever Infectious?" *LMG*, 9 (1832), 503–05. An epidemic in Manchester, 1830–31.

T. Ogier Ward, notice, *LMG*, 14 (1834), 815–16. Case in Birmingham, 1834.

Epidemic of "Puerperalfriesel" in 1836 in Baden village of Gerichtstetten, report in letter of Dr. Hermann Wertheim of 5 September 1837 in folder 236/16088 in Generallandesarchiv in Karlsruhe.

R. Yates Ackerley, "Remarks on the Nature and Treatment of Puerperal Fever," *LMG*, NS, ii (1838), 463–66. Case from an epidemic in London, 1838.

James Reid, "Report of Parochial Lying-in Cases . . . 1839 to 1840," *LMG*, NS, i (1841), 233–39. One case, London, 1839.

James Reid, "Obstetric Report of Cases," *LMG*, NS, i (1845), 1324–32. Case in London, 1842.

W. B. Kesteven, "A Case of Puerperal Uterine Phlebitis," *LMG*, NS, 11 (1850), 926–30. Case in London, 1850.

Matthew Jennette, "On Inflammation and Abscess of the Uterine Appendages," *LMG*, NS, 11 (1850), cases on pp. 275–76. Three cases in Birkenhead, 1844, 1850.

Frederick J. Brown, "Case of Puerperal Phlebitis," *LMG*, NS, 13 (1851), 418–21. Case in Rochester (Eng.), 1850.

Zandyck, *Etude sur la fièvre puerpérale . . . à Dunkerque* (Paris, 1856), three of the cases on pp. 7–19. Epidemic in 1854.

Schulten, "Ergebnisse einiger Blutuntersuchungen in Puerperalkrankheiten," *Virchows Archiv für pathologische Anatomie*, 14 (1858), 501–09.

Schulten, "Einiges über contagiöse Puerperalkrankheiten," *Virchows Archiv für pathologische Anatomie*, 17 (1859), 228–38. Both reports concern the same epidemic in a village in Rheinhessen in the 1850s.

Anon., *Generalbericht der Sanitäts-Verwaltung im Königreiche Bayern*, II (1863), 82, and III (1868), 58–59. 1860/61 epidemic in Schwaben; 1862–63 epidemics around Eggenfelden and Fürth.

Ch. Fichot, *Une Epidémie de fièvre puerpérale à Pont-Saint-Ours* (Nevers, 1879). I took three cases, pp. 16–17, apparently in 1879.

Adolf Weber, *Bericht über hundert in der Landpraxis operativ behandelte Geburten* (Munich, 1901), p. 16. Two cases from Alsfeld area in 1890s.

Arthur v. Magnus, "Über reine puerperale Staphylokokkenpyämie," *ZBG*, 26 (1902), 868–73. 1901 case in Königsberg.

Harold Bailey, "A Report of Five Years' Activities of . . . Bellevue Hospital," *AJO-G*, 16 (1928), 462–68. 1922–24 cases in New York City.

INFECTIONS ACQUIRED IN HOSPITAL

Peu, *Pratique accouchemens*, pp. 268–69. A general account, Paris, 1664.

J. P. Xaviero Fauken, *Das in Wien im Jahre 1771 . . . Fäulungsfieber* (Vienna, 1772), pp. 61–69. Vienna, 1746, 1770. The title of the book refers to a non-obstetrical epidemic.

Henriette Carrier, *Origines de la Maternité de Paris* (Paris, 1888), pp. 41–42. Paris, 1746, 1778.

John Leake, *Practical Observations on the Child-Bed Fever*, 5th ed. (London, 1781), II, 161–99. Nine cases, 1768–70, London, most of them in epidemics.

Jacques-René Tenon, *Mémoires sur les Hôpitaux de Paris* (Paris, 1788), pp. 243–45. General account of epidemics, 1774–86.

Francis Home, *Clinical Experiments* (London, 1782), 71–77. Two cases in Edinburgh, 1774.

Osiander, *Beobachtungen*, pp. 55–70. Five cases in Kassel, 1781.

Doublet, "Mémoire sur le fièvre à laquelle on donne le nom de fièvre puerpérale," *Journal de médecine*, November, 1782, 2–5. General account, Paris, 1781.

Dejean, et al., *Mémoire sur la maladie qui a attaqué . . . les femmes en couche* (Soissons, 1783), pp. 6–9. General account, Paris, ca. 1782.

Alphonse Leroy, *Essai sur l'histoire naturelle de la grossesse* (Geneva, 1787), pp. 142–49. General account, Paris, mid-1780s.

Lukas Boër, *Abhandlungen und Versuche geburtshilflichen Inhalts* (Vienna, 1792), II, 132–36, 176–77. Vienna; four cases, 1790–91.

Johann Friedrich Osiander, *Bemerkungen über die französische Geburtshülfe* (Hanover, 1813), 247–51, 261–66. Three cases, Paris, 1810.

Franz Karl Nägele, *Schilderung des Kindbettfiebers . . . zu Heidelberg* (Heidelberg, 1812). I took the first six cases, pp. 20–23; epidemic in 1811–12.

Robert Gooch, *An Account of Some of the Most Important Diseases Peculiar to Women* (London, 1829), pp. 40–58, 90–93. General account, London, 1812–20; one case from 1820s.

Ad. Elias von Siebold, *Versuch . . . Darstellung des Kindbettfiebers* (Frankfurt/M., 1826). I took five of the Berlin deaths in March, 1825, pp. 148–68.

Robert Collins, *A Practical Treatise on Midwifery Containing the Result of 16,654 Births Occurring in the Dublin Lying-In Hospital* (Boston, 1841). I took only the first four deaths among the many he reports for Dublin, 1826–31, pp. 254–60.

Lee, "Severe Affections," pp. 663–65. Two cases, London, 1829.

Dormann, "Nachrichten über die Ereignisse in der Herzoglich-Nassauischen Hebammenlehr . . . Anstalt," *Medicinische Jahrbücher für das Herzogtum Nassau*, 3 (1845), 113–28. Three cases, Hadamar, 1830, 1832, 1838.

Meigs, "Introductory Essay," *History Puerperal Fever*, pp. 26–28. One case, Philadelphia, 1830.

Daniel Tyerman, "Case of Difficult Labour," *LMG*, 12 (1833), 704. One case, London, 1833.

Edward Rigby, "General Lying-In Hospital: Midwifery Reports," *LMG*, 17 (1836), 121–22. Two cases, London, 1834.

James Reid, notice, *LMG*, NS, ii (1838), 371–72, and i (1841), 270–71. One case, London, 1837; 1841 epidemic.

Eugène Fabre, *Clinique d'accouchements . . . de Marseille* (Paris, 1840), pp. 51–57, 77–82. Two cases, Marseille, evidently 1839.

James Reid, notice, *LMG*, NS, i (1845), 1324–32. Three cases, London, 1843–44.

Carl Heymer, *Beiträge zum Puerperalfieber* (Würzburg: med. diss., 1847). I took only two cases in this 1847 Würzburg epidemic, pp. 31–37.

D.-N. Bonnet, *Treize années de pratique à la Maternité de Poitiers* (Poitiers, 1857), pp. 114–23. General account, 1849–50.

Emile Thierry, *Des maladies puerpérales observées à l'hôpital Saint-Louis en 1867* (Paris, 1868), passim. General account, 1867.

J. S. Parry, report, *AJO*, 7 (1874–75), 162–65. Two cases, Philadelphia, 1870, 1873.

Franz Torggler, *Bericht über die Thätigkeit der . . . Klinik zu Innsbruck* (Prague, 1888). pp. 153–55. Fifteen cases, 1881–85.

Hermann Pfannenstiel, "Kasuistischer Beitrag zur Ätiologie des Puerperalfiebers," *ZBG,* 12 (1888), 617–27. Breslau epidemic, 1887.
Paul Bar, *La Maternité de l'hôpital St-Antoine . . . du 18 mai 1897 au 1er janvier 1900* (Paris, 1900), pp. 159–60. Six cases.
Ploeger, "Bericht über die Geburten . . . Frauenklinik in Berlin während 15 Jahren," *ZGH,* 53 (1905), 253–58. Thirty-one cases, 1890–1902.
Sanders, "Wochenbetts- und Säuglingsstatistik," *ZGH,* 66 (1910), 1–18. Six cases, Berlin, 1907–09.
Bailey, "Report of Five Years." Four cases, New York City, 1922–24.
W. A. Defoe, "An Account of an Epidemic of Puerperal Sepsis," *Edinburgh Obstetrical Society, Transactions,* 84 (1925), 133–39. 1924 epidemic in Toronto.

Estimating the Mortality from Postpartum Sepsis

Official statistics before 1930, which were based on vital registration of causes of death, are largely valueless in studying the frequency of sepsis. Various problems made the registration seriously incomplete.

As table 6.C (page 314) shows, around 15 percent of all puerperal deaths were put in incorrect categories in official publications, because the doctor signing the death certificate had failed to note that the death occurred in connection with a pregnancy. Appearing as "intestinal obstruction" or some such thing, they had no chance even to be considered as maternal sepsis deaths. Stanley Warren, commenting on the offical registration of maternal deaths around 1900 in Maine, said that, "although it is impossible for me to prove the statement by actual figures, I believe that the statistics given in our State Report . . . are incomplete; that is, they tell the truth, but not the whole truth. Puerperal deaths, caused in all human probability by sepsis, are returned to local Health Boards as due to peritonitis, exhaustion, pelvic abscess, etc. when the certificate should read, 'Cause of Death, Puerperal Septicemia.' "[1] A study done in 1911 by the U.S. Census Bureau changed about 10 percent of the deaths reported as "peritonitis" to "puerperal sepsis."[2] Things improved when printed death certificates began to include a space for any "unrelated cause which was regarded as having contributed in important degree to the death." This change was instituted in England and Wales, for example, in 1927.[3] Scotland after 1929 required the general practitioner to put "P" on certificates where a pregnancy existed at the time or within four previous weeks.[4]

Yet even if the doctor who certified the death had properly noted a puerperal association, statistical officials might well have put the death in some other category. Thus, when pneumonia was the terminal symptom in puerperal sepsis, the death might have been classed under "lung diseases." A fatal urinary tract infection might end up in the "acute nephritis" group, and so forth. Thus, until Georges Widal proposed his test for typhoid fever in 1896, "a considerable number" of puerperal fever deaths in England were considered "enteric fever" (typhoid fever). "Furthermore, many puerperal deaths in the past were attributed to scarlet fever, . . . bronchitis, influenza. These are a few examples of how fatalities from puerperal fever were explained away."[5]

After the classification of maternal deaths started to become more sophisticated, these fatalities become classified as "associated with pregnancy but unrelated to it." These so-called "unrelated" deaths pose severe problems. They are stamped "maternal" and so don't escape our view entirely. But how many were the result of genital infection? How many predated the delivery? And how many were genuinely contracted postpartum through some nongenital route? This is not so much a problem of medical "cheating"—which is to say of doctors trying to avoid the reproach of having "given a patient puerperal fever"—as it is a problem of the doctors of the time having insufficient knowledge about the etiology of postpartum infection. Puerperas who died of pneumonia two weeks postpartum, and who did not exhibit the obvious symptoms of peritonitis (tympanites, high fever, racing pulse), were honestly thought to have died of a lung infection independent of the childbirth. Some of the diphtheria and typhoid fever deaths may be legitimate, because these infectious diseases were, after all, commonly encountered in the general population. Mothers who died of perforated gastric ulcer or of cancer during the puerperium legitimately belong in the "independent" category. And some of the chronic heart and kidney disease deaths were legitimate, too, especially given the high incidence of group A streptococcal infections in the general population (rheumatic fever, acute glomerulonephritis).

But a careful Scottish study in the early 1930s found that only 2.5 percent of 2,500 maternal deaths "had no connection, save one of time, with pregnancy." Another 1.4 percent were aggravated by the pregnancy (deaths from Hodgkin's disease, ulcerative colitis, and the like.)[6] So 5 percent may be taken as a reasonable estimate of "unrelated" deaths in the pre-antibiotic period, and higher levels may be regarded suspiciously. Thus, it was unlikely that 17 percent of the maternal deaths in 1929–34 in Wales were really due to "associated" causes—that is, to conditions existing antepartum.

The review committee which reassessed them reduced "associated" deaths by one half.[7] This committee went carefully over each antepartum history and concluded that the "associated" diagnoses of heart disease, gynecological disease, and influenza in particular had been overused.[8]

Another problem was the British tendency to place some sepsis deaths in the column called "accidents of childbirth" rather than in the "sepsis" column. Thus, the diagnosis "phlegmasia alba dolens" whether of septic

origin or not was, before 1921, automatically put under "all other puerperal causes" and excluded from "puerperal fever."[9] People simply misunderstood the infectious origin of much thromboembolism and confused
postpartum urinary-tract-infection with the "toxemias" of pregnancy.
Other classification problems further diminish the accurate reporting of
sepsis—for example, when after 1911 the English shifted "mastitis" deaths
from sepsis to "all other puerperal causes."[10]

As a result of these various flaws, official sepsis statistics before 1900
are much too low. In 1933, Munro Kerr stated explicitly "that the early
figures [on puerperal fever for England] underestimate the mortality relative to that of the present, many deaths associated with pregnancy and
childbirth having been omitted."[11] A student of Dutch sepsis registration
around 1900 considered the official statistics "as not deserving of
confidence."[12] A study of sepsis deaths in the 1880s in Neuchâtel Canton
in Switzerland judged them 20 percent underregistered.[13]

Official statistics on puerperal sepsis after about 1910, on the other
hand, are probably too high because they include septic abortions (this
problem is discussed in chapter 8). But I want to observe here that after
so many women began to die of septic abortions, the bias in "maternal
sepsis" shifts from underreporting to *overreporting*. The English, for example, listed only a tiny percentage of induced abortion deaths in the
"abortion" category—namely, those in which a coroner's jury had reached
a verdict of "homicide" or "suicide." Until 1930 the English Registrar
General included postabortive sepsis under "puerperal sepsis."[14] And even
after that date it is unlikely that all abortive sepsis deaths found their
way into the new "postabortive sepsis" category.

As a result of these problems, the powerful long-term decline in sepsis
mortality has been completely obscured in official statistics. First, in the
nineteenth century too few deaths were reported as septic, making rates
unreasonably low. Then early in the twentieth century, after the decline
in full-term sepsis, abortions made it seem as though "deaths from puerperal infection" were continuing as before at a constant level.

To replace the official statistics, I have tried to construct time series
by aggregating local studies. In such studies the maternal deaths are normally listed individually, making it possible to exclude the abortions,
to include the appropriate "independent" deaths, and so forth.

The "independent" deaths from heart and lung diseases, and the "nonseptic" deaths from phlegmasia alba dolens, embolism, and nephritis
pose a special problem, however. Did they arise from a puerperal
infection?

The number of maternal deaths genuinely owing to organic heart disease was very small. Otfried Fellner estimated that only 0.9 percent of the women with mitral stenosis or mitral insufficiency, who gave birth in Vienna's University Women's Clinic actually died of the condition.[15] (A careful antepartum exam revealed a large number of mothers with heart disease.) Hence mortality series containing a relatively large number of "heart disease" victims should be regarded suspiciously, for the underlying cause of the cardiac arrest in most cases was likely to have been a septicemia contracted intrapartum. Similarly, septic processes often involved the lungs. For example, in 222 autopsies in 1829 at Paris's Maternité, pleuritis was found in 19 percent of the mothers, pneumonia or other lung alterations in an additional 12 percent.[16] Hence, beware of "pneumonia" as an "unrelated" cause of death.

When insufficient detail forces an estimate, I have tended to assume, in the absence of any reference to the existence of the condition antepartum, that all lung disease except tuberculosis and all heart failure deaths arose from some infectious process. I have also tended to share the Scottish Maternal Mortality review committee's view that, in regard to deaths from "pyelitis," "cystitis," and other urinary tract conditions, "there must obviously be grave doubts as to whether some of these cases were not actually due . . . to the pregnancy under consideration," unless diagnosed antepartum.[17]

Phlegmasia alba dolens and thromboembolism create other problems, in the absence of a post-mortem confirmation of the diagnosis (and in 22 of the 28 "maternal embolism" deaths studied by the English maternal mortality review committee, an autopsy did not take place).[18] For example, upon checking back, they found one "embolism" death due to gas gangrene.[19] The apparent decline in deaths from phlegmasia alba dolens and embolism—once a common diagnosis—was "probably due to the frequent acknowledgement of its septic origin."[20] In truth, there is little reason for suspecting a change in the level of nonseptic thromboembolic disease over the years, save for such innovations in patient management as early ambulation. My own feeling is that the vast majority of phlegmasia alba dolens and embolism deaths were, in fact, septic. And this view receives some confirmation from a doubling in Scotland of cases diagnosed following the First World War (up from 20 deaths per 100,000 births in 1918 to 39 in 1921, to 49 in 1927). Likely explanation: doctors were using the diagnosis of "embolism" on septic abortions.[21] It is further interesting that the review committee for Wales considered more than a quarter of the phlegmasia alba dolens and embolism deaths in 1929–34 to be the result of sepsis; another 12 percent were assigned to hemorrhage or toxemia; the remainder to "trauma."[22]

1. Stanley Warren, "The Prevalence of Puerperal Septicemia in Private Practice," *AJO*, 51 (1905), 309.

2. Cited in Grace L Meigs, *Maternal Mortality . . . in the United States* (Washington: U.S. Department of Labor, Children's Bureau, pub. no. 19, 1917), p. 39.

3. Great Britain, Ministry of Health, *Report on an Investigation into Maternal Mortality* (London, 1937), p. 35.

4. J. M. Munro Kerr, *Maternal Mortality and Morbidity* (Edinburgh, 1933), p. 4.

5. Ibid., pp. 4, 63.

6. Charlotte Douglas and Peter L. McKinlay, *Report on Maternal Morbidity and Mortality in Scotland* (Edinburgh: Department of Health for Scotland, 1935), pp. 203–10.

7. Great Britain, Ministry of Health, *Report on Maternal Mortality in Wales* (London, 1937), p. 47.

8. Ibid., p. 153.

9. Douglas and McKinlay, *Report Maternal Mortality* [6], contains a convenient chart (p. 302) showing how various causes of puerperal death have been shifting among reporting categories over the years.

10. Ibid., p. 302.

11. Munro Kerr, *Maternal Mortality* [4], p. 4.

12. Catharine van Tussenbroek, "Kindbett-Sterblichkeit in den Niederlanden," *Archiv für Gynäkologie*, 95 (1911–12), p. 38.

13. Edmond Weber, *Beiträge zur Mortalitäts-Statistik an septischen puerperalen Prozessen* (Berne: med. diss., 1890), p. 21.

14. Douglas and McKinlay, *Report Maternal Mortality* [6], p. 302.

15. Otfried Fellner, *Die Beziehungen innerer Krankheiten zu Schwangerschaft, Geburt und Wochenbett* (Leipzig, 1903), pp. 73–75, 85. Of the 30,600 births in his series, only 94 women were diagnosed with organic heart disease, though Fellner estimated that over 700 parturients had some kind of defect. Of this considerable number of women at risk, only 6 actually died of heart disease.

16. Dr. Tonnellé, "Des Fièvres puerpérales," *Archives générales de médecine*, 22 (1830), 487.

17. Douglas and McKinlay, *Report Maternal Mortality* [6], p. 72.

18. Great Britain, *Maternal Mortality*, p. 163.

19. Ibid., p. 34.

20. Ibid., p. 52.

21. Douglas and McKinlay, *Report Maternal Mortality* [6], p. 57.

22. Great Britain, *Maternal Mortality Wales* [7], p. 152.

Sources for Calculating Full-Term Sepsis Mortality (1860–1939)

Unless otherwise stated, rates calculated from the following sources exclude deaths from abortion, from perforated uteri, and from caesarean sections. I have made an effort to include, when appropriate, fatalities deemed at the time to be "non-obstetrical" in nature. In hospital data I have tried to keep track of fatally ill mothers transferred out to medical wards. Similarly, hospital statistics presented here exclude mothers infected on admission.

The figures in parentheses at the end of each entry are the number of sepsis deaths per 1,000 deliveries.

HOSPITAL (1860–69)

Emma L. Call, "The Evolution of Modern Maternity Technic," *AJO*, 58 (1908), 400. I have accepted her definition of "sepsis"; New England Hospital for Women (20 per 1,000 births).

Louis Hirigoyen, *Compte-Rendu de la clinique obstétricale de l'hôpital Saint-André de Bordeaux* (Bordeaux, 1880), pp. 28–30. A list describes each maternal death (19.6 per 1,000).

Queirel, *Histoire de la maternité de Marseille* (Marseille, 1889), p. 44. The data I have assigned to the 1860s cover 1827–67. I have taken as septic the following: deaths from peritonitis, septicemia, pneumonia, pleurisy, enteritis, "cerebral affection," phlebitis, ic-

terus, erysipelas, scarlet fever, miliary and intermittent fever, and measles (40.8 per 1,000).
Catharine van Tussenbroek, "Kindbett-Sterblichkeit in den Niederlanden," *Archiv für Gynäkologie*, 95 (1911–12), 44. Amsterdam Lying-In Hospital in 1865. I have accepted her definition of *Infektion* (40 per 1,000).
Louis Sentex, *Compte-Rendu des faits observés à la clinique d'accouchements de . . . Bordeaux* (Bordeaux, 1863), pp. 24–27. For 1859–63. In addition to the obvious, I have counted as septic numerous cases of "enteritis," erysipelas, and the like (35.4 per 1,000).

HOSPITAL (1870–79)

For data from Tussenbroek, "Kindbett," Hirigoyen, *Saint-André de Bordeaux*, and Call, "Modern Technic," see under HOSPITAL (1860–69). The rates are 48, 24.3, and 4.7 per 1,000, respectively.

G. Eustache, *Clinique d'accouchements . . . de Lille* (Lille, 1889), pp. 27–28 for 1877–81. I took the 6 maternal deaths clearly associated with infection (9.3 per 1,000).

HOSPITAL (1880–89)

For data from Call, "Modern Technic," Eustache, "Clinique de Lille," Queirel, *Maternité Marseille*, and Tussenbroek, "Kindbett," see under Hospital (1860–69). The rates are 1.6, 7.0, 19.0, and 10 per 1,000, respectively.

F. Ahlfeld, "Beiträge zur Lehre vom Resorptionsfieber . . . ," *ZGH*, 27 (1893), 497–500. Data on the Marburg Lying-In Hospital in 1883–93. From a list of maternal deaths, I have taken those obviously from sepsis (4.7 per 1,000).
Robert Boxall, "Mortality in Childbed," *JOB*, 7 (1905), 326–27. The York Road Hospital (General Lying-in Hospital); a list of deaths (2.9 per 1,000).
Georges Duval, *De la Morbidité de la Charité* (Lille, 1899), pp. 39–60. 1878–89 data. I have included various cases of "pulmonary congestion," "gangrene of the vulva," and so forth (22.2 per 1,000).
Camillo Fürst, *Klinische Mittheilungen über Geburt und Wochenbett . . . Wien* (Vienna, 1883). I have included various cases of endocarditis, bronchitis, and so on. He specifically followed mothers who died in the medical wards after being transferred out (10.3 per 1,000).
Jacob Genneper, *Die Geburten und puerperalen Todesfälle der Bonner Frauenklinik 1885–94* (Bonn: med. diss., 1894), p. 6. I have included 1 embolus of a pulmonary artery, 5 *vitum cordis*, 4 pneumonia, 3 typhus, and 1 diptheritis, in addition to 17 *puerperale Infektion* deaths (8.5 per 1,000).
Adolphe Pinard, *Du Fonctionnement de la maternité de Lariboisière . . . 1882–1889* (Paris, 1889), pp. 24–25, 37. Deaths listed (3.3 per 1,000).

HOSPITAL (1890–99)

For data from Boxall, "Childbed," Call, "Modern Technic," Duval, *Morbidité Charité*, Genneper, *Frauenklinik*, and Tussenbroek, "Kindbett," see HOSPITAL (1880–89). The rates are 0.2, 1.0, 1.2, 8.5, and 60, respectively.

Paul Bar, *La Maternité de l'hôpital St-Antoine* (Paris, 1900), pp. 159–160. A list for 1897–99 (3.8 per 1,000).
C. de Marval, *Ueber Mortalität und Morbidität des Puerperalfiebers . . . zu Basel . . . 1887–1896* (Basel: med. diss., 1897), p. 25. The fourteen infection cases include two pneumonia and one nephritis (3.7 per 1,000).
Koblanck, "Zur puerperalen Infektion," *ZGH*, 34 (1896), 269–270. Data for Berlin's University "Frauenklinik," 1888–95. I have included in the thirty-eight sepsis deaths attributable to hospital infection, eight from "nephritis" and fourteen from other "medical" causes such as "Apoplexio," pneumonia, embolus, and so forth (4.6 per 1,000).
Porak and Macé *Statistique du service d'accouchement de la Charité* (Paris, 1898), pp. 10–11 for 1895–97. The four infections include a pneumonia death (1.6 per 1,000).
H. Schimmel, "Bericht über die geburtshilfliche Abteilung der Universitäts-Frauenklinik

Würzburg," *ZGH*, 87 (1924), 421, for 1889–1900. I am taking as given the number in
the source of "infections acquired in hospital" (0.8 per 1,000).
F. von Winckel corresponded with a number of clinics and reported their maternal mortality
in *Handbuch der Geburtshülfe*, I(i)–III(iii) (Wiesbaden, 1903–07), III(ii), p. 340, plus
notes on subsequent pages. The three clinics with sufficiently detailed data to let us
exclude caesarean-sections, abortions, and those infected outside, and to include suspicious
"medical" deaths, were:

Budapest (1894–1903)	1.4 per 1,000
Basel (1896–1901)	0.2 per 1,000
Leipzig (1892–1904)	1.1 per 1,000

HOSPITAL (1900–1909)

For data from Boxall, "Childbed," Schimmel, "Würzburg," and Tussenbroek, "Kindbett,"
see HOSPITAL (1890–99). The sepsis mortality rates are 0.4, 0.0, and 0.0, respectively.
From Winckel: Kiel (10 per 1,000), for Lausanne and for Basel 0.0.

Constantin J. Bucura, "Geburtshülfliche Statistik der Klinik Chrobak," *Archiv für Gynäkologie*, 77 (1906), 453–83. Vienna, 1903–4; some of the maternal deaths are listed (1.1
per 1,000).
Henri Ferré, *Fonctionnement de la Maternité de Pau* (Pau, 1909), p. 4. 1905–07; in addition
to one "infection" death stated as such, I have assigned to sepsis: 1 erysipelas death, 1
auto-infection chez une albuminurique," and 1 death *par pneumonie chez une albumin-
rique* (4.2 per 1,000).
I. L. Hill, "The Statistics of One Thousand Cases of Labor," *AJO*, 54 (1906), 47. For the
Cornell Medical College in New York City, *ca.* 1905 (no maternal deaths).
Sanders, "Wochenbetts- und Säuglingsstatistik," *ZGH*, 66 (1910), 1–18. The Virchow Hospital in Berlin, 1907–09. Deaths listed (4.5 per 1,000).

HOSPITAL (1910–19)

For data from Schimmel, "Würzburg," see HOSPITAL (1900–1909) (0.6 per 1,000).

James A. Harrar, "Clinical Report of the Work of the First Division of the Lying-In Hospital
for the Year 1912," *Bulletin of the Lying-In Hospital of the City of New York*, 9 (1914),
215–16. A list; all 3 sepsis deaths occurred after obstetric operations (2.7 per 1,000).
M. Rothbaum, "Vergleich der mütterlichen und kindlichen Mortalität," *MGH*, 110 (1940),
93. Zurich 1912–13; maternal deaths listed. I have considered as septic a long string of
deaths from "anemia-nephritis-enteritis," "meningitis purulenta," "myocarditis," "gall-
stones-phlegmonosa," "uremia," and the like, in addition to 1 acknowledged death from
"sepsis" (4.8 per 1,000).
Samuel J. Scadron, "The Maternal Mortality in 34,900 Deliveries," *AJO-G*, 27 (1934),
128–133. Data for the Jewish Maternity Hospital in New York, 1909–20. I have accepted
his definition of "sepsis," subtracting from his totals the caesarean-section deaths (0.9
per 1,000).

HOSPITAL (1920–29)

For data from Scadron, "Maternal Mortality," and Schimmel, "Würzburg," see HOSPITAL
(1910–19). The sepsis mortality rates per 1,000 deliveries are, respectively, 0.5 and 0.0.

W. Bickenbach, "Über die Müttersterblichkeit bei klinischer Geburtshilfe," *ZBG*, 64 (1940),
830 (for Göttingen, 1925–29); all 3 sepsis deaths followed operations (0.7 per 1,000).
F. J. Browne, "Antenatal Care and Maternal Mortality," *Lancet*, 2 July 1932, pp. 1–4 (data
on 8 London hospitals, *ca.* 1926–30; hospital "C" omitted). I have taken as given the
30 deaths he calls septic; caesarean-sections omitted (0.7 per 1,000).
Charles W. Frank, "Obstetric Mortality: An Analysis of 2268 Maternity Cases at the Bronx
Hospital," *AJO-G*, 21 (1931), 708–14. No sepsis deaths.

S. A. Gammeltoft, "The Importance of Ante-natal Care," *Acta Obstetricia et Gynecologica Scandinavica*, 5 (1926), 365. Copenhagen, 1917–25. In addition to 24 diagnosed cases of puerperal infection (some of who arrived in the hospital already septic), I have included 7 "embolism" deaths, 5 nonchronic nephritis deaths, 2 pernicious anemia deaths (diagnosed postpartum), 1 "parotitis," 1 cerebral abscess, and 1 "pneumococcal meningitis" deaths (2.7 per 1,000).

J. Severy Hibben, "Statistical Survey of Obstetrics in Pasadena," *AJO-G*, 10 (1935), 843–47. No sepsis deaths in 1924; mainly hospital deliveries.

R. W. Holmes, et al., "Factors and Causes of Maternal Mortality," *JAMA*, 93 (1929), 1445. Minneapolis, 1925–28. I have added 9 embolism deaths to the 20 sepsis deaths acknowledged in hospital confinements (1.1 per 1,000).

Carl H. Ill, "An Analysis of Obstetric Work Done in Essex County, N.J. Hospitals . . . 1927–1929," *AJO-G*, 22 (1931), 129–33. In addition to acknowledged sepsis deaths, I have included 6 pneumonia cases, 1 pleurisy, 1 pyeliti-phlebitis, 1 phlegmonous gastritis, 2 emboli, et cetera (0.9 per 1,000).

Clifford B. Lull, "An Analysis of One Thousand Obstetric Case Histories," *AJO-G*, 24 (1932), 75–86 (from Philadelphia in the 1920s; no deaths from sepsis).

James Raglan Miller, "The Use of Mortality Statistics in Rating Maternity Service," *AJO-G*, 25 (1933), 580. To the 10 acknowledged sepsis deaths I have added 5 from heart disease and 5 from pneumonia.

Hans Nevinny, "Über zehn Jahre Klinikgeburten," *ZGH*, 107 (1933–34), 96–97. Innsbruck, 1922–31. To 3 puerperal sepsis cases, I have added 3 "scarlet fever" deaths, 1 lung embolism associated with thrombosis, 1 perichondritis and mediastinitis death on the twelfth day, and 1 thrombosis of the carotid artery on the sixteenth day (1.1 per 1,000).

Ernst Puppel, "Über Totgeburten, Frühsterblichkeit und mütterliche Mortalität in den Jahren 1925–1931," *Archiv für Gynäkologie*, 150 (1932), 263–64 (Mainz, 1925–1931). Both sepsis deaths followed operations (0.4 per 1,000).

Meyer Rosensohn, "Obstetric Mortality: An Analysis of the Cases at the [New York] Lying-In Hospital in 1924," *AJO-G*, 11 (1926), 97. In addition to 1 sepsis death after a uterine rupture, I have included an embolism death (0.4 per 1,000).

Scottish Board of Health, *Maternal Mortality: Report on Maternal Mortality in Aberdeen, 1918–1927* (Edinburgh, 1928), p. 47, table VII. The deaths called "septic" in booked hospital deliveries exclude fatalities from phlegmasia alba dolens, phlebitis, and embolism (normally included in the figures I report here) because that category also included such evidently nonseptic causes of death as uncontrollable vomiting (4.5 per 1,000).

Stephen E. Tracy, "A Review of One Thousand and One Obstetric Cases," *AJO-G*, 16 (1928), 51–56. No sepsis deaths in the Jewish Maternity Hospital in Philadelphia, 1925–26.

HOSPITAL (1930–39)

For data from Bickenbach, "Müttersterblichkeit," and Rothbaum, "Vergleich," see HOSPITAL (1920–29) and (1910–19). Sepsis mortality rates from these sources were, respectively, 0.1 and 2.4 per 1,000 deliveries.

Clarence C. Briscoe, "A Ten-Year Analysis of Puerperal Sepsis Deaths in Philadelphia," *AJO-G*, 45 (1943), 145 (for 1932–42). Rates accepted as given in source; abortions excluded.

M. Edward Davis, "A Review of the Maternal Mortality at the Chicago Lying-In Hospital, 1931–1945," *AJO-G*, 51 (1946), 497. To the 16 deaths from genital infections before 1939, I have added 5 from pneumonia and 2 from meningitis, although it is unclear from the source when these "non-genital" infections took place (0.9 per 1,000).

Felicitas Denker-Hauser, "Über die Müttersterblichkeit bei klinischer Geburtshilfe," *ZBG*, 66 (1942), 791. Data for Rostock, 1934–40. All 3 sepsis deaths followed operations (0.4 per 1,000).

A. Edeling, "Zur Frage der Anstaltsentbindungen," *ZBG*, 65 (1941), 1700 (for Dessau, 1933–40); maternal deaths listed (0.4 per 1,000).

H. Husslein, "Zur Frage Haus- oder Anstaltsgeburt," *ZBG*, 64 (1940), 1957 (for Prague, 1935–39); 7 deaths acknowledged as septic and 1 pneumonia (0.8 per 1,000).

J. Irving Kushner, "A Critical Analysis of the First 3060 Cases Delivered at the Bronx

Hospital," *AJO-G,* 32 (1936), 877 (for 1932–34); no sepsis deaths apart from caesarean sections.

H. I. McClure, "Maternal Mortality in Hospital Practice," *JOB,* NS, 44 (1937), 1001–02 (for Belfast, 1927–36). In addition to 3 acknowledged puerperal sepsis deaths, I include 1 sepsis after eclampsia, 2 from "heart disease" ("the patients suddenly collapsed within a few days after delivery and died in 48 hours"), and 2 deaths from pyelonephritis, not diagnosed antepartum (0.9 per 1,000).

New York Academy of Medicine, *Maternal Mortality in New York City: A Study of All Puerperal Deaths 1930–1932* (New York, 1933), pp. 85, 141. 265 septicemia deaths (excluding caesarean sections) plus 70 deaths from phlegmasia alba dolens (1.4 per 1,000).

Mario Nizza, "La Mortalità materna per cause ostetriche," *Ginecologia,* 4 (1938), 9. For Turin, 1935–37. I accept his definition of "sepsis" (0.4 per 1,000).

Obstetrical Society of Boston, "Maternal Mortality in Boston . . . 1933–1935," *NEJM,* 14 January 1937, 45. Figures for "sepsis" as given in source; caesarean sections and abortions excluded (0.9 per 1,000).

Lazar Stark, "Auswertung von 1000 Anstaltsgeburten," *MGH,* 89 (1931), 161 (for Breslau, *ca.* 1930). One apparent sepsis death from "orbital phlegmone," which could represent a distant metastasis (1 per 1,000).

Else Theisen, "Betrachtungen über Anstalts- und Hausgeburten," *ZBG,* 64 (1940), 307. No sepsis deaths in spontaneous deliveries. (Unclear how many occurred in operative deliveries; she says that the operative death rate is higher in *home* deliveries than in hospital.)

HOME (1860–69)

For Tussenbroek, "Kindbett," see HOSPITAL (1860–69) (7.8 per 1,000).

Alfred Hegar, *Die Sterblichkeit während Schwangerschaft, Geburt und Wochenbett unter Privatverhältnissen* (Freiburg, 1868), 7–16. For 34,500 midwife-assisted births in the Oberrheinkreis of Baden, 1864–66, I estimated 107 infection deaths, half of them associated with obstetric operations (3.1 per 1,000).

E. Marchal, *Etude sur la mortalité des femmes en couches dans la ville de Metz* (Metz, 1867), p. 8. For the 7,500 births in 1856–65, I calculate 47 maternal deaths from infection, including 27 from peritonitis or puerperal fever, 7 *affections aiguës des voies respiratoires,* 3 *affections du coeur,* 4 typhoid fever, 1 scarlet fever, 1 enteritis, 1 dysentery, 1 "sudden death 8 days later," and 2 anémie compliquant l'état puerpéral (6.2 per 1,000).

HOME (1870–79)

For Tussenbroek, "Kindbett," see HOSPITAL (1860–69)(3.5 per 1,000).

Samuel W. Abbott, "A Summary of Obstetric Cases Reported by Members of the Middlesex East District Medical Society," *Boston Medical and Surgical Journal,* 107 (1882–83), 5 (for Boston area, 1875–81). I have ascribed to genital sepsis: four peritonitis, 2 septicemia, 3 embolism, a rheumatic endocarditis, an erysipelas, a renal disease, a uremia, and several others (5.6 per 1,000).

H. H. Atwater, "Analysis of One Thousand Cases of Midwifery in Private Practice," *AJO,* 12 (1879), 285 (for Burlington, Vt., 1870s). The 4 probable infection deaths include 3 "puerperal fever" and 1 "hydrothrorax." (4.4 per 1,000).

HOME (1880–89)

For Pinard, *Lariboisière,* and Tussenbroek, "Kindbett," see HOSPITAL (1880–89) and (1860–69), respectively. Sepsis mortality for Pinard's Lariboisière Hospital's home-delivery service in 1883–88 was 1.8 per 1,000; in Tussenbroek's Amsterdam, 4.2 per 1,000.

Franz Unterberger, "Die Sterblichkeit im Kindbett im Grossherzogtum Mecklenburg-Schwerin in den Jahren 1886–1909," *Archiv für Gynäkologie,* 95 (1911–12), 133. Among 163 probable infection deaths for 1886–87, I have included a number of "pneumonia," "pleuritis," and "nephritis" cases (4.5 per 1,000)

HOME (1890–99)

For Tussenbroek, "Kindbett," see HOSPITAL (1860–69) (1.6 per 1,000).

Philipp Ehlers, *Die Sterblichkeit "Im Kindbett" in Berlin und in Preussen, 1867–1896* (Stuttgart, 1900), p. 50. Berlin, 1895–96; I am accepting his own definition of "sepsis," but he will not have been too far below the mark because he checked back to the circumstances surrounding a number of maternal deaths. The vast majority of births in Berlin in these years were at home (2.6 per 1,000).

HOME (1900–1909)

For Tussenbroek, "Kindbett," and Unterberger, "Mecklenburg-Schwerin," see HOSPITAL (1860–69) and HOME (1880–89). The rates for this decade are, respectively, 1.1 and 1.9 per 1,000.

James A. Harrar, "The Results and Technique of the Lying-In Hospital Out-Patient Service in 45,000 Confinements," *Bulletin of the Lying-In Hospital of the City of New York,* 6 (1909), 60–61. (for 1895–1909). In addition to 36 deaths from "bacteremia" and "sapremia," I have counted as sepsis of genital origin: 8 pneumonia deaths, 6 cardiac, 4 uremia, 3 embolism, 2 acute nephritis, 1 "fever and ecchymotic rash," and 1 erysipelas. By Harrar's account, deaths from sepsis decline from 1.2 per 1,000 in the first 10,000 deliveries to 0.2 in the most recent 5,000 (1.4 per 1,000).

HOME (1910–19)

W. R. Nicholson, "Remarks" on maternal mortality in Philadelphia, 1915, in *AJO,* 73 (1916), 514. In addition to the 5 cases of acknowledged sepsis, I have included 3 embolism deaths, 1 phlebitis, 1 endocarditis, 1 phlebitis-and-endocarditis, and 1 pneumonia (0.9 per 1,000).
Stroeder, "Zur Notwendigkeit der Trennung der Puerperalfieber-Erkrankungen und -Todesfälle post abortum und derjenigen post partum maturum . . . ," *ZBG,* 36 (1912), 1185 (Hamburg, 1910–11). Mortality from sepsis in full-term births taken as given in source. Although some hospital births are intermingled, the vast majority will have been home births (1.7 per 1,000).

HOME (1920–29)

For data on Aberdeen, see Scottish Health Board, *Maternal Mortality,* in HOSPITAL (1920–29); for Minneapolis, see Holmes, "Factors and Causes," in HOSPITAL (1920–29). The rates were, respectively, 1.2 and 0.7 per 1,000.

John S. Fairbairn, "Observations on the Maternal Mortality in the Midwifery Service of the Queen Victoria's Jubilee Institute," *BMJ,* 8 January 1927, pp. 48–49 (for England, 1924–25). In addition to 40 acknowledged deaths from puerperal sepsis, I have included 33 from "influenza, pneumonia or bronchitis"; 24 from embolism and thrombosis; 11 from "cardiac disease, sometimes with bronchitis"; 3 from "cerebral hemorrhage"; and 1 from "congestion of the lungs" (0.7 per 1,000).
F. W. Jackson, "A Five-Year Survey of Maternal Mortality in Manitoba, 1928–32," *Canadian Public Health Journal,* 25 (1934), 104–05. Included in the 126 estimated full-term deaths from sepsis are 34 fatalities from phlegmasia alba dolens, embolism, and sudden death; excluded were 48 maternal deaths from "other," unspecified causes, some of which were doubtlessly genital sepsis (1.8 per 1,000).
A communication from Marian Ross, Secretary of the Frontier Nursing Service in Wendover, Kentucky, to J. M. Munro Kerr, *Maternal Mortality and Morbidity* (Edinburgh, 1933), pp. 248–49. 0 sepsis deaths in the 1920s until 1931.
W. H. F. Oxley, "Maternal Mortality in Rochdale," *BMJ,* 16 February 1935, p. 306 (for 1929–31). I have added 3 embolism deaths to the 10 from sepsis; the number of "unrelated" maternal deaths is not given, so this rate is a minimum (3.5 per 1,000).

HOME (1930–39)

For data from Briscoe, "Ten-Year Analysis," the New York Academy of Medicine, *Maternal Mortality*, Nizza, "Mortalità Materna," and Theisen, "Hausgeburten," see HOSPITAL (1930–39). The sepsis mortality rates are 1.2, 1.0 and 0.5 and 0.0, respectively.

Henry Buxbaum, "Out-Patient Obstetrics," *AJO-G*, 31 (1936), 409–19 (out-patient department of Chicago Maternity Center, 1932–34); a list of maternal deaths, all autopsied; 6 sepsis (0.9 per 1,000).

A survey done by "N. Conti and Pohlen" of maternal mortality in Germany in midwife deliveries, cited in H. Husslein, "Zur Frage Haus- oder Anstaltsgeburt," *ZBG*, 64 (1940), 1958. *Tod durch Puerperalsepsis* given as 0.8 per 1,000.

SUPPLEMENTARY TABLES

TABLE 6.A

Maternal Mortality from Sepsis in the Period of Traditional Midwifery

	Number of Maternal Sepsis Deaths per 1,000 Deliveries
Northeim (1618–1775)[1]	7.1
Ravensberg (1782–92)[2]	10.8
Neumark Brandenburg (1789–98)[3]	6.6
Kurmark Brandenburg (1789–98)[4]	7.4
Königsberg (1790)[5]	14.0
Königsberg (1794–95)[6]	7.9
A Berlin hospital: ward and home service (1829–35)[7]	11.2
A Baden county (1864–66)[8]	3.1
Redditch (England), a private practice (1834–42)[9]	5.3
Metz (1856–65)[10]	6.2
Average of Rates	8.0

NOTE: Data for Northeim, Ravensberg, the Brandenburgs, and Königsberg distinguish only between mothers dead "while giving birth" (*Kreissenden*) and "in the puerperium" (*Wöchnerinnen*). I have assumed that the latter category are sepsis deaths, on the logic that the other major categories of obstetric mortality—hemorrhage, eclampsia, and shock—result in death shortly after the onset. Among primiparous mothers dying in the 1920s in Massachusetts, for example, 52 percent of the eclampsia fatalities occurred within twenty-four hours after the end of delivery. None of the infection fatalities died that quickly. Mary F. DeKruif, "A Study of 370 Deaths of Primiparae," *NEJM*, 27 December 1928, 1305.

[1] From Boris Schaefer, *Die Wöchnerinnensterblichkeit im 18ten Jahrhundert* (Berlin: med. diss., 1923), pp. 48–49. Deaths to *Wöchnerinnen* represented 83 percent of all maternal deaths.

[2] Ibid., p. 51. *Wöchnerinnen* had 85 percent of all maternal deaths.

[3] Ibid., p. 56. *Wöchnerinnen* have 71 percent of all maternal deaths.

[4] Ibid., p. 55. *Wöchnerinnen* have 77 percent of all maternal deaths.

[5] Wilhelm Walter, *Die Sterblichkeit in Königsberg . . . 1790 und 1791* (Kiel: med. diss., 1917), pp. 46–48. One death "in der Geburt";

25 deaths in "Wochenbett"; some of the "Wochenbett" deaths are probably not from infection.

[6] Paul Strassen, *Die Sterblichkeit in Königsberg . . . 1794 und 1795*
(Kiel: med. diss., 1919), p. 18. One death in "Kindbett"; 30 deaths in
"Wochenbett."

[7] H. Wollheim, *Versuch einer medicinischen Topographie und Statistik von Berlin* (Berlin, 1844), pp. 342–43 (data from the inpatient
and domestic delivery services of the "Königliche Entbindungsanstalt").
Of the 38 maternal deaths, I have considered the following as septic: 7
puerperal fever, 3 *Nervenfieber*, 2 abdominal typhus, 3 inflammation
and gangrene of the uterus, 4 putrefaction of the uterus and phlebitis,
1 phlegmasia alba dolens, 1 apoplexy, 1 mania, and 1 lung gangrene.
They represented 61 percent of all maternal deaths.

[8] Alfred Hegar, *Die Sterblichkeit während Schwangerschaft, Geburt
und Wochenbett* (Freiburg, 1868), pp. 7–16 (Oberrheinkreis, mostly
midwife-assisted deliveries). Of 187 total maternal deaths, I have considered the following septic: 24 peritonitis, 80 various pelvic infections
(which exclude 6 ruptured uteri), 2 "albuminuria-hydrops," and 1 peri-
tonitis-myoma. They represent 57 percent of all maternal deaths. All
gestations were full- or near-term.

[9] H. E. Collier, "A Study of the Influence of Certain Social Changes
Upon Maternal Mortality and Obstetrical Problems, 1834–1927," *JOB*,
37 (1930), 29. In 565 consecutive cases, 3 probable sepsis (his only
maternal deaths).

[10] E. Marchal, *Étude sur la mortalité des femmes en couches dans
la ville de Metz* (Metz, 1867), p. 8. Of 68 total maternal deaths, I
have assigned the following to sepsis: 27 peritonitis or puerperal fever,
2 "anemia" (hemorrhage is listed separately), 7 acute lung infections,
3 heart disease, 4 typhoid fever, 1 enteritis, 1 dysentery, 1 scarlet fever,
and 1 sudden death 8 days later (embolism?). These 47 probable infection
deaths represent 69 percent of all maternal mortality.

In defense of my assumption that deaths occurring in the puerperium
stemmed, in the period in question, largely from sepsis, let me offer
the following additional local cases, where listings of causes of death
were obtained:

Hamburg (1826): A minimum of 81 percent of all deaths were from
infection, because of 27 total maternal deaths, 22 were from puerperal
fever. "Uebersicht des Gesundheitszustandes der Stadt Hamburg," *Maga-
zin der ausländischen Literatur der gesamten Heilkunde,* March-April,
1829, pp. 329–30.

Geneva (1838–55): 65 percent of all deaths were probably from sepsis.
Among 91 total maternal deaths, there were 48 puerperal fever, 5 anascara
or phlegmasia alba dolens, 3 pneumonia, and 2 vaginal gangrene. Fr.
Oesterlen, *Handbuch der medicinischen Statistik* (Tübingen, 1865),
pp. 669–70.

Towns of Denmark (1876–85): a minimum of 71 percent of all maternal
deaths were from "puerperal fever." *Denmark: Its Medical Organization,
Hygiene and Demography* (Copenhagen, 1891), p. 428.

TABLE 6.B

Bacteria Responsible for Postpartum Bloodstream Infections (1909–46) *

	Number of Mothers†	Laboratory Findings	Percentage
Hamburg General Hospital (1909–10)[1]	14	hemolytic streptococcus	21
		anaerobic streptococcus	36
		E. coli	21
		other	21
			100
Vienna (1912–17)[2]	86	hemolytic streptococcus	65
		"non-hemolytic" streptococcus	28
		staphylococcus	3
		other	4
			100
Berlin (1920s)[3]	244	hemolytic streptococcus	23
		anaerobic streptococcus	22
		staphylococcus	35
		other and mixed	19
			100
St. Louis (1924–34)[4]	22	hemolytic streptococcus	25
		anaerobic streptococcus	33
		staphylococcus	17
		other	25
			100
London Queen Charlotte-Isolation Hospital (1930–38)[5]	213	hemolytic streptococcus	62
		anaerobic streptococcus	17
		E. coli	7
		staphylococcus	5
		other	9
			100
London, Queen Charlotte-Maternity Hospital (1930–39)[6]	31	hemolytic streptococcus	29
		anaerobic streptococcus	13
		staphylococcus	16
		clostridia	16
		other	26
			100
New York, Lying-In Hospital (1935–43)[7]	98	hemolytic streptococcus	6
		anaerobic streptococcus	22
		other streptococcus	39
		E. coli	14
		staphylococcus	7
		other	12
			100
Melbourne, Women's Hospital (1941–46)[8]	53	hemolytic streptococcus	9
		anaerobic streptococcus	57
		other streptococcus	8
		E. coli	11
		other	15
			100

* All cultures grown aerobically and anaerobically.

† The "number of mothers" is sometimes the number of cultures that were positive.

[1] Hugo Schottmüller, "Zur Bedeutung einiger Anaëroben in der Pathologie, insbesondere bei puerperalen Erkrankungen," *Mitteilungen aus den Grenzgebieten der Medizin und Chirurgie,* 21 (1910), 450–90 (data on 14 full-term infected puerperas on p. 490). He calls the aerobic streptococcus *S. erysipelas.*

[2] Josef Halban and Robert Köhler, *Die pathologische Anatomie des Puerperalprozesses* (Vienna, 1919), pp. 162–63. All cases were fatal. Blood samples in 17 additional fatal cases were "sterile," even after repeated cultures. The investigators recovered anaerobic streptococci only one time, even though their anaerobic techniques seem to have been meticulous.

[3] Kurt Sommer, "Die puerperale Sepsis," *ZGH,* 94 (1929), 484. Of the 244 mothers with postpartum infections, most died. Blood findings from 42 were classed "sterile"—a finding that weakens one's confidence in the reliability of the laboratory procedures.

[4] Otto H. Schwarz and T. K. Brown, "Puerperal Infection due to Anaerobic Streptococci," *AJO-G,* 31 (1936), 379–87. Of full-term mothers with fatal infections, 10 had "sterile" samples. Only 4 of the 22 deaths were associated with spontaneous deliveries. The others all followed from caesarean sections or major operations.

[5] For 1930–32, from L. C. Rivett, et al., "Puerperal Fever. A Report Upon 533 Cases Received at the Isolation Block of Queen Charlotte's Hospital," *Proceedings of the Royal Society of Medicine,* 26 (1932–33), 1161–75 (includes only mothers with peritonitis or septicemia whose blood cultures were positive). For 1933–38, from G. F. Gibberd, "Puerperal Sepsis, 1930–1965," *JOB,* 73 (1966), 1–10. The author does not state how the samples were cultured, and I am only assuming that both aerobic and anaerobic cultures were made of the blood. A series of percentages follows his caption, "Organisms responsible for fatal sepsis."

[6] Ibid. I have averaged together percentages for 1930–34 and 1935–39. Again, the provenance of the samples and modes of culturing them are unclear.

[7] R. Gordon Douglas and Ione F. Davis, "Puerperal Infection," *AJO-G,* 51 (1946), 352–68. Of 295 patients with postpartum infections, the hospital took 524 cultures. From the 90 that were positive, 98 different organisms were grown. The high proportion of "Alpha strep" cultures is a result of repeated samples from patients with subacute bacterial endocarditis.

[8] Arthur M. Hill, "The Diagnosis, Prevention and Treatment of Puerperal Infection," *Medical Journal of Australia,* 35 (1948), 227–35.

TABLE 6.C

Maternal Deaths: Percentage in Which the Death Certificate Was Misleading (failing to mention that a pregnancy had preceded the death)

	Percentage
Denmark (1882–89)[1]	16
Berlin (1885–92)[2]	25
Berlin (1895–96)[3]	41
Aberdeen (1918–27)[4]	13
Wales (1929–34)[5]	3
England (1934)[6]	4
Average	15

[1] E. Ingerslev, "Die Sterblichkeit an Wochenbettfieber in Dänemark und die Bedeutung der Antiseptik für dieselbe," *ZGH,* 26 (1893), 457.

[2] Philipp Ehlers, *Die Sterblichkeit "Im Kindbett" in Berlin und in Preussen, 1877–1896* (Stuttgart, 1900), pp. 30–33.

[3] Ibid.

[4] J. Parlane Kinloch, et al., *Maternal Mortality . . . in Aberdeen, 1918–1927, with Special Reference to Puerperal Sepsis* (Edinburgh, 1928; Scottish Board of Health), p. 8.

[5] Great Britain, Ministry of Health, *Report on Maternal Mortality in Wales* (London, 1937), p. 46.

[6] Great Britain, Ministry of Health, *Report on an Investigation into Maternal Mortality* (London, 1937), p. 34.

TABLE 8.A

Percentage of All Maternal Sepsis Deaths That
Were Caused by Infected Abortion in the 19th and
20th Centuries

Year	Percentage
Switzerland[1]	
1901–09	18
1910–19	34
1920–29	33
1930–39	45
Hamburg[2]	
1875–79	7
1880–89	15
1890–94	22
1901–09	52
1910–19	73
1920–27	83
Berlin[3]	
1885–87	19
1895–96	34
1910–12	67
1920–26	79
Magdeburg[4]	
1924–27	72
Germany[5]	
1926–28	57
1931–33	54
1934–38	42
Four Dutch Cities[6]	
1885	5
1895	19
1900	29
Towns in West	
Riding of Yorkshire[7]	
1923–29	33
England and Wales[8]	
Early 1930s	21
Scotland[9]	
1931–35	13
1936–38	18
Oregon[10]	
1927–28	64
Manitoba[11]	
1928–32	29

Ontario[12]	
1933–34	38
Minneapolis[13]	
1925–28	53
Washington, D.C.[14]	
1937–40	24
United States	
(15-state survey)[15]	
1927–28	45

[1] *Statistisches Jahrbuch der Schweiz*, 1945, pp. 124–25.

[2] Hamburg (1875–94) from Philipp Ehlers, *Die Sterblichkeit "Im Kindbett" in Berlin und in Preussen, 1877–1896* (Stuttgart, 1900), p. 48 (I have assumed that all deaths from abortion were septic). Hamburg (1901–27), Hans Nevermann, "Zur Frage der Mortalität durch Schwangerschaft, Geburt und Wochenbett," *ZBG*, 52 (1928), 2356 (only septic abortions included).

[3] Berlin (1885–96) from Ehlers, *Sterblichkeit*, pp. 33, 43 (I have assumed that all abortion deaths were septic). Berlin (1910–12) from Sigismund Peller, *Fehlgeburt und Bevölkerungsfrage* (Stuttgart, 1930), p. 159. Berlin (1922–26) from E. Roesle, "Die Ergebnisse der Magdeburger Fehlgeburtenstatistik," *Statistisches Jahrbuch der Stadt Magdeburg, 1927*, p. 140.

[4] Roesle, *Jahrbuch Magdeburg*, p. 138 (*Ansässige Frauen* only).

[5] Germany (1926–28) from Max Hirsch, *Mutterschaftsfürsorge* (Leipzig, 1931), p. 154. Germany (1931–38) from E. Philipp, "Der heutige Stand der Bekämpfung der Fehlgeburt," *ZBG*, 64 (1940), 231.

[6] Catharine van Tussenbroek, "Kindbett-Sterblichkeit in den Niederlanden," *Archiv für Gynäkologie*, 95 (1911–12), 50, 68. I am assuming that all abortion deaths were due to infection—Amsterdam, Rotterdam, s'Gravenhage, and Utrecht.

[7] Janet Campbell, ed., *High Maternal Mortality in Certain Areas* (London, Ministry of Health, Reports on Public Health and Medical Subjects, no. 68, 1932), pp. 24–44 (tabulated from data on 5 towns).

[8] J. M. Munro Kerr, *Maternal Mortality and Morbidity* (Edinburgh, 1933), p. 46. He summarizes the report of a departmental committee on maternal mortality; quoting from the report, "Sepsis following abortion accounts for 21.2 percent of maternal deaths from puerperal sepsis."

[9] Scotland (1931–33) from Charlotte A. Douglas and Peter L. McKinlay, *Report on Maternal Morbidity and Mortality in Scotland* (Edinburgh: Department of Health for Scotland, 1935), p. 54. Scotland (1934–38) from Scotland, Registrar General, *Annual Reports*, 1934–38. Full-term sepsis statistics include deaths from "puerperal phlegmasia alba dolens, embolism," most of which are likely to have been septic.

[10] Raymond E. Watkins, "A Five-Year Study of Abortion," *AJO-G*, 26 (1933), 161.

[11] F. W. Jackson, "A Five-Year Survey of Maternal Mortality in Manitoba, 1928–1932," *Canadian Public Health Journal*, 25 (1934), 105. Among the 126 full-term sepsis deaths are 34 from phlegmasia alba dolens, and so forth.

[12] J. T. Phair and A. H. Sellers, "A Study of Maternal Deaths in the Province of Ontario," *Canadian Public Health Journal*, 25(1934), 566.

[13] R. W. Holmes, et al., "Factors and Causes of Maternal Mortality," *JAMA*, 9 November 1929, p. 1445 "Fifty-three percent of the deaths from puerperal septicemia occurred under the 5th month."

[14] Beatrice Bishop Berle, "An Analysis of Abortion Deaths in the District of Columbia for the Years 1938, 1939, 1940," *AJO-G*, 43 (1942), 820.

[15] Frances C. Rothbert, "A Study of Maternal Mortality in 15 States," *AJO-G*, 26 (1933), 280–81 They excluded "criminal" abortions from this study: that is, presumably those in which a second party was known to be involved. Nevertheless, over half of the nontherapeutic abortions in the series were induced.

NOTES

Abbreviations Used in Notes

AJO	*American Journal of Obstetrics*
AJO-G	*American Journal of Obstetics and Gynecology (after 1920)*
BMJ	*British Medical Journal*
JAMA	*Journal of the American Medical Association*
JOB	*Journal of Obstetrics and Gynaecology of the British Empire (after 1961 "of the British Commonwealth")*
LMG	*London Medical Gazette*
MGH	*Monatsschrift für Geburtshilfe und Gynäkologie*
NEJM	*New England Journal of Medicine*
ZBG	*Zentralblatt für Gynäkologie*
ZGH	*Zeitschrift für Geburtshilfe (-hülfe) und Gynäkologie*

The name of the publisher is given only for books published after 1945. The numbers in brackets refer to the original complete citation of a particular reference in each chapter.

Chapter 1

1. In addition to my own, Edward Shorter, *The Making of the Modern Family* (New York: Basic Books, 1975), see Lawrence Stone, *The Family, Sex and Marriage in England, 1500–1800* (New York: Harper & Row, 1977); and Jean-Louis Flandrin, *Familles: Parenté, maison, sexualité dans l'ancienne société* (Paris: Hachette, 1976). Points of view contrary to my own may be found in Michael Mitterauer and Reinhard Sieder, *Vom Patriarchat zur Partnerschaft: Zum Strukturwandel der Familie* (Munich: Beck, 1977); and Louise A. Tilly and Joan W. Scott, *Women, Work, and Family* (New York: Holt, Rinehart & Winston, 1978). For an overview of the various squabbling doctrines, see Michael Anderson, *Approaches to the History of the Western Family, 1500–1914* (London: Macmillan, 1980).

2. Lionel Tiger, *Men in Groups* (London: Nelson, 1969).

3. Alexandre Bouët, *Breiz Izel ou vie des Bretons dans l'Armorique,* new ed. Reprint of the 1835 ed. (Quimper, 1918), p. 278.

4. Ernst Schlee, "Sitzordnung beim bäuerlichen Mittagsmahl," *Kieler Blätter zur Volkskunde*, 8 (1976), 6–9.

5. Eugène Olivier, *Médecine et santé dans le pays de Vaud au XVIIIᵉ siècle, 1675–1798*, 2 vols. (Lausanne, 1939), I, 578.

6. Yves Castan, *Honnêteté et relations sociales en Languedoc, 1715–1780* (Paris: Plon, 1974), pp. 164, 171, 172.

7. Alain Corbin, *Archaïsme et modernité en Limousin au XIXᵉ siècle*, 2 vols. (Paris: Rivière, 1975), I, 282–83 ("La fumelle de chez nous a fait ceci").

8. Quoted in Martine Segalen, "Le mariage, l'amour et les femmes dans les proverbes populaires francais (suite)," *Ethnologie française*, 6 (1976), 70.

9. Marta Wohlgemuth, *Die Bäuerin in zwei badischen Gemeinden* (Karlsruhe, 1913), pp. 111–12.

10. See Hans Fehr, *Die Rechtsstellung der Frau und der Kinder in den Weistümern* (Jena, 1912), p. 57 ("Der Mann ist des Weibes Vogt und Meister").

11. Ibid., pp. 57–60.

12. Lisbeth Burger, *Vierzig Jahre Storchentante: Aus dem Tagebuch einer Hebamme* (Breslau, 1936), p. 178; see also p. 247.

13. Eduard Dann, *Topographie von Danzig* (Berlin, 1835), p. 155.

14. Christoph Gottlieb Büttner, *Vollständige Anweisung wie . . . ein verübter Kindermord auszumitteln sey* (Königsberg, 1771), p. 180.

15. Johann Storch, *Von Weiberkranckheiten*, 8 vols. (Gotha, 1746–53), V, 245–47.

16. Segalen, "Proverbes" [8], p. 74.

17. Elfriede Moser-Rath, "Frauenfeindliche Tendenzen im Witz," *Zeitschrift für Volkskunde*, 74 (1978), 54n67.

18. Shorter, *Modern Family* [1].

19. Segalen, "Proverbes" [8], pp. 76–77.

20. Ibid., p. 77.

21. Françoise Loux, "Certaines pratiques à l'égard de l'enfant mort peuvent apparaître étranges ou marquées d'indifférence; elles ont en réalité un but précis," *Le Jeune enfant et son corps dans la médecine traditionnelle* (Paris: Flammarion, 1978), p. 257; see also pp. 19–20.

22. Adolf Müller, *Beiträge zu einer hessischen Medizingeschichte des 15.–18. Jahrhunderts* (Darmstadt, 1929), p. 19 ("Kühverrecke grosser Schrecke, Weibersterbe kein Verderbe").

23. Ludwig Büttner, *Fränkische Volksmedizin* (Erlangen, 1935), p. 214 ("Weiber sterben, kein Verderben, Gaul verrecken, das macht Schrecken").

24. Jacques Cambry, *Voyage dans le Finistère ou état de ce département en 1794 et 1795*, 3 vols. (Paris, an VII–1799), II, 11.

25. Quoted in Guy Arbellot, *Cinq paroisses du Vallage, XVIIᵉ–XVIIIᵉ* (Paris: Ecole des Hautes Etudes en Science Sociales, thèse 3ᵉ cycle, 1970), p. 274n1.

26. Rudolf Dohrn, "Erfahrungen bei Prüfungen und dem Nachexamen der Hebammen," *ZBG*, 30 (1906), 908.

27. Burger, *Storchentante* [12], p. 26.

28. Max Thorek, *A Surgeon's World: An Autobiography* (Philadelphia, 1943), pp. 80–81.

29. Anne Amable Augier du Fot, *Catéchisme sur l'art des accouchemens* (Soissons, 1775), p. xv.

30. Dr. Flügel, *Volksmedizin und Aberglaube im Frankenwalde* (Munich, 1863), pp. 47–48.

31. Maria Bidlingmaier, *Die Bäuerin in zwei Gemeinden Württembergs* (Tübingen: staatswiss. diss., 1918), p. 173. I am grateful to David Sabean for this reference.

32. Burger, *Storchentante* [12], pp. 53–55.

33. Charles White, *A Treatise on the Management of Pregnant and Lying-In Women* (London, 1772), pp. 251–52.

34. Segalen, "Proverbes" [8], p. 71 ("Quand la poule recherche le coq, l'amour ne vaut pas une noix").

35. Burger, *Storchentante* [12], pp. 90–91.

36. Rudolf Temesváry, *Volksbräuche und Aberglauben in der Geburtshilfe und der Pflege des Neugebornen in Ungarn* (Leipzig, 1900), p. 101.

37. Michael Zuckerman, "William Byrd's Family," *Perspectives in American History*, 12 (1979), 270–71.

38. Bud Berzing, ed., *Sex Songs of the Ancient Letts* (New York: University Books, 1969), pp. 37, 66, 81, 86, respectively. I owe this reference to the kindness of Andrejs Plakans.

39. E. Pelkonen. *Über volkstümliche Geburtshilfe in Finnland* (Helsinki, 1931), p. 90.

40. The songs are scattered throughout Berzing, *Sex Songs* [38], but see especially pp. 255–62.

41. Ibid., p. 257.

42. Pelkonen, *Geburtshilfe Finnland* [39], p. 56 ("mit dem Hinterteil wird gedroschen, mit dem Munde gesät"). See also Christian Gotthilf Salzmann, *Über die heimlichen Sünden der Jugend*, 2nd ed. (Frankfurt, 1794), p. 54 ("Bey dem Zanken der Eheleute macht oft die Frau dem Manne den Vorwurf, dass er ihr nicht ehelich beywohne und doch von ihr verlange, dass sie ihm ——").

43. G. H. Fielitz, "Beobachtungen über verschiedene Hindernisse und Schwierigkeiten bei Ausübung der Geburtshülfe," *Johann Christ. Starks Archiv für die Geburtshülfe*, 2(1) (1789), 58.

44. Dr. Martin, *Mémoires de médecine* (Paris, 1835), pp. 282–86.

45. Guillaume de la Motte, *Traité complet des acouchemens* (1715; rpt. Leiden, 1729), p. 293.

46. Adrian Wegelin, "Allgemeine Uebersicht des dritten Hunderts künstlicher Entbindungen," *J. C. Stark's Neues Archiv für die Geburtshülfe*, 3 (1804), 91–93.

47. Fehr, *Weistümer* [10], p. 2.

48. Ian Maclean, *The Renaissance Notion of Woman* (Cambridge: Cambridge University Press, 1980), p. 105n54.

49. Jacques Solé, *L'Amour en Occident à l'Epoque moderne* (Paris: Michel, 1976), pp. 87–92.

50. Jean L. Liébaut, *Thrésor des remèdes secrets pour les maladies des femmes* (Paris, 1597), p. 529.

51. Robert Burton, *Anatomy of Melancholy*, 3 vols. (1621; rpt. London: Dent/Everyman, 1932), III, 55.

52. Segalen, "Proverbes" [8], pp. 48, 63.

53. These new attitudes are well chronicled in Carl N. Degler, *At Odds: Women and the Family in America from the Revolution to the Present* (New York: Oxford University Press, 1980), pp. 249–79; and Randolph Trumbach, *The Rise of the Egalitarian Family: Aristocratic Kinship and Domestic Relations in Eighteenth-Century England* (New York: Academic, 1978), pp. 87–113 and passim.

54. Shorter, *Modern Family* [1], ch. 3.

55. Emmanuel Le Roy Ladurie, *Montaillou: The Promised Land of Error*, Eng. trans. Barbara Bray (New York: Random House/Vintage, 1979), chs. 10–12.

56. Berzing, *Sex Songs* [38], pp. 89, 199.

57. Ibid., pp. 245–46.

58. Ibid., p. 86.

59. Ibid., pp. 230, 274.

60. Ibid., p. 46.

61. De la Motte, *Traité* [45], pp. 11–12.

62. Ibid., p. 71.

63. Margaret Hagood, *Mothers of the South: Portraiture of the White Tenant Farm Woman* (1939; rpt. New York: Norton, 1977), pp. 118, 166–67.

64. Marie Stopes, *"The First Five Thousand": Being the First Report of the First Birth Control Clinic in the British Empire* (London, 1925), p. 47.

65. Emma Goldman, *Living My Life*, 2 vols. (1931; rpt. New York: Dover, 1970), I, 186.

66. Burger, *Storchentante* [12], p. 93.

67. Wohlgemuth, *Bäuerin Baden* [9], pp. 112–15.

68. Bidlingmaier, *Bäuerin Württemberg* [31], pp. 167–68.

69. Women's Co-operative Guild, *Maternity: Letters from Working-Women* (1915; rpt. New York: Garland, 1980), pp. 48–49, 67.

Chapter 2

1. Rose Frisch, "Menstrual Cycles: Fatness as a Determinant of Minimum Weight for Height Necessary for their Maintenance or Onset," *Science*, 185 (1974), 949–51.

2. Francis E. Johnston et al., "Critical Weight at Menarche: Critique of a Hypothesis," *American Journal of Diseases of Children*, 129 (1975), 19–23; James Trussell, "Menarche and Fatness," *Science*, 200 (1978), 1506–9 (see Frisch's reply in "Menstrual Cycles," [1], pp. 1510–13); and W. Z. Billewicz et al., "Comments on the Critical Metabolic Mass and the Age of Menarche," *Annals of Human Biology*, 3 (1976), 51–59.

3. Lennart Jacobson, "On the Relationship Between Menarcheal Age and Adult Body Structure," *Human Biology*, 26 (1954), 130, table 1, found relationships between "fat factor" and body weight. Francis E. Johnston reviews the literature in "Control of Age at Menarche," *Human Biology*, 46 (1974), 159–71. See also J. C. Van Wieringen, "Secular Growth Changes," in Frank Falkner and J. M. Tanner, eds. *Human Growth*, 2 vols. (New York: Plenum, 1978), II, 451–52.

4. Darrel Amundsen and Carol Jean Diers, "The Age of Menarche in Classical Greece and Rome," *Human Biology*, 41 (1969), 125–32, and "The Age of Menarche in Medieval Europe," *Human Biology*, 45 (1973), 363–69; the quote is from the latter article, p. 368.

5. The source is "Quarinonius," quoted in Leona Zacharias and Richard J. Wurtman, "Age at Menarche: Genetic and Environmental Influences," *NEJM*, 17 April 1969, p. 873.

6. Edward Shorter, "L'Age des premières règles en France, 1850–1950," *Annales: Economies, Sociétés, Civilisations*, 36 (1981), 497, table 1.

7. J. E. Brudevoll et al., "Menarcheal Age in Oslo During the Last 140 Years," *Annals of Human Biology*, 6 (1979), 411, figure 1. Bengt-Olov Ljung et al., "The Secular Trend in Physical Growth in Sweden," *Annals of Human Biology*, 1 (1974), 253, figure 11.

8. See most recently J. M. Tanner and P. B. Eveleth, "Variability between Populations in Growth and Development at Puberty," in S. R. Berenberg, ed., *Puberty: Biologic and Psychosocial Consequences* (Leiden: Kroese, 1975), p. 269, figure 8.

9. See G. H. Brundtland, "Menarcheal Age in Norway: Halt in the Trend towards Earlier Maturation," *Nature*, 241 (1973), 478; and T. C. Dann and D. F. Roberts, "End of the Trend? A 12-year Study of Age at Menarche," *BMJ*, 4 August 1973, pp. 265–67.

10. See D. J. Frommer, "Changing Age of the Menopause," *BMJ*, 8 August 1964, pp. 349–51.

11. Much interesting data on the "secular trend" will be found in J. M. Tanner, *Growth at Adolescence*, 2nd ed. (Oxford: Blackwell, 1962), p. 149; and Phyllis B. Eveleth and J. M. Tanner, *Worldwide Variation in Human Growth* (Cambridge: Cambridge University Press, 1976), pp. 260–61. For 1830s Belgian data on an apparently middle-class population, see Lambert A. J. Quetelet, *A Treatise on Man*, Eng. trans. (Edinburgh, 1842), p. 64. For 1971–74 U.S. data, see Department of Health, Education, and Welfare, *Weight and Height of Adults 18–74 Years of Age: United States, 1971–74* (Hyattsville: National Center for Health Statistics, 1979; DHEW pub. no. [PHS] 79-1659), table 15, p. 28.

12. Wilhelm Ludwig Willius, *Beschreibung der natürlichen Beschaffenheit in der Marggravschaft Hochberg* (Nürnberg, 1783), pp. 192–94.

13. These examples are from Lily Weiser-Aall, "Die Speise des Neugeborenen," in Edith Ennen and Günter Wiegelmann, eds. *Festschrift Matthias Zender*, 2 vols. (Bonn: Röhrscheid, 1972), I, 543–44.

14. Franz Xaver Mezler, *Versuch einer medizinischen Topographie der Stadt Sigmaringen* (Freiburg, 1822), p. 155.

15. Example from Lucienne A. Roubin, *Chambrettes des Provençaux: Une Maison des hommes en Méditerranée septentrionale* (Paris: Plon, 1970), p. 130 (Commune of La Mûre, toward 1912).

16. Marta Wohlgemuth, *Die Bäuerin in zwei badischen Gemeinden* (Karlsruhe, 1913), p. 76.

17. Weiser-Aall, "Speise des Neugeborenen" [13], I, p. 543.

18. Gertrud Herrig, *Ländliche Nahrung im Strukturwandel des 20. Jahrhunderts: Untersuchungen im Westeifeler Reliktgebiet am Beispiel der Gemeinde Wolsfeld* (Meisenheim: Hain, 1974), p. 99n210.

19. From Derek Oddy and Derek Miller, eds. *The Making of the Modern British Diet* (London: Croom Helm, 1976), p. 220, quoting from "The Sixth Report of the Medical Officer of the Privy Council," 1864.

20. Quoted in Hans J. Teuteberg and Günter Wiegelmann, *Der Wandel der Nahrungsgewohnheiten unter dem Einfluss der Industrialisierung* (Göttingen: Vandenhoeck, 1972), p. 325.

21. Moritz T. W. Bromme, *Lebensgeschichte eines modernen Fabrikarbeiters* (1905; rpt. Frankfurt: Athenäum, 1971), p. 351.

22. This chronology is from the British Pediatric Association, *Report on the Incidence of Rickets in War-Time* (London: Ministry of Health, Reports on Public Health, no. 92 1944), p. 7.

23. On the reliability with which these various symptoms recur, see Alfred F. Hess and Lester J. Unger, "Infantile Rickets: The Significance of Clinical, Radiographic and Chemical Examinations in its Diagnosis and Incidence," *American Journal of Diseases of Children,* 24 (1922), 328, 337.

24. Percivall Willughby, *Observations in Midwifery* (1863; rpt. East Ardsley: S. R. Publishers, 1972), p. 16. Willughby's manuscript stemmed from the seventeenth century.

25. Quoted in J. Lawson Dick, *Rickets* (New York, 1922), p. 63.

26. August Hirsch, *Handbuch der historisch-geographischen Pathologie,* 2nd ed. (Stuttgart, 1886), III, 516–17.

27. James R. Smyth, "Miscellaneous Contributions to Pathology and Therapeutics," *LMG,* NS, 1 (1843–44), 328; Smyth also mentioned other "causes," such as damp habitation.

28. Dr. Rame, *Essai historique et médical sur Lodève* (Lodève, 1841), pp. 62–63.

29. Dr. Olivet, "Essai sur la topographie médicale de la ville de Montereau, Haut-Yonne," February 1819. Manuscript is in the collection "Société de l'école de médecine de Paris, mémoires OP," of the Paris Académie de Médecine.

30. Francis Ivanhoe, "Was Virchow Right about Neanderthal?" *Nature,* 227 (1970), 578; see also H. Grimm, "Über Rachitis und Rachitis-Verdachtsfälle im ur- und frühgeschichtlichen Material," *Zeitschrift für die gesamte Hygiene und ihre Grenzgebiete,* 18 (1972), 451–55.

31. Grimm, ibid.

32. Poul Norlund, *Wikingersiedlungen in Grönland* (Leipzig, 1937), pp. 122–23.

33. Dr. Brouzet, *Essai sur l'éducation médicinale des enfans* (Paris, 1754), II, 213–14.

34. See Calvin Wells, "Prehistoric and Historical Changes in Nutritional Diseases," *Progress in Food and Nutrition Science,* 1 (1975), 752–53; and Paul A. Janssens, *Palaeopathology: Diseases and Injuries of Prehistoric Man* (London: Baker, 1970), p. 66.

35. For example, Jean-Marie Munaret, *Le Médecin des villes et des campagnes,* 3rd ed. (Paris, 1862), pp. 446–47; Fritz Kipping, *Über die ätiologische Bedeutung der äusseren Lebensbedingungen für die Häufigkeit des engen Beckens* (Freiburg: med. diss., 1911), pp. 13, and 44–45 on urban-rural; and Victor Fossel, *Volksmedicin und medicinischer Aberglaube in Steiermark* (Graz, 1886), p. 83.

36. P. J. Lesauvage, *Essai topographique et médical sur Bayonne et ses environs* (Paris, 1825), pp. 120–21; Jürdens, "Versuch einer medizinischen Topographie der Stadt Hof," *Journal der practischen Arzneykunde,* 6 (1798), 843–44; Fr. Wilhelm Lippich, *Topographie . . . Laibach* (Laibach, 1834), p. 183; on Lyon, Dr. Martin, *Mémoires de médecine* (Paris, 1835), p. 4; Friedrich Julius Morgen, *Beiträge zu einer medizinischen Topographie . . . Memel* (Memel, 1843), p. 228; Jakob Christian Schäffer, *Versuch einer medizinischen Ortsbeschreibung der Stadt Regensburg* (Regensburg, 1787), p. 44, who says it afflicts mainly poor children; and Hermann Wasserfuhr, *Untersuchungen über die Kindersterblichkeit in Stettin* (Stettin, 1867), p. 22.

37. Dr. W. Fordyce, quoted in Dick, *Rickets* [25], p. 315.

38. Johann Jakob Rambach, *Versuch einer physisch-medizinischen Beschreibung von Hamburg* (Hamburg, 1801), p. 176.

39. Dr. Wunderlich, *Versuch einer medizinischen Topographie der Stadt Sulz am Neckar* (Tübingen, 1809), p. 61.

40. Franz Alois Stelzig, *Versuch einer medizinischen Topographie von Prag,* 2 vols. (Prague, 1824), II, 67.

41. Dr. Ludwig Mauthner in 1841, quoted in Gustav Otruba, "Lebenserwartung und Todesursachen der Wiener," *Jahrbuch des Vereines für Geschichte der Stadt Wien,* 15–16 (1959–60), 214.

42. Isambard Owen, "Reports of the Collective Investigation Committee . . . ," *BMJ*, 19 January 1889, p. 114.

43. Janet Campbell et al., *High Maternal Mortality in Certain Areas* (London: Ministry of Health, Reports on Public Health, no. 68, 1932), pp. 28–29.

44. John L. Morse, "The Frequency of Rickets in Infancy in Boston and Vicinity," *JAMA*, 24 March 1900, p. 724.

45. British Pediatric Association, *Incidence Rickets* [22], p. 4, citing a report by Dr. Chisholm.

46. Cited in Carl Coerper, "Beitrag zur Rachitisfürsorge," *Zeitschrift für Säuglings-und Kleinkinderschutz*, 15 (1923), 335–36.

47. Dick, *Rickets* [25], pp. 58–59.

48. On pelvic deformities from rickets in infants, see Theodor Hoffa, "Die Entstehung des rachitischen Beckens," *Monatsschrift für Kinderheilkunde*, 27 (1923–24), esp. 436.

49. Robert M. Bernard, "The Shape and Size of the Female Pelvis," *Transactions of the Edinburgh Obstetrical Society*, in the *Edinburgh Medical Journal*, 59 (1952), 2, table 1. On the difficulties in labor of this sample of short women, see D. B. Stewart and R. M. Bernard, "A Clinical Classification of Difficult Labour and Some Examples of its Use," *JOB*, 61 (1954), 322–23.

50. William Smellie, *Treatise on the Theory and Practice of Midwifery* (London, 1752), p. 82.

51. For example, Pierre Dionis, *Traité général des accouchemens* (1718). On Dionis, see Heinrich Fasbender, *Geschichte der Geburtshilfe* (Jena, 1906), pp. 187–88.

52. Harold E. Harrison, in Henry L. Barnett and Arnold H. Einhorn, *Pediatrics*, 15th ed. (New York: Appleton-Century-Crofts, 1972), p. 205.

53. Brouzet, *Essai éducation médicinale* [33], II, 215.

54. See Joseph B. DeLee, *Principles and Practice of Obstetrics*, 6th ed. (Philadelphia, 1933), pp. 720, 733.

55. Ibid., p. 718; and Louis M. Hellman and Jack A. Pritchard, *Williams Obstetrics*, 14th ed. (New York: Appleton-Century-Crofts, 1971), p. 897; the percentages are based on 48,000 cases in the Obstetrical Statistical Co-operative.

56. Franz von Winckel, *Handbuch der Geburtshülfe*, 3 vols. (Wiesbaden, 1903–07), II, 1874.

57. Joseph Daquin, *Topographie médicale de la ville de Chambéry* (Chambéry, 1787), pp. 79, 82.

58. Carl Schreiber, *Physisch-medicinische Topographie . . . Eschwege* (Marburg, 1849), pp. 164–65.

59. E. D. Plass and H. J. Alvis, "A Statistical Study of 129,539 Births in Iowa," *AJO-G*, 28 (1934), 297.

60. See the summary of Ernesto Pestalozza's paper in *ZBG*, 20 (1896), 1090.

61. F. Ahlfeld, *Berichte und Arbeiten aus der geburtshülflich . . . Klinik zu Giessen, 1881–1882* (Leipzig, 1883), p. 10.

62. J. Whitridge Williams, "A Statistical Study of the Incidence and Treatment of Labor Complicated by Contracted Pelvis," *AJO-G*, 11 (1926), 737, table 1.

63. Von Winckel, *Handbuch* [56], III, 1870.

64. See Aaron J. Ihde, "Studies on the History of Rickets, II: The Roles of Cod Liver Oil and Light," *Pharmacy in History*, 17 (1975), 13–20.

65. Willughby, *Observations* [24], pp. 109–10.

66. Stephen Kern, *Anatomy and Destiny: A Cultural History of the Human Body* (Indianapolis: Bobbs-Merrill, 1975), p. 10.

67. Samuel Thomas Soemmerring, *Über die Schädlichkeit der Schnürbrüste* (Leipzig, 1788), pp. 104–05, 160–61; Soemmerring lists previous critics of the corset on pp. 96–97.

68. Axel Hansen, "Die Chlorose im Altertum," [*Sudhoff's*] *Archiv für die Geschichte der Medizin*, 24 (1931), 184.

69. Paul Diepgen, *Frau und Frauenheilkunde in der Kultur des Mittelalters* (Stuttgart: Thieme, 1963), p. 207.

70. Lawrence Stone, *The Family, Sex and Marriage in England, 1500–1800* (New York: Harper & Row, 1977), pp. 445–46.

71. John. Jac. Günther, *Versuch einer medicinischen Topographie von Köln am Rhein* (Berlin, 1833), pp. 113–15; Morgen, *Topographie Memel* [36], p. 130; and Paul M. Zettwach, *Über die fehlerhafte Ernährung der Kinder in Berlin* (Berlin, 1845), p. 6.

72. Leopold Fleckles, *Die herrschenden Krankheiten des schönen Geschlechtes . . . in grossen Städten* (Vienna, 1832), p. 14.

73. John S. Haller, Jr., and Robin M. Haller, *The Physician and Sexuality in Victorian America* (Urbana: University of Illinois Press, 1974), pp. 146–74.

74. Christoph Raphael Schleis von Löwenfeld, *Medizinische Ortsbeschreibung der Stadt Schwandorf im Nordgau* (Sulzbach, 1799), p. 29.

75. Joseph Steiner, *Versuch einer medizinischen Topographie vom Landgerichtsbezirke Parckstein und Weyden in der obern Pfalz* (Sulzbach, 1808), p. 62; F. J. Werfer, *Versuch einer medizinischen Topographie der Stadt Gmünd* (Gmünd, 1813), p. 80, and Eugène Bougeatre, *La Vie rurale dans le Mantois* (Meulan, 1971).

76. Bougeatre, ibid., p. 41.

77. Soemmerring, *Schädlichkeit Schnürbrüste* [67], p. 149.

78. Eugène Olivier, *Médecine et santé dans le Pays de Vaud aux XVIIIᵉ siècle*, 2 vols. (Lausanne, 1939), I, 565.

79. Munaret, *Médecin des villes et des campagnes* [35], p. 419.

80. Wohlgemuth, *Bäuerin badische Gemeinden* [16], p. 93; and Maria Bidlingmaier, *Die Bäuerin in zwei Gemeinden Württembergs* (Tübingen: staatswiss. diss., 1918), p. 111.

81. Bidlingmaier, ibid., p. 111. ("Das Korsett verschmäht die Bäuerin, während es die jungen Mädchen meistens sonntags tragen").

82. Dr. W. H. Sheehy, note in *Lancet*, 18 February 1871, p. 256. I am indebted to a seminar paper by K. Vertesi, "On the Theoretical and Methodological Errors of 19th Century Physicians Writing on the Detrimental Effects of the Corset," 1981, for this and other references.

83. Gerhart S. Schwarz, "Society, Physicians, and the Corset," *Bulletin of the New York Academy of Medicine*, 55 (1979), 556–57.

84. Gerhart S. Schwarz, *NEJM:* letters of 15 March 1973, p. 584; 21 June 1973, p. 1359; 5 July 1973, p. 46; 27 September 1973, p. 698; and Schwarz's letter of 10 October 1974, p. 802.

Chapter 3

1. World Health Organization, *Traditional Birth Attendants* (Geneva: World Health Organization, 1979), p. 7. "Between 60 percent and 80 percent of all births are attended by TBAs."

2. Brigitte Jordan, *Birth in Four Cultures* (Montreal: Eden Press, 1978), p. 95n3.

3. Catherine M. Scholten, " 'On the Importance of the Obstetrick Art': Changing Customs of Childbirth in America, 1760 to 1825," *William and Mary Quarterly*, 3rd ser., 34 (1977), 433.

4. In Gustav Klein, ed., *Eucharius Rösslin's "Rosengarten"* (Munich, 1910), p. 8. The first German edition, *Der Swangern Frauwen und Hebammen Rosegarten*, appeared in Worms in 1513, and the first English edition, *The Byrth of Mankynde*, appeared in 1540 in London. Translation is mine. The German original:

> Ich meyn die Hebammen alle sampt
> Die also gar kein wissen handt
> Darzu durch ihr Hynlessigkeit
> Kind verderben weit und breit.

5. For a convenient sampling of these criticisms, see Jacques Gélis, "Sages-femmes et accoucheurs: l'obstétrique populaire aux XVIIᵉ et XVIIIᵉ siècles," *Annales: Economies, Sociétés, Civilisations*, 32 (1977), 927–57; and Mireille Laget, "La Naissance aux siècles classiques. Pratique des accouchements et attitudes collectives en France aux XVIIᵉ et XVIIIᵉ siècles," 958–92.

6. Elseluise Haberling, however, cited some who did read manuals in *Beiträge zur Geschichte des Hebammenstandes: Der Hebammenstand in Deutschland von seinen Anfängen bis zum Dreissigjährigen Krieg* (Berlin, 1940), pp. 57–58.

7. For a full description of these remarkable professional organizations, see ibid., pp. 42–44 and passim.

8. Johann Ferdinand Roth, *Fragmente zur Geschichte der Bader, Barbierer, Hebammen,*

Erbaren Frauen und Geschwornen Weiber in der freyen Reichsstadt Nürnberg (Nürnberg, 1792), p. 35.

9. Ibid., p. 35.

10. Heinrich Fasbender, *Geschichte der Geburtshilfe* (Jena, 1906), p. 81.

11. Ibid., p. 81n6.

12. Alois Nöth, *Die Hebammenordnungen des XVIII. Jahrhunderts* (Würzburg: med. diss., 1931).

13. Georg Burckhard, *Die deutschen Hebammenordnungen von ihren ersten Anfängen bis auf die Neuzeit* (Leipzig, 1912), p. 34.

14. Haberling, *Hebammenstand* [6], p. 29.

15. Ibid., p. 29.

16. Ida Wehrli, *Das öffentliche Medizinalwesen der Stadt Baden im Aargau* (Aagau, 1927), p. 95.

17. Alexandre Faidherbe, *Les Accouchements en Flandre avant 1789* (Lille, 1891), pp. 17–18.

18. Jean-Pierre Goubert, *Malades et médecins en Bretagne, 1770–1790* (Paris: Klincksieck, 1974), p. 163.

19. Haberling, *Hebammenstand* [6], p. 90.

20. Burckhard, *Hebammenordnungen* [13], p. 34.

21. Friedrich Osiander, *Beobachtungen . . . Krankheiten der Frauenzimmer und Kinder und die Entbindungswissenschaft betreffen* (Tübingen, 1787), pp. 181–82.

22. Dr. Goldschmidt, *Volksmedicin im Nordwestlichen Deutschland* (Bremen, 1854), pp. 92–93.

23. J. B. Gebel, *Aktenstücke die Möglichkeit der gänzlichen Blattern-ausrottung . . . betreffend* (Breslau, 1802), pp. 130–31.

24. Percivall Willughby, *Observations in Midwifery* (1863; rpt. East Ardsley. S. R. Publishers, 1972), p. 29.

25. Ibid., p. 9.

26. H. Krauss, "Zur Geschichte des Hebammenwesens im Fürstentum Ansbach," [*Sudhoff's*] *Archiv für die Geschichte der Medizin*, 6 (1912), 65–66.

27. Joseph Berthelot, *Topographie de . . . Bressuire (en 1786)* (Bressuire, 1887), p. 15.

28. Laget, "Naissance" [5], p. 976.

29. Anne Amable Augier du Fot, *Catéchisme sur l'art des accouchemens pour les sages-femmes de la campagne* (Soissons, 1775), p. xi.

30. Gebel, *Aktenstücke* [23], p. 130.

31. Haberling, *Hebammenstand* [6], pp. 16–17.

32. Ibid., pp. 36–37.

33. Egon Schmitz-Cliever, *Die Heilkunde in Aachen* (Aachen: Sonderdruck Zeitschrift Aachener Geschichtsverein, Bd. 74/75, 1963), p. 59.

34. H. Deichert, *Geschichte des Medizinalwesens im Gebiet des ehemaligen Königreichs Hannover* (Hannover, 1908), pp. 91–92.

35. Jacob Rüff, *Ein schön lustig Trostbüchle . . .* (Zurich, 1554). This judgment about the relatively greater value of Rüff's textbook is from Haberling, *Hebammenstand* [6], pp. 94–101. On Zurich's midwifery legislation see Eugène Olivier, *Médecine et santé dans le pays de Vaud au XVIIIᵉ siècle, 1675–1798*, 2 vols. (Lausanne, 1939) I, 276.

36. On Amsterdam, see Catharine van Tussenbroek, "Das Hebammenwesen in den Niederlanden," *Gynäkologische Rundschau*, 6 (1912), 255; on Darmstadt, Adolf Müller, *Beiträge zu einer hessischen Medizingeschichte des 15.–18. Jahrhunderts* (Darmstadt, 1929), pp. 17–18; and on Bavaria, Alexander von Hoffmeister, *Das Medizinalwesen im Kurfürstentum Bayern* (Munich: Fritsch, 1975), p. 84.

37. Nöth, *Hebammenordnungen* [12], pp. 58–59.

38. Gélis, "Sages-femmes" [5], p. 953n30.

39. François Lebrun, *Les Hommes et la mort en Anjou* (Paris: Mouton, 1971), p. 212n53.

40. Goubert, *Malades Bretagne* [18], p. 162, for an example of Brittany.

41. Jean Donnison, *Midwives and Medical Men: A History of Inter-Professional Rivalries and Women's Rights* (New York: Schocken, 1977), p. 6. Read story from Donnison; see also James H. Aveling, *English Midwives, Their History and Prospects* (1872; rpt. London: Elliott, 1967), p. 88.

42. J. M. Munro Kerr, ed., *Historical Review of British Obstetrics and Gynaecology*,

1800–1950 (Edinburgh: Livingstone, 1954), p. 278. On eighteenth-century regulations in Edinburgh, see, however, R. E. Wright-St. Clair, "Early Essays at Regulating Midwives," *New Zealand Medical Journal*, 63 (1964), 725.

43. Herbert Thoms, *Chapters In American Obstetrics* (Springfield, Ill., 1933), pp. 7–8.
44. Deichert, *Medizinalwesen Hannover* [34], p. 92.
45. Fasbender, *Geschichte Geburtshilfe* [10], p. 85; and Nöth, *Hebammenordnungen* [12], passim.
46. Haberling, *Hebammenstand* [6], p. 106.
47. Fasbender, *Geschichte Geburtshilfe* [10], p. 85.
48. Marcel Fosseyeux, *L'Hôtel-Dieu de Paris au XVIIe et au XVIIIe siècle* (Paris, 1912), pp. 286, 402. For a description of the delivery service in the Hôtel Dieu, see Jacques-René Tenon, *Mémoires sur les hôpitaux de Paris* (Paris, 1788), p. 230ff.
49. Hermann Freund, "Das Hebammenwesen," in Joseph Krieger, ed., *Topographie der Stadt Strassburg* (Strasbourg, 1889), p. 306. The date is often given incorrectly as "1728"; see, for example, Gélis, "Sages-femmes" [5], p. 955n48.
50. On Würzburg's school, see Joseph Horsch, *Versuch einer Topographie der Stadt Würzburg* (Arnstadt, 1805), pp. 384–85; on Berlin, F. C. Wille, *Über Stand und Ausbildung der Hebammen im 17. und 18. Jahrhundert in Chur-Brandenburg* (Berlin, 1934), p. 121; on Neuötting, Hoffmeister, *Medizinalwesen Bayern* [36], pp. 84–85; on Basel, Hans Jenzer, "Die Gründung der Hebammenschulen in der Schweiz im 18. Jahrhundert," *Gesnerus*, 23 (1966), 69. The Coblence "school" was a three-month course; what clinical facilities existed is unclear from the account in E. François, "La Population de Coblence au XVIIIe siècle," *Annales de démographie historique*, 1975, pp. 314–15.
51. Laget, "Naissance" [5], p. 985; Goubert, *Malades Bretagne* [18], p. 165 (on the first midwife courses in Brittany) and p. 168ff. (on Madame du Coudray's tour). Jacques Gélis published a map of training courses for midwives in France founded between 1750 and 1800: "Regard sur l'Europe médicale des Lumières: la collaboration internationale des accoucheurs et la formation des sages-femmes au XVIIIe siècle," in Arthur Imhof, ed. *Mensch und Gesundheit in der Geschichte* (Husum: Matthiesen, 1980), p. 288.
52. G. V. Jägerschmidt, "Hygienische Ortsbeschreibung des Badischen Physikats Rötteln und Sausenberg" (1760), in Generallandesarchiv, Karlsruhe, manuscript no. 394 of Hausfideikommiss. I owe a copy of this manuscript to the kindness of Arthur Imhof.
53. Dietrich Tutzke, "Über statistische Untersuchungen als Beitrag zur Geschichte des Hebammenwesens im ausgehenden 18. Jahrhundert," *Centaurus*, 4 (1956), 353.
54. "Soll den Hebammen der Gebrauch des Mutterrohres in der geburtshilflichen Praxis verboten werden?" *Wiener Medizinische Presse*, offprint from no. 5 (1890), p. 4.
55. Tutzke, "Statistische Untersuchungen" [53], p. 354.
56. C. F. Senff, *Über Vervollkommnung der Geburtshülfe* (Halle, 1812), p. 41.
57. Rudolf Dohrn, "Erfahrungen bei Prüfungen und dem Nachexamen der Hebammen," *ZBG*, 30 (1906), 904–05.
58. Gélis, "Sages-femmes" [5], map on p. 935. See, however, the description of a midwife election in the Sarlat diocese, in Georges Rocal, *Le Vieux Périgord* (Paris, 1927), p. 45.
59. Rembert Watermann, *Vom Medizinalwesen des Kurfürstentums Köln* (Neuss: Gesellschaft für Buchdruckerei, 1977), p. 136.
60. Jean-Marie Munaret, *Le Médecin des villes et des campagnes*, 3rd ed. (Paris, 1862), p. 399.
61. Bern. Christ. Faust, *Gedanken über Hebammen und Hebammenanstalten auf dem Lande* (Frankfurt/M., 1784), pp. 34–35. See also Osiander's polemic on the uneducability of any midwife candidate over thirty (*Krankheiten Frauenzimmer* [21], pp. 168–71).
62. H. G. Gernet, *Geschichte des Hamburgischen Landphysicats von 1818 bis 1871* (Hamburg, 1884), p. 63.
63. Bertel von Bonsdorff, *The History of Medicine in Finland* (Helsinki: Finnish Society of Sciences, 1975), p. 215.
64. Alain Corbin, *Archaïsme et modernité en Limousin aux XIXe siècle*, 2 vols. (Paris: Rivière, 1975), I, 92–93; and Bernard Edeine, *La Sologne*, 2 vols. (Paris: Mouton, 1974), II, 585.
65. Dohrn, "Erfahrungen" [57], p. 908.
66. Goubert, *Malades Bretagne* [18], pp. 171–72.
67. Friedrich Julius Morgen, *Beiträge zu einer medicinischen Topographie des Kreises und der Stadt Memel* (Memel, 1843), p. 49.

68. Marcelle Bouteiller, *Médecine populaire d'hier et d'aujourd'hui* (Paris: Maisonneuve, 1966), p. 23.
69. Moritz von Willich, *Erfahrungen und Bemerkungen über die Krankheiten auf der Insel Rügen* (n.p., 1805), pp. 18–19.
70. Johann Adolph Behrends, *Der Einwohner in Frankfurt am Mayn in Absicht auf seine Fruchtbarkeit, Mortalität und Gesundheit geschildert* (Frankfurt/M., 1771), pp. 228–29.
71. Eduard Otto Dann, *Topographie von Danzig* (Berlin, 1835), p. 279.
72. Johann Gottfried Ebel, *Schilderung des Gebirgsvolkes vom Kanton Glarus* (Leipzig, 1802), p. 291.

Chapter 4

1. Suzanne Arms, *Immaculate Deception: A New Look at Women and Childbirth in America* (Boston: Houghton Mifflin, 1975), p. 8.
2. Florence E. F. Barnes, ed., *Ambulatory Maternal Health Care* (n.p.: American Public Health Association: Committee on Maternal Health Care, 1978), p. 18.
3. R. de Westphalen, *Petit dictionnaire des traditions populaires messines* (Metz, 1934), p. 328.
4. H. Höhn, "Sitte und Brauch bei Geburt, Taufe und in der Kindheit," *Württembergische Jahrbücher* (1909), p. 256.
5. Aloys Winterling, *Die bäuerliche Lebens-und Sittengemeinschaft der hohen Rhön* (Cologne, 1939), p. 88.
6. Barbara Ehrenreich and Deirdre English, *Witches, Midwives, and Nurses: A History of Women Healers*, 2nd ed. (Old Westbury, N.Y.: The Feminist Press, 1973), pp. 15–17.
7. Ibid., p. 19 and passim.
8. Guillaume Mauquest de la Motte, *Traité complet des acouchemens*, rev. ed. (1715; rpt. Leiden, 1729), pp. 64–65.
9. Franz Strohmayr, *Versuch einer physisch-medicinischen Topographie von . . . St. Pölten* (Vienna, 1813), pp. 117–18.
10. Ibid., p. 117.
11. Friedrich Colland, *Untersuchung der gewöhnlichen Ursachen so vieler frühzeitig-todtgebohrner . . . Kinder* (Vienna, 1800), p. 9.
12. *Bavaria: Landes-und Volkskunde des Königreichs Bayern*, vol. 1: *Ober- und Niederbayern* (Munich, 1860), p. 463. The "Zentner" figure does not include blood lost from blistering.
13. See the exchange of letters between Dr. Koestlin and Dr. Israel in *Zeitschrift für Medizinalbeamte*, 23 (1910), 561–64.
14. Lily Weiser-Aall, "Die Speise des Neugeborenen," in Edith Ennen and Günter Wiegelmann, eds., *Festschrift Matthias Zender*, 2 vols. (Bonn: Ludwig Röhrscheid, 1972) I, 543n62.
15. For examples of indulgence, see Westphalen, *Petit Dictionnaire* [3], p. 327; Freddy Sarg, *La Naissance en Alsace* (Strasbourg: Oberlin, 1974), pp. 12–13; and Yvonne Verdier, *Façons de dire, façons de faire* (Paris: Gallimard, 1979), pp. 49–52.
16. Hans Fehr, *Die Rechtstellung der Frau und der Kinder in den Weistümern* (Jena, 1912), p. 5.
17. On Franconia, see Christian Pfeufer, "Über das Verhalten der Schwangeren . . . auf dem Lande," *Jahrbuch der Staatsarzneikunde*, 3 (1810), 49; on Périgord, see R. Beaudry, "Alimentation et population rurale en Périgord au XVIIIᵉ siècle," *Annales de démographie historique*, 1976, pp. 52–53.
18. Weiser-Aall, "Speise des Neugeborenen" [14], p. 543.
19. Gertrud Herrig, *Ländliche Nahrung im Strukturwandel des 20. Jahrhunderts* (Meisenheim: Hain, 1974), p. 215.
20. Dr. Zengerle, "Auszug . . . statistisch-medicinischen Topographie des Oberamtsbezirks Wangen," *Medicinisches Correspondenz-Blatt des württembergischen ärztlichen Vereins*, 18 (1848), 256.
21. Herrig, *Ländliche Nahrung* [19], p. 215n43, sometime in the early twentieth century.
22. Marta Wohlgemuth, *Die Bäuerin in zwei badischen Gemeinden* (Karlsruhe, 1913), calculated from table on pp. 116–23.

23. Maria Bidlingmaier, *Die Bäuerin in zwei Gemeinden Württembergs* (Tübingen: Staatswiss. diss., 1918), p. 267.

24. Louis Caradec, *Topographie médico-hygiénique du département du Finistère* (Brest, 1860), p. 78.

25. Pfeufer, "Verhalten Schwangeren" [17], p. 48.

26. Dr. Märkel, "Medicinisch-topographische und ethnographische Beschreibung des Physicats-Bezirkes Roding, 1860," manuscript in "Bestand: Landgerichtsarzt Roding," no. 2, in Bayerisches Staatsarchiv, Amberg.

27. See the "Rural Child Welfare Series" of the Children's Bureau of the U.S. Department of Labor, Frances Sage Bradley and Margaretta A. Williamson, *Rural Children in Selected Counties of North Carolina* (1918), p. 34: Viola I. Paradise, *Maternity Care and the Welfare of Young Children in a Homesteading County in Montana* (1919), p. 58; and Helen M. Dart, *Maternity and Child Care in Selected Rural Areas of Mississippi* (1921), p. 38. These have been conveniently reprinted by the Arno Press (New York, 1972).

28. E. Pelkonen, *Über volkstümliche Geburtshilfe in Finnland* (Helsinki, 1931), p. 88.

29. Höhn, "Geburt" [4], p. 258.

30. Westphalen, *Petit dictionnaire* [3], p. 327; "descende et décolle bien."

31. Heinz Küstner, *Fortpflanzungsschädigung der erwerbstätigen Frau und ihre Abhilfe* (Leipzig, 1930), pp. 48, 55–58.

32. Bonnie S. Worthington, "Nutrition in Pregnancy," *Birth and the Family Journal*, 6 (1979), 184.

33. Women's Co-operative Guild, *Maternity: Letters from Working-Women* (London, 1915), pp. 22, 53.

34. Herbert Thoms, *Chapters in American Obstetrics* (Springfield, Ill., 1933), p. 10.

35. De la Motte, *Traité* [8], pp. 428–29.

36. Jean-Marie Munaret, *Le Médecin des villes et des campagnes* (Paris, 1862), p. 396.

37. On older-younger women, see Reinhard Worschech, *Frauenfeste und Frauenbräuche in vergleichender Betrachtung mit besonderer Berücksichtigung Frankens* (Würzburg: phil diss., 1971), p. 183n236 for example from Dithmarschen.

38. Bernhard Christian Faust, *Gedanken über Hebammen und Hebammenanstalten auf dem Lande* (Frankfurt/M., 1784), p. 31n14.

39. Alois Nöth, *Die Hebammenordnungen des XVIII. Jahrhunderts* (Würzburg: med. diss., 1931), p. 117.

40. Adams Walther, "Zur Hebammenfrage," *ZBG*, 8 (1884), 306.

41. Christoph Raphaël Schleis von Löwenfeld, *Warum ist die Sterblichkeit der neugebohrnen Kinder so gross?* (Sulzbach, 1794), p. 53.

42. Munaret, *Médecin des villes* [36], p. 400.

43. Daniel Fabre and Jacques Lacroix, *La Vie quotidienne des paysans du Languedoc au XIXe siècle* (Paris: Hachette, 1973), p. 91.

44. Bernard Edeine, *La Sologne: Contribution aux études d'ethnologie métropolitaine*, 2 vols. (Paris: Mouton, 1974), II, 586 ("Puisque tu as été à la façon, tu s'ras à la récolte").

45. Medieval views summarized in Elseluise Haberling, *Beiträge zur Geschichte des Hebammenstandes: Der Hebammenstand in Deutschland von seinen Anfängen bis zum Dreissigjährigen Krieg* (Berlin, 1940), p. 67.

46. Ibid., p. 67.

47. Heinrich Fasbender, *Geschichte der Geburtshilfe* (Jena, 1906), p. 38.

48. Alfred Martin, "Gëbarlage der Frau . . . ," [*Sudhoff's*] *Archiv für die Geschichte der Medizin*, 10 (1917), 211.

49. Haberling, *Geschichte Hebammenstandes* [45], p. 69.

50. Max Höfler, *Der Isar-Winkel aerztlich-topographisch geschildert* (Munich, 1891), p. 187.

51. Friedrich Julius Morgen, *Beiträge zu einer medicinischen Topographie . . . Memel* (Memel, 1843), pp. 49–50.

52. Pfeufer, "Verhalten Schwangeren" [17], p. 51.

53. Carl Müller, *Volksmedizinisch-geburtshilfliche Aufzeichnungen aus dem Lötschental* (Berne: Hans Huber, 1969), p. 70.

54. Edeine, *Sologne* [44], II, 584.

55. Rose-Claire Schüle, "L'Accouchement dans le Valais central de 1850 à 1950," *Gesnerus*, 36 (1979), p. 57.

56. Rudolf Temesváry, *Volksbräuche und Aberglauben in der Geburtshilfe . . . in Ungarn* (Leipzig, 1900), pp. 46–47.

57. Roberto Caldeyro-Barcia, "The Influence of Maternal Position on Time of Spontaneous Rupture of the Membranes, Progress of Labor, and Fetal Head Compression," *Birth and the Family Journal*, 6 (1979), 7–15.

58. Percivall Willughby, *Observations in Midwifery* (1863; rpt. East Ardsley: S. R. Publishers, 1972), p. 14, see also pp. 73–75, 160.

59. C. E. Fischer, *Bemerkungen über die englische Geburtshülfe* (Göttingen, 1797), p. 32.

60. Charles White, *A Treatise on the Management of Pregnant and Lying-In Women* (London, 1772), p. 290.

61. "Concluding Report of Infant Mortality Committee," *Obstetrical Society of London, Transactions*, 12 (1870), p. 390.

62. *Lancet* note, 17 April 1875, p. 563.

63. See Jean Paul Stucky, *Der Gebärstuhl: Die Gründe für sein Verschwinden im deutschen Sprachbereich* (Zurich: Juris, 1965), p. 34 and passim.

64. Willughby, *Observations* [58], p. 22.

65. Ibid., p. 21.

66. Moritz Gerhard Thilenius, *Kurzer Unterricht für die Hebammen und Wöchnerinnen auf dem Lande* (Kassel, 1769), p. 38.

67. Nöth, *Hebammenordnungen* [39], p. 17.

68. Müller, *Aufzeichnungen Lötschental* [53], p. 77.

69. J. H. Wigand, *Beyträge zur . . . Geburtshülfe* (Hamburg, 1800), p. 78.

70. Ibid., p. 82.

71. Jane B. Donegan, *Women and Men Midwives: Medicine, Morality, and Misogyny in Early America* (Westport: Greenwood, 1978), p. 10.

72. Leo Eloesser et al., *Pregnancy, Childbirth and the Newborn: A Manual for Rural Midwives*, 3rd English ed. (Ninos Héroes: Instituto Indigenista Interamericano, 1973), pp. 40–46.

73. For example, Jack A. Pritchard and Paul C. MacDonald, *Williams Obstetrics*, 16th ed. (New York: Appleton-Century-Crofts, 1980), pp. 405–35.

74. C. F. Senff, *Über Vervollkommnung der Geburtshülfe* (Halle, 1812), p. 89.

75. Schleis von Löwenfeld, *Warum Sterblichkeit* [41], p. 52n.

76. Wigand, *Beyträge* [69], p. 74.

77. Adolf Müller, *Beiträge zu einer hessischen Medizingeschichte* (Darmstadt, 1929), p. 18.

78. Nöth, *Hebammenordnungen* [39], p. 43 (" . . . den Frauen-Leib von einander reissen . . .").

79. Ibid., p. 154.

80. Ibid., p. 160.

81. Ibid., p. 175.

82. Louise Bourgeois, *Observations diverses sur la sterilité* (Paris, 1626), pp. 47–48.

83. L. S. ("Nicolas") Saucerotte, *Examen de plusieurs préjugés et usages abusifs concernant les femmes enceintes* (Strasbourg, 1777), p. 16 ("Je veux parler des attouchemens continuels et peu ménagés qu'elles font aux femmes qui sont dans les maux, en s'efforcant de dilater mal-à-propos l'orifice de la matrice, dans la fausse vue de hâter le travail").

84. Jacques Mesnard, *Le Guide des accoucheurs* (Paris, 1753), pp. 336–37 (" . . . en dilatant le vagin de la malade du côté de son anus, et en lui repoussant le coccyx en arrière . . .").

85. Schüle, "L'Accouchement" [55], pp. 56, 59.

86. Willughby, *Observations* [58], p. 20.

87. Ibid., p. 119.

88. Fasbender, *Geschichte Geburtshilfe* [47], p. 39.

89. Summarized in Haberling, *Geschichte Hebammenstand* [45], pp. 69–70.

90. Jean L. Liébaut, *Thrésor des remèdes secrets pour les maladies des femmes* (Paris, 1597), p. 882.

91. Fasbender, *Geschichte Geburtshilfe* [47], p. 214.

92. Quote is from Willughby, *Observations* [58], p. 39.

93. F. Ahlfeld, "Die geburtshilflichen Operationen in der Hebammenpraxis," *ZBG*, 14 (1890), 260.

94. Saucerotte, *Examen préjugés* [83], p. 25.

95. Augustus Bozzi Granville, *A Report of the Practice of Midwifery at the Westminster General Dispensary during 1818* (London, 1819), p. 203.

96. Nöth, *Hebammenordnungen* [39], p. 160.

97. Müller, *Aufzeichnungen Lötschental* [53], p. 106.

98. Edmund Chapman, *A Treatise on the Improvement of Midwifery*, 2nd ed. (London, 1735), p. 124.

99. Bourgeois, *Observations* [82], pp. 175–76, 182–83.

100. A. F. Nolde, *Notizen zur Kultur Geschichte der Geburtshülfe in dem Herzogthum Braunschweig* [Erfurt, 1807), p. 91.

101. Henrich Ernest Justi, "Etwas über die sehr nothwendige Verbesserung des Hebammenwesens in Sachsen," *Johann Christ. Starks Archiv für die Geburtshülfe*, 1 (ii) (1787), 43–45.

102. On the remote history of these doctrines see Fasbender, *Geschichte Geburtshilfe* [47], p. 766 and passim.

103. Nöth, *Hebammenordnungen* [39], p. 24.

104. Francis Ramsbotham, *The Principles and Practice of Obstetric Medicine and Surgery* (London, 1841), pp. 195–96. See also Charles D. Meigs, *Obstetrics*, 5th ed. (Philadelphia, 1867), p. 352; and Fleetwood Churchill, *On the Diseases of Women*, new Amer. ed. (Philadelphia, 1852), p. 543.

105. Alain Mathiot, *Pratique obstétricale à Lyon à la fin du XVIIIe et au XIXe siècles* (Lyon: med. diss., 1975), p. 77.

106. See Wohlegemuth, *Bäuerin badischen Gemeinden* [22], p. 124; and G. Lammert, *Volksmedizin und medizinischer Aberglaube in Bayern* (Würzburg, 1869), p. 173.

107. Josefine Biedermann, *Die weise Frau: Ernste und heitere Erlebnisse aus 30-jähriger Praxis* (Graz, 1934), p. 58.

108. Women's Co-operative Guild, *Maternity* [33], p. 32.

109. In the discussion following a paper by Victor Bonney, "The Continued High Maternal Mortality of Child-bearing," *Proceedings of the Royal Society of Medicine. London*, 12 (1918–19), 103.

110. Ramsbotham, *Obstetric Medicine* [104], p. 196.

111. Dr. Rieger, manuscript "Topographie des Physikats-Bezirkes Cadolzburg," 1860, in Bayerische Staatsbibliothek, Cod. Germ. 6874.

112. Letter of 1784, cited in Jacques Gélis, "Sages-femmes et accoucheurs: l'obstétrique populaire aux XVIIe et XVIIIe siècles," *Annales: Economies, Sociétés, Civilisations*, 32 (1977), 952n8.

113. Dr. Wunderlich, *Versuch einer medicinischen Topographie der Stadt Sulz am Neckar* (Tübingen, 1809), p. 50.

114. Thilenius *Unterricht Hebammen* [66], pp. 6–7.

115. Emil Schleiniger, *Die Gesundheitsverhältnisse der Bevölkerung des Eifischtales* (Basel: med. diss., 1938), p. 18.

116. Caradec, *Topographie Finistère* [24], p. 78.

117. Mathias Macher, *Medizinisch-statistische Topographie . . . Steiermark* (Graz, 1860), p. 107. See also Anton Elsener, *Medizinisch-topographische Bemerkungen über einen Theil des Urnerlandes* (Altdorf, 1811), p. 85, who says second day, and Wilhelm Brenner-Schaeffer, *Darstellung der sanitätlichen Volks-Sitten . . . der Oberpfalz* (Amberg, 1861), p. 14, who says two to three days for "some" mothers.

118. Pfeufer, "Verhalten der Schwangeren" [17], p. 54.

119. P. J. Schneider, *Versuch einer medizinisch statistischen Topographie von Ettlingen* (Karlsruhe, 1818), pp. 131–32n.

120. Catherine M. Scholten, " 'On the Importance of the Obstetrick Art': Changing Customs of Childbirth in America, 1760 to 1825," *William and Mary Quarterly*, 3rd ser., 34 (1977), p. 434.

121. Ann Oakley, "A Case of Maternity: Paradigms of Women as Maternity Cases," *Signs*, 4 (1979), 607–31.

Chapter 5

1. An entry in 1813 quoted in Carl N. Degler, *At Odds: Women and the Family in America from the Revolution to the Present* (New York: Oxford Univ. Press, 1980), p. 59.

2. W. B. Kesteven, "A Case of Puerperal Uterine Phlebitis," *LMG*, NS, 11 (1850), 926.

3. Women's Co-operative Guild, *Maternity: Letters from Working-Women* (1915; rpt. New York: Garland, 1980), p. 166.

4. Zandyck, *Etude sur la fièvre puerpèrale . . . qui a regné à Dunkerque* (Paris, 1856), pp. 37–38.

5. Erwin Richter, "Verschiedenes von unbekannteren Volksheilbräuchen in bayerischen Mirakelbüchern," *Münchener medizinische Wochenschrift,* 25 December 1953, p. 1401.

6. Freddy Sarg, *La Naissance en Alsace* (Strasbourg: Oberlin, 1974), p. 29.

7. Victor Fossel, *Volksmedicin und medicinischer Aberglaube in Steiermark* (Graz, 1886), p. 52.

8. Keith Thomas, *Religion and the Decline of Magic* (New York: Scribner's, 1971), p. 28.

9. H. Höhn, "Sitte und Brauch bei Geburt, Taufe und in der Kindheit," *Württembergische Jahrbücher,* 1909, p. 257 ("Ist vollends der Aschermittwoch trübe, so sterben in demselben Jahre alle Wöchnerinnen").

10. Mireille Laget, "La Naissance aux siècles classiques: pratique des accouchements et attitudes collectives en France aux XVIIe et XVIIIe siècles," *Annales ESC,* 32 (1977), 967.

11. Fr. Scholz, "Fahrlässige Tödtung einer Gebärenden," *Vierteljahrsschrift für gerichtliche und öffentliche Medicin,* NF, 6 (1867), 327–28.

12. Runzler, "Auszug aus den Acten einer Untersuchung gegen einen Chirurgen und eine Hebamme . . . . ," *Zeitschrift für die Staatsarzneikunde,* 25 Ergänzungsheft (1838), 173 ("O mein Gott, jetzt muss ich sterben, jetzt reisst ihr mir den Bauch ab! Ich bitt ums Blut Christi willen, lasst mich nur ein wenig verschnaufen!").

13. Among the sources for these midwives' and doctors' estimates of frequency see: Ludwig Formey, *Versuch einer medicinischen Topographie von Berlin* (Berlin, 1796), p. 122 ("Unter hundert Geburten kann man höchstens 4 bis 6 schwere und widernatüliche im Durchschnitt annehmen"); Gottlieb von Ehrhart, *Physisch-medizinische Topographie . . . Memmingen* (Memmingen, 1813), p. 108, end table VII ("schlimme Niederkünfte" in 1743 deliveries); Jak. Kriechbanner, "Medizinische Topographie des königlich bairischen Landgerichts Tölz, 1805," ms. in Staatsarchiv München, Gesundheitsamt Tölz, no. 68; Joseph Steiner, *Versuch einer medizinischen Topographie vom Landgerichtsbezirke Parckstein und Weyden in der obern Pfalz* (Sulzbach, 1808), pp. 57, 352 ("schwere regelmässige Geburten" plus 13 "regelwidrige Geburten" in 2,300 deliveries); John S. Fairbairn, "Observations on the Maternal Mortality in the Midwifery Service of the Queen Victoria's Jubilee Institute," *BMJ,* 8 January 1927, p. 48 (16,221 "calls for difficulty or delay in labour" in 104,000 deliveries; 24,000 calls to a doctor generally); Maria Bidlingmaier, *Die Bäuerin in zwei Gemeinden* (Tübingen: staatswiss. diss., 1918), p. 176 (based on 475 labors); and J. Lane-Claypon, "Preliminary Report by the Medical Officer . . . in Lancashire," *in Forty-Third Annual Report of the Local Government Board, 1913–14 Containing a Third Report on Infant Mortality,* London, Cd. paper no. 7511, 1914, pp. 149–68 (7,313 births "for which medical aid sought" among 54,000 total births notified by midwives; doctors' booked cases excluded).

14. Cited by Doris Haire, "The Cultural Warping of Childbirth," in John Ehrenreich, ed., *The Cultural Crisis of Modern Medicine* (New York: Monthly Review Press, 1978), p. 194.

15. "Labor usually is not prolonged." Jack A. Pritchard and Paul C. MacDonald, *Williams Obstetrics,* 16th ed. (New York: Appleton-Century-Crofts, 1980), p. 802.

16. Marie Lachapelle, *Pratique des accouchemens,* 3 vols. (Paris, 1825), II, end table.

17. Ibid.

18. Rudolf Beck, *Geburten und Geburtshilfe in ländlichen Verhältnissen: eine statistische Studie aus den Geburtstabellen des Amtes Sursee über die letzten 39 Jahre* (Basel, med. diss., 1930), p. 19. I have taken *unregelmässige Schädellage* to mean "occiput-posterior." "Head," of course, means vertex or top of the skull.

19. Fleetwood Churchill conveniently compiles large statistical series on presentations.

On the Theory and Practice of Midwifery, 3rd ed. (Philadelphia, 1848), pp. 386–404. See also the studies by Davis (on London) (see notes to table 5.3), Spiegelberg (on Baden) *Text Book of Midwifery*, 2 vols., Eng. trans. (London, 1887–88), Büttner (on Mecklenburg) (see notes to table 5.3), Hecker (on the Munich Maternity Hospital) (see notes to table 5.3), Collins (on Dublin's Rotunda Hospital) (see notes to table 5.3), and Hirsch (citing statewide statistics from Baden) (see notes to table 5.4). In addition may be mentioned Alfred Velpeau, *Traité complet de l'art des accouchemens* (Paris, 1835), I, cxxvii, citing Madame Boivin's results in Paris's Maison royale de santé, around 1800–12; Anselm Martin, *Die neue Gebär-Anstalt* (Munich, 1857), pp. 171–75 on results in Munich for 1783–1856; Siegfried Rosenfeld, "Zum Schutze der Gebärenden," *ZGH*, 57 (1906), 156, for data on Austria by province, 1898–1902; James W. Markoe, "Observations and Statistics on Sixty Thousand Labors Occurring in the Service of the Society of the Lying-In Hospital of the City of New York," *Bulletin of the Lying-in Hospital*, 6 (1909), 104, for New York for the years 1890–1909; and Great Britain, Ministry of Health, *Report on Maternal Mortality in Wales*, (London, Cmd. paper no. 5423, 1937), p. 66, for presentations in midwife-assisted deliveries in Wales, 1934.

20. See the citation to Rosenfeld, "Zum Schutze" [19], p. 156.

21. Bidlingmaier, *Bäuerin* [13], p. 176.

22. Cited in Louis M. Hellman and Jack A. Pritchard, eds., 14th ed. *Williams Obstetrics* (New York: Appleton-Century-Crofts, 1971), p. 396.

23. Trent Busby, "Duration of Labor," *AJO-G*, 55 (1948), 850.

24. Ferdinand August Ritgen, *Jahrbücher der Entbindungsanstalt zu Giessen*, 2 (1820), end tables (Average: 15.4 hours). I omitted from the averages a labor of 226 hours and one of 261 hours. Ritgen breaks the 109 labors down into five separate periods and gives the duration of each period. Dormann, "Nachrichten über die Ereignisse in der . . . Entbindungsanstalt zu Hadamar," *Medicinische Jahrbücher für das Herzogthum Nassau*, 3 (1845), 89–92 (Average: 16 hours). Data concern 379 "natural" deliveries only and therefore tend to understate overall durations. John George Metcalf, "Statistics in Midwifery," *American Journal of Medical Sciences*, NS, 6 (1843), 330 (Average: 19 hours). The numerical values for these 300 cases should not be taken too exactly because Metcalf tended to group his cases at 12 hours, 24 hours and 36 hours. The longest labor is 90 hours. Otto Spiegelberg, *Midwifery* [19], p. 186. 506 cases, time period unclear (Average: 17 hours for primiparas, 11 for multiparas).

Spiegelberg doubts the reliability of some "statistics that are not uncommonly quoted as showing a shorter average duration," that he attributes to "the difficulty of exactly fixing the commencement of labor" I, 186. He might well have been referring to Robert Collins's commonly cited statistics on the Rotunda Hospital of Dublin in the 1820s in *A Practical Treatise of Midwifery* (Boston, 1841). According to Collins, 22 percent of the 15,850 cases of which the duration was recorded lasted one hour or less. Unbelievably low durations similarly turn up in Lachapelle's series for 1811 in the Paris Maison d'accouchement: 15 percent of all labors lasting 2 hours or less, with the average duration of labor being 6.5 hours. *Pratique* [16], I, 147.

25. Augustus Granville, *Report of the Practice of Midwifery at the Westminster General Dispensary during 1818* (London, 1819), p. 22.

26. T. N. A. Jeffcoate, "Prolonged Labour," *Lancet*, 8 July 1961, p. 62, fig. 3.

27. Hellman and Pritchard, *Obstetrics* [22], p. 840.

28. Jeffcoate, "Prolonged Labour" [26], p. 61.

29. Guillaume Mauquest de la Motte, *Traité complet des acouchemens*, rev. ed. (1715; rpr. Leiden, 1729), p. 182.

30. Quoted in Margaret J. Hagood, *Mothers of the South* (1939; rpt. New York: Norton, 1977), p. 115.

31. De la Motte, *Traité* [29], pp. 377–78.

32. See, for example, Dorothée Chellier, *Voyage dans l'Aurès: Notes d'un médicin envoyé en mission chez les femmes arabes* (Tizi-Ouzou, 1895), pp. 17–18. L. Raynaud, *Etude sur l'hygiène et la médecine au Maroc* (Algiers, 1902), p. 138.

33. John Roberton, "Observations on Parturition," *LMG*, 11 (1833), 42, cites testimony of two South Seas' missionaries.

34. Edward Ford, "Notes on Pregnancy and Parturition in the D'Entrecasteaux Islands," *Medical Journal of Australia*, 16 Nov. 1940, p. 500.

35. Louise Bourgeois, *Observations diverses sur la sterilité* (Paris, 1626), p. 48.

36. A seventeenth-century manuscript, Percivall Willughby, *Observations in Midwifery* (1863; rpt. East Ardsley: S. R. Publishers, 1972), p. 158.

37. Cited in Laget, "Naissance" [10], p. 977.

38. Moritz Gerhard Thilenius, *Kurzer Unterricht für die Hebammen und Wöchnerinnen auf dem Lande* (Kassel, 1769), pp. 2, 8.

39. François Mauriceau, *Observations sur la grossesse et l'accouchement* (Paris, 1694), pp. 45–46.

40. W. R. Wilde, "A Short Account of the Superstitions and Popular Practices Relating to Midwifery . . . in Ireland," *Monthly Journal of Medical Science*, NS, 35 (1849), 721–22.

41. Rudolf Temesváry, *Volksbräuche und Aberglauben in der Geburtshilfe . . . in Ungarn* (Leipzig, 1900), p. 54.

42. Ibid., p. 54.

43. See Friedrich A. Flückiger, *Pharmacographia: A History of the Principal Drugs of Vegetable Origin met with in Great Britain and British India*, 2nd ed. (London, 1879), p. 740; and Gerhard Madaus, *Lehrbuch der biologischen Heilmittel*, (1938; rpt. Hildesheim: Olms, 1976), III, 2503.

44. G. Lammert, *Volksmedizin und medizinischer Aberglaube in Bayern* (Würzburg, 1869), p. 166.

45. Christian Pfeufer, "Ueber das Verhalten der Schwangeren, Gebährenden und Wöchnerinnen auf dem Lande," *Jahrbuch der Staatsarzneikunde*, 3 (1810), 52–53.

46. Wilde, "Short Account" [40], p. 722.

47. Willughby, *Observations* [36], pp. 156–57; the procedure failed, moreover.

48. K. B. Wiklund, *Lappische Heilkunde* (Oslo, 1932), p. 155.

49. See de la Motte, *Traité* [29], p. 270.

50. Wiklund, *Lappische Heilkunde* [48], p. 155.

51. E. Pelkonen, *Über volkstümliche Geburtshilfe in Finnland* (Helsinki, 1931), p. 160.

52. Anon., *Kurzgefasste Gedanken von dem verderbten Zustande der Hebammen*, (Lübeck, 1752), pp. 7–8.

53. G. H. Fielitz, "Beobachtungen über verschiedene Hindernisse und Schwierigkeiten bei Ausübung der Geburtshülfe," *Johann Christ. Starks Archiv für die Geburtshülfe*, 2(1) (1789), 69–70.

54. Pelkonen, *Geburtshilfe Finnland* [51], p. 163.

55. De la Motte, *Traité* [29], p. 365.

56. Alois Nöth, *Die Hebammenordnungen des XVIII. Jahrhunderts* (Würzburg: med. diss., 1931), p. 23, summarized various eighteenth-century midwife ordinances. Elseluise Haberling showed how sophisticated was the skilled urban midwives' treatment of this complication, compared to the doctors of the time. *Beiträge zur Geschichte des Hebammenstandes . . . von seinen Anfängen bis zum Dreissigjährigen Krieg* (Berlin, 1940), pp. 75–76.

57. For one example among many see H. Krauss, "Zur Geschichte des Hebammenwesens im Fürstentum Ansbach," [*Sudhoff's*] *Archiv für die Geschichte der Medizin*, 6 (1912), 67–68, "Schwobacher Amtsbericht" of 13 January 1745.

58. Augier du Fot, *Catéchisme sur l'art des accouchemens pour les sages-femmes de la campagne* (Soissons, 1775), p. xii.

59. Schwarz, "Nachricht von einem merkwürdigen Geburtsfalle . . . , " *Zeitschrift für die Staatsarzneikunde*, 3 (1823), 143–44.

60. Willughby, *Observations* [36], p. 164.

61. Barbara Ehrenreich and Deirdre English, *For Her Own Good: 150 Years of the Experts' Advice to Women* (New York: Anchor, 1979), pp. 8–9.

62. This account from Heinrich Fasbender, *Geschichte der Geburtshilfe* (1906; rpt. Hildesheim: Olms, 1964), pp. 124–25.

63. These references from Haberling, *Geschichte des Hebammenstandes* [56], p. 99.

64. Nöth, *Hebammenordnungen* [56], p. 144.

65. I. G. Oberteufer, "Beobachtungen verschiedener merkwürdiger widernatürlicher Geburtsfälle," *Johann Christ. Starks Neues Archiv für die Geburtshülfe*, 2 (1801), 447–50.

66. Adolf Weber, *Bericht über Hundert in der Landpraxis operativ behandelte Geburten* (Munich, 1901), p. 17.

67. De la Motte, *Traité* [29], pp. 522–23.

68. Höfling, "Zur medicinischen Statistik von Kurhessen," *Zeitschrift für die staatliche Arzneikunde*, 21 (1841), 462–68.

69. C. F. Danz and C. F. Fuchs, *Physisch-medicinische Topographie des Kreises Schmalkalden* (Marburg, 1848), p. 257.

70. Rudolf Beck, *Geburten und Geburtshilfe in ländlichen Verhältnissen: eine statistische Studie aus den Geburtstabellen des Amtes Sursee über die letzten 39 Jahre* (Basel: med. diss., 1930), pp. 35–37.

71. Otto Büttner, "Mecklenburg-Schwerins Geburtshilfe im Jahre 1904," *ZGH*, 61 (1908), 193–94.

72. John Hall Davis, *Parturition and Its Difficulties with Clinical Illustrations and Statistics of 13,783 Deliveries* (London, 1865), p. 339.

73. Quoted in Claude E. Heaton, "Obstetrics in Colonial America," *American Journal of Surgery*, NS, 45 (1939), 607.

74. Edmund Chapman, *A Treatise on the Improvement of Midwifery*, 2nd ed. (London, 1735), p. vi.

75. Runzler "Auszug" [12], 183.

76. Dohrn, "Ueber die operativen Befugnisse der preussischen Hebammen," *Deutsche medizinische Wochenschrift*, 16 (1890), 140.

77. For a résumé of this familiar story see Walter Radcliffe, *Milestones in Midwifery* (Bristol: Wright, 1967), pp. 30–45.

78. Jean-Marie Munaret, *Le Médecin des villes et des campagnes* (Paris, 1862), p. 412.

79. Lisbeth Burger, *Vierzig Jahre Storchentante: Aus dem Tagebuch einer Hebamme* (Breslau, 1936), pp. 20–21.

80. Herbert R. Spencer, *The History of British Midwifery from 1650 to 1800* (1927; rpt. New York: AMS, 1978), p. 73n74a.

81. See Davis, *Parturition* [72], p. 339.

82. Max Hirsch, *Fruchtabtreibung und Präventivverkehr im Zusammenhang mit dem Geburtenrückgang* (Würzburg, 1914), p. 73.

83. See, for example, Jacques Gélis, "Sages-femmes et accoucheurs: l'obstétrique populaire aux XVIIe et XVIIIe siècles," *Annales ESC*, 32 (1977), 949; and Louis Caradec, *Topographie médico-hygiènique du département du Finistère* (Brest, 1860), p. 337.

84. Friedrich B. Osiander, *Beobachtungen, Abhandlungen und Nachrichten welche vorzüglich Krankheiten der Frauenzimmer und Kinder und die Entbindungswissenschaft betreffen* (Tübingen, 1787), pp. 177–78.

85. Ernest Gray, ed., *Man Midwife: The Further Experiences of John Knyveton, M.D.* (London, 1946), p. 41.

86. Jean Donnison, *Midwives and Medical Men: A History of Inter-Professional Rivalries and Women's Rights* (New York: Schocken, 1977), p. 22.

87. Quoted in James H. Aveling, *English Midwives, Their History and Prospects* (1872; rpt. London: Elliott, 1967), p. 128.

88. Johann F. Osiander, *Bemerkungen über die französische Geburtshülfe* (Hanover, 1813), pp. 91–92.

89. Hirsch, *Fruchtabtreibung* [82], p. 72.

90. K. Schreiber, "Ein Beitrag zur Statistik der Geburtshülfe mit besonderer Beziehung auf Kurhessen," *Neue Zeitschrift für Geburtskunde*, 11 (1842), 196.

91. For various series, see Hirsch, *Fruchtabtreibung* [82], p. 73; and Max Hirsch, "Der Weg der operativen Geburtshilfe in bevölkerungspolitischer Beleuchtung," *Archiv für Frauenkunde*, 13 (1927), 208–09.

92. Joseph DeLee, *Principles and Practice of Obstetrics*, 6th ed. (Philadelphia, 1933), p. 1111.

93. Adrian Wegelin, "Allgemeine Uebersicht des dritten Hunderts künstlicher Entbindungen," *Johann Christ. Stark's Neues Archiv für die Geburtshülfe*, 3 (1804), 155–57.

94. The debate about saving the life of the mother or the infant has still not found its historian. But for a brief overview, see Haberling, *Geschichte des Hebammenstandes* [56], p. 26; positions are taken by Churchill, *Theory Midwifery* [19], p. 317; Edmund Chapman, *A Treatise on the Improvement of Midwifery*, 2nd ed. (London, 1735), p. 156; and de la Motte, *Traité* [29], pp. 335, and 527ff.

95. Beck, *Geburten ländlichen Verhältnissen* [18], p. 40.

96. Ernst Zürcher, *Die geburtshülfliche Landpraxis* (Trogen, 1887), p. 9.

97. Churchill, *Theory Midwifery* [19], pp. 353–54.

98. Haberling, *Geschichte des Hebammenstandes* [56], pp. 78–79.

99. Wilde, "Superstitions Midwifery" [40], p. 724.

100. Willughby, *Observations* [36], p. 55; see another case on p. 56.

101. De la Motte, *Traité* [29], p. 269.

102. Du Fot, *Catéchisme* [58], p. xii.

103. Jean-Louis Baudelocque, cited in paraphrase by Osiander, *Franz. Geburtshülfe* [88], p. 160.

104. H. Deichert, *Geschichte des Medizinalwesens . . . Hannover* (Hanover, 1908), p. 94.

105. Thilenius, *Unterricht Hebammen* [38], p. 91.

106. See various maternal mortality series for Paris hospitals in Léon LeFort, *Des Maternités* (Paris, 1866), pp. 24–30.

107. Willughby, *Observations* [36], p. 81.

108. For a recent review, see Dorothy Nortman, "Parental Age as a Factor in Pregnancy Outcome and Child Development," *Reports on Population / Family Planning*, no. 16 (August, 1974), p. 1 ff.

109. See most recently Jacques Dupâquier, *La Population rurale du Bassin Parisien à l'époque de Louis XIV* (Paris: Editions de l'école des hautes études en sciences sociales, 1979), p. 364, for data on a sample of nine villages in the seventeenth and eighteenth centuries.

110. See the sample data in Derek Llewellyn-Jones, "The Effect of Age and Social Status on Obstetric Efficiency," *JOB*, 72 (1965), 197.

111. Franz Torggler, *Bericht über die Thätigkeit der geburtshilflich-gynäkologischen Klinik zu Innsbruck* (Prague, 1888), pp. 110–13.

112. Wegelin, "Allgemeine Uebersicht" [93], pp. 141–42; p. 127 for the age distribution of the thirty-five primiparas.

113. Pritchard and MacDonald, *Obstetrics* [15], p. 488, fig. 21–1A.

114. Burger, *Storchentante* [79], pp. 154–55.

115. De la Motte, *Traité* [29], p. 282.

116. Mireille Laget counted the references in "Naissance," [10], p. 970.

117. Joseph Schneider, *Versuch einer Topographie der Residenzstadt Fulda* (Fulda, 1806), p. 206.

118. Pelkonen, *Geburtshilfe Finnland* [51], p. 292.

119. Osiander, *Beobachtungen Krankheiten* [84], pp. 174–75.

120. Hellman and Pritchard, *Obstetrics* [22], p. 609.

121. De la Motte, *Traité* [29], p. 331.

122. Nöth, *Hebammenordnungen* [56], p. 121.

123. Bourgeois, *Observations* [35], p. 67.

124. Chapman, *Treatise Midwifery* [74], pp. 98–100.

125. On the history, see Fasbender, *Geschichte Geburtshilfe* [62], pp. 745–63.

126. Hirsch, "Weg operativen Geburtshilfe" [91], p. 210.

127. Hermann Fehling, *Entwicklung der Geburtshilfe und Gynäkologie im 19. Jahrhundert* (Berlin, 1925), p. 112; see also the discussion of H. Küstner's paper, "Die Zunahme der geburtshilflichen Komplikationen in den letzten Jahren," in *ZBG*, 50 (1926), 3402–03.

128. Willughby, *Observations* [36], p. 205.

129. Fleetwood Churchill, "Report of Cases of Convulsions Occurring in Puerperal Women," *LMG*, 15 (1835), 107–08.

130. Nortman, "Parental Age" [108], graphs on p. 19.

131. Mauriceau, *Observations grossesse* [39], p. 3.

132. Fleetwood Churchill, *On the Diseases of Women*, new Amer. ed. (Philadelphia, 1852), p. 491.

133. Carl Müller, *Volksmedizinisch-geburtshilfliche Aufzeichnungen aus dem Lötschental* (Berne: Huber, 1969), p. 60.

134. Gray, *Man Midwife* [85], pp. 80–81.

135. Laget, "Naissance" [10], p. 970.

136. Pfeufer, "Verhalten der Schwangeren" [45], pp. 52–53.

137. James H. Ferguson, "Mississippi Midwives," *Journal of the History of Medicine*, 5 (1950), 94.

138. Alma Thomas (pseud. Anneliese Bergsteiger), *Erinnerungen einer Hebamme*, (Osterwieck, 1941), p. 31.

139. Women's Co-operative Guild, *Maternity* [3], pp. 36–37.

140. Hirsch, "Weg operativen Geburtshilfe" [91], p. 211.

141. Dorothy Long, *Medicine in North Carolina*, 2 vols. (Raleigh: North Carolina Medical Society, 1972), II, 663–64.

142. Churchill, *Diseases* [132], p. 499.

143. DeLee, *Principles of Obstetrics* [92], p. 396.

144. Pritchard and MacDonald, *Obstetrics* [15], p. 687.

145. J. M. Munro Kerr et al., eds., *Historical Review of British Obstetrics and Gynaecology, 1800–1950* (Edinburgh: Livingstone, 1954), p. 156.

146. See Charles White, *Treatise on the Management of Pregnant and Lying-In Women* (London, 1772), p. 340.

147. David Levine and Keith Wrightson, *Poverty and Piety in an English Village, Terling, 1525–1700* (New York: Academic Press, 1979), p. 58.

148. John Demos, *A Little Commonwealth* (New York: Oxford Univ. Press, 1970), p. 66.

149. John Jewett, "Changing Maternal Mortality in Massachusetts," *NEJM*, 28 February 1957, p. 397.

150. Frederick Irving, "Modern Trends in the Artificial Termination of Pregnancy and Labor," *AJO-G*, 40 (1940), 621.

151. Arno Trübenbach, *Dorfsippenbuch von Grossurleben und Kleinurleben nebst . . . Wiegleben* (Langensalza, 1941) p. 240, table 37.

152. Sigismund Peller, "Studies on Mortality Since the Renaissance," *Bulletin of the History of Medicine*, 13 (1943), 443.

153. Arthur Imhof, "Die Übersterblichkeit verheirateter Frauen im fruchtbaren Alter," *Zeitschrift für Bevölkerungswissenschaft*, (1979), 504, table 6.

154. See Dupâquier, *Population bassin parisien* [109], p. 347, table 140, which summarizes the available French "family reconstitution" studies.

155. Claude Bruneel, *La Mortalité dans les campagnes: Le Duché de Brabant aux XVIIᵉ et XVIIIᵉ siècles* (Louvain: Editions Nauwelaerts, 1977), p. 456n8.

156. Peller, "Studies on Mortality" [152], 446.

157. *Denmark: Its Medical Organization, Hygiene and Demography* (Copenhagen, 1891), pp. 428–30; for towns only.

158. Maternal deaths in Sweden are from Friedrich Hendriks, "On the Vital Statistics of Sweden from 1749–1855," *Journal of the Statistical Society of London*, 25 (1862), 167. Number of deliveries are taken from Gustav Sundbärg, *Bevölkerungsstatistik Schwedens, 1750–1900* (1967; rpt. Stockholm: Statistiska Centralbyran, 1970), p. 127.

159. Thomas R. Forbes, "The Regulation of English Midwives in the Eighteenth and Nineteenth Centuries," *Medical History*, 3 (1971), 354.

160. Friedrich Colland, *Untersuchung der gewöhnlichen Ursachen so vieler frühzeitig-todtgebohrner und der grossen Sterblichkeit neugebohrner Kinder* (Vienna, 1800), p. 90n.

161. For Swiss data, see *Statistisches Jahrbuch der Schweiz*, 1945, p. 124; 1979, p. 67.

162. Edmond Weber, *Beiträge zur Mortalitäts-Statistik an septischen puerperalen Prozessen* (Berne: med. diss., 1890), end table I.

163. Brennecke, *Die soziale Bewegung auf geburtshilflichem Gebiete während der letzten Jahrzehnte* (Halle a.S., 1896), pp. 42–44.

164. Otto Walter, *Geschichte des Hebammenwesens im Grossherzogthum Mecklenburg-Schwerin* (Rostock: med. diss., 1883), pp. 62–67; and Franz Unterberger, "Die Sterblichkeit im Kindbett im Grossherzogtum Mecklenburg-Schwerin in den Jahren 1886–1909," *Archiv für Gynäkologie*, 95 (1911–12), 132.

165. For Iceland, see Gunnlaugur Snaedel et al., "Obstetric and Perinatal Medicine in Iceland, 1881–1971," *Acta Obstetricia et Gynacologica Scandinavica*, suppl. 45 (1975), 14–15. Data on Belgium and Sweden are taken from annual volumes of their respective statistical yearbooks. Overall data for England, 1891–1930, presented in Donnison, *Midwives* [86], p. 188.

166. Mary Dublin, "Maternal Mortality and the Decline of the Birth Rate," *Annals of the American Academy of Political and Social Sciences*, 188 (Nov. 1936), 107–16.

167. Linda Berry, "Age and Parity Influences on Maternal Mortality: United States, 1919–1969," *Demography*, 14 (1977), 297–310.

168. Edward Jow-Ching Tu, "Cohort Maternal Mortality: New York, 1917–1972," *American Journal of Public Health*, 69 (1979), 1052–55.

169. Janet Campbell, *Maternal Mortality* (London: Reports on Public Health, no. 25, 1924), p. 9.

170. Great Britain, Ministry of Health, *Report on an Investigation into Maternal Mortality* (London, 1937), p. 111.

171. Ibid., p. 136.

172. J. M. Winter, "Infant Mortality, Maternal Mortality, and Public Health in Britain in the 1930s," *Journal of European Economic History*, 8 (1979), 455.

173. Hugo Ehrenfest, ed., *Fetal, Newborn, and Maternal Morbidity and Mortality* (New York, 1933), p. 96.

Chapter 6

1. Ad. Elias von Siebold, *Versuch einer pathologisch-therapeutischen Darstellung des Kindbettfiebers* (Frankfurt/M., 1826), p. 102.

2. Francis Adams, ed., *The Genuine Works of Hippocrates*, 2 vols. (London, 1849), I, 378–79; Epidemics, Book I, case XI.

3. Notice, *AJO*, 7 (1874–75), 164.

4. Guy Thuillier, *Pour une histoire du quotidien au XIXe siècle en Nivernais* (Paris: Mouton, 1977), p. 86n39, quoting Dr. Fichot.

5. Freddy Sarg, *La Naissance en Alsace* (Strasbourg: Oberlin, 1974), p. 39.

6. Victor Fossel, *Volksmedicin und medicinischer Aberglaube in Steiermark* (Graz, 1886), p. 60.

7. J. Matthews Duncan, *On the Mortality of Childbed and Maternity Hospitals* (Edinburgh, 1870), p. 7.

8. Zandyck, *Etude sur la fièvre puerpérale . . . qui a régné à Dunkerque* (Paris, 1856), p. 69.

9. Rudolf Temesváry, *Volksbräuche und Aberglaube in der Geburtshilfe . . . in Ungarn* (Leipzig, 1900), p. 96.

10. Mortiz Gerhard Thilenius, *Kurzer Unterricht für die Hebammen und Wöchnerinnen auf dem Lande* (Kassel, 1769), p. 74.

11. Guillaume Mauquest de la Motte, *Traité complet des acouchemens*, rev ed. (Leiden, 1729), pp. 228–29.

12. Robert Bland, *Some Calculations of the Number of Accidents of Deaths Which Happen in Consequence of Parturition* (London, 1781), p. 8.

13. William Squire, "Puerperal Temperatures," *Obstetrical Society of London, Transactions*, 9 (1867), 133.

14. Stanley P. Warren, "The Prevalence of Puerperal Septicemia in Private Practice," *AJO*, 51 (1905), 306.

15. Richard L. Sweet and William J. Ledger, "Puerperal Infectious Morbidity," *AJO-G*, 117 (1973), 1098.

16. See, for example, Arthur M. Hill, "Why Be Morbid? Paths of Progress in the Control of Obstetric Infection, 1931 to 1960," *Medical Journal of Australia*, 25 Jan. 1964, 103.

17. Dormann, "Nachrichten über die Ereignisse . . . Entbindungsanstalt zu Hadamar," *Medicinische Jahrbücher für das Herzogthum Nassau*, 3 (1845), 101.

18. Frank H. Jackson, "Puerperal Sepsis," *AJO*, 54 (1906), 21.

19. Alexander Miller, "Presidential Address—Twenty Years' Obstetric Practice," *Glasgow Medical Journal*, ser. 5, 51 (1899), 219–21.

20. Robert Lee, "On Puerperal Fever and Crural Phlebitis," in Charles Meigs, ed., *The History, Pathology, and Treatment of Puerperal Fever* (Philadelphia, 1842), p. 222.

21. Walter Sigwart, "Die Pathologie des Wochenbetts," in Josef Halban and Ludwig Seitz, eds., *Biologie und Pathologie des Weibes* (Berlin, 1927), VIII, 459, 477.

22. Rudolf Beck, *Geburten und Geburtshilfe in ländlichen Verhältnissen* (Basel: med. diss., 1930), p. 53.

23. Tonnellé, "Des fièvres puerpérales," *Archives générales de médecine*, 22 (1830), 482.

24. Josef Halban and Robert Köhler, *Die pathologische Anatomie des Puerperalprozesses* (Vienna, 1919), pp. 160–62.

25. D. Berry Hart and A. H. Freeland Barbour, *Manual of Gynecology* (Edinburgh, 1886), p. 164.

26. Great Britain, Ministry of Health, *Report on an Investigation into Maternal Mortality* (London, 1937), p. 179.

27. Francis Home, *Clinical Experiments, Histories and Dissections* (London, 1782), pp. 71–77, 86.

28. A study by "Dr. Ferguson" cited in Fleetwood Churchill, *On the Theory and Practice of Midwifery*, 3rd ed. (Philadelphia, 1848), p. 497.

29. Alphonse Leroy, *Essai sur l'histoire naturelle de la grossesse et de l'accouchement* (Geneva, 1787), p. 146.

30. De la Motte, *Traité* [11], pp. 629–30.

31. Charles White, *A Treatise on the Management of Pregnant and Lying-In Women*, 2nd ed. (London, 1777), pp. 283–84.

32. Augustus B. Granville, *A Report of the Practice of Midwifery at the Westminster General Dispensary During 1818* (London, 1819), p. 163.

33. David Charles and Maxwell Finland, *Obstetric and Perinatal Infections* (Philadelphia: Lea & Febiger, 1973), p. 264.

34. Joseph B. DeLee, *The Principles and Practice of Obstetrics*, 6th ed. (Philadelphia, 1933), p. 931.

35. G. F. Gibberd, "Puerperal Sepsis, 1930–1965," *JOB*, NS, 73 (1966), 2. See also de la Motte, *Traité* [11], p. 579.

36. J. M. Munro Kerr, *Maternal Mortality and Morbidity* (Edinburgh, 1933), p. 50.

37. Robert Lee, "Cases of Severe Affections of the Joints After Parturition," *LMG*, 3 (1829), 664–65.

38. Percivall Willughby, *Observations in Midwifery* (a seventeenth-century manuscript) (1863; rpt. East Ardsley: S. R. Publishers, 1972), pp. 220–22.

39. Women's Co-operative Guild, *Maternity: Letters from Working-Women* (London, 1915), pp. 39–40.

40. Joseph DeLee, *Obstetrics* [34], p. 935.

41. William Godwin, *Memoirs of the Author of a Vindication of the Rights of Woman* (London, 1798), pp. 173–99, and Kenneth Neill Cameron, ed., *Shelley and his Circle, 1773–1822* (Cambridge: Harvard Univ. Press, 1961), I, 186–96.

42. William T. Lusk, "Puerperal Fever," in William Pepper, ed., *A System of Practical Medicine* (Philadelphia, 1885), I, 1008.

43. Women's Co-operative Guild, *Maternity* [39], p. 173.

44. James Young, "Maternal Mortality from Puerperal Sepsis," *BMJ*, 9 June 1928, p. 967.

45. Matthew Jennette, "On Inflammation and Abscess of the Uterine Appendages," *LMG*, NS, 11 (1850), 275–76.

46. On these events, see William J. Sinclair, *Semmelweis: His Life and his Doctrine* (Manchester, 1909), pp. 360–61. For a modern account of growing understanding of the streptococcus, see Harry F. Dowling, *Fighting Infection: Conquests of the Twentieth Century* (Cambridge: Harvard Univ. Press, 1977), pp. 55–69. Louis Pasteur tells the story in *Bulletin de l'académie de médecine*, 2nd ser., 8 (1879), 271–74.

47. Hugo Schottmüller, "Zur Bedeutung einiger Anaëroben in der Pathologie, insbesondere bei puerperalen Erkrankungen," *Mitteilungen aus den Grenzgebieten der Medizin und Chirurgie*, 21 (1910), 450–90.

48. August Hirsch reviews the older literature in *Handbuch der historisch-geographischen Pathologie*, 2nd ed., 3 vols. (Stuttgart, 1881–86), III, 327–28.

49. Lukas Boër, *Abhandlungen und Versuche geburtshilflichen Inhalts* (Vienna, 1807), II, 140.

50. Paul Delaunay, *La Maternité de Paris* (Paris: 1909), pp. 146, 149, 159.

51. Robert Storrs, Notice, *LMG*, NS, i (1845), 1087–88.

52. F. von Winckel, *Handbuch der Geburtshülfe*, 3 vols. (Wiesbaden, 1903–07), III, 396.

53. Arthur Hill, "The Diagnosis, Prevention and Treatment of Puerperal Infection," *Medical Journal of Australia*, 21 February 1948, p. 231.

54. Charles H. Rammelkamp, "Hemolytic Streptococcal Infections," in George W. Thorn

et al., eds., *Harrison's Principles of Internal Medicine*, 8th ed. (New York: McGraw-Hill, 1977), p. 818.

55. Gilles R. G. Monif, *Infectious Diseases in Obstetrics and Gynecology* (New York: Harper & Row, 1974), p. 134.

56. Sherwood L. Gorbach and John G. Bartlett, "Anaerobic Infections," *NEJM*, 23 May 1974, p. 1179.

57. Willughby, *Observations* [38], p. 172.

58. Fordyce Barker, *The Puerperal Diseases* (New York, 1878), p. 305.

59. Lucas Boër, *Abhandlungen und Versuche geburtshilflichen Inhalts* (Vienna, 1804), II, p. 90.

60. J. Wernitz, "Über die Misserfolge der Antisepsis beim Puerperalfieber," *ZBG*, 18 (1894), 1064.

61. Gorbach and Bartlett, "Anaerobic Infections" [56], p. 1183. Richard L. Sweet, "Anaerobic Infections of the Female Genital Tract," *AJO-G*, 122 (1975), 892.

62. Ibid., pp. 896–97; and Arthur M. Hill, "Post-Abortal and Puerperal Gas Gangrene," *JOB*, NS, 43 (1936), 201–51.

63. Johann Friedrich Osiander, *Bemerkungen über die französische Geburtshülfe* (Hanover, 1813), pp. 259–66.

64. Georg Wilhelm Christoph Consbruch, *Medicinische Ephemeriden nebst einer medicinischen Topographie der Grafschaft Ravensberg* (Chemnitz, 1793), p. 139.

65. This list from Sweet, "Anaerobic Infections" [61], p. 892.

66. See Heinrich Fasbender, *Geschichte der Geburtshilfe* (Jena, 1906), p. 591.

67. A. K. Chalmers, *The Health of Glasgow, 1818–1925* (Glasgow, 1930), p. 262.

68. Joan Taylor and H. D. Wright, "The Nature and Sources of Infection in Puerperal Sepsis," *JOB*, NS, 37 (1930), 228.

69. Burtis B. Breese and Caroline Breese Hall, *Beta Hemolytic Streptococcal Diseases* (Boston: Houghton Mifflin, 1978), p. 36 and passim.

70. John F. Jewett et al., "Childbed Fever: A Continuing Entity," *JAMA*, 7 October 1968, pp. 344–50.

71. Philip B. Mead et al., "Group A Streptococcal Puerperal Infection: Report of an Epidemic," *Obstetrics and Gynecology*, 32 (1968), 460–64.

72. Jean Donnison, *Midwives and Medical Men: A History of Inter-Professional Rivalries and Women's Rights* (New York: Schocken Books, 1977), p. 190 and passim.

73. Richard W. Wertz and Dorothy C. Wertz, *Lying-In: A History of Childbirth in America* (New York: Free Press, 1977), p. 128.

74. J. M. Munro Kerr, *Maternal Mortality* [36], pp. 82, 105.

75. Charles A. White and Franklin P. Koontz, "Beta-Hemolytic Streptococcus Infections in Postpartum Patients," *Obstetrics and Gynecology*, 41 (1973), 27.

76. B. P. Watson, "Puerperal Infection," *AJO-G*, 40 (1940), 585.

77. George W. Kosmak, in the "Discussion" of another paper. *AJO-G*, 7 (1924), 726.

78. Sanders, "Wochenbetts- und Säuglingsstatistik," *ZGH*, 66 (1910), 5–6.

79. Carl Müller, *Volksmedizinisch-geburtshilfliche Aufzeichnungen aus dem Lötschental* (Berne: Hans Huber, 1969), pp. 72–75, 115.

80. Young, "Maternal Mortality" [44], p. 968.

81. Josefine Biedermann, *Die weise Frau: Ernste und heitere Erlebnisse aus 30-jähriger Praxis* (Graz, 1934), p. 32.

82. K. B. Wiklund, *Lappische Heilkunde* (Oslo, 1932), p. 162; vol. 20 of a series of publications edited by J. Qvigstad.

83. Charlotte A. Douglas and Peter L. McKinlay (Department of Health for Scotland), *Report on Maternal Morbidity and Mortality in Scotland* (Edinburgh, 1935), pp. 179–180.

84. Ferdinand August Ritgen, *Jahrbücher der Entbindungsanstalt zu Giessen* (Giessen, 1820), II, passim.

85. Calculated from data in Adolphe Pinard, *Du Fonctionnement de la Maternité de Lariboisière* (Paris, 1889), passim. To heighten the contrast, I omitted the mothers with temperatures between 38.0 and 38.9.

86. Otto Büttner, "Mecklenburg-Schwerins Geburtshilfe im Jahre 1904," *ZGH*, 61 (1908), 198.

87. Müller, *Aufzeichnungen* [79], p. 72.

88. E. Radtke, "Ursachen und Bekämpfung des Kindbettfiebers," *Veröffentlichungen aus dem Gebiete der Medizinalverwaltung*, 1 (1912), 29.

89. Douglas and McKinlay, *Maternal Mortality Scotland* [83], p. 182.

90. Franz Unterberger, "Die Sterblichkeit im Kindbett . . . Mecklenburg-Schwerin," *Archiv für Gynäkologie*, 95 (1911–12), 136.

91. Janet Campbell, *Maternal Mortality* (London: Great Britain, Ministry of Health, Reports on Public Health, no. 25, 1924), p. 110.

92. J. Whitridge Williams contributing to a "Discussion on Puerperal Sepsis," *JOB*, NS, 32 (1925), 242.

93. Hill, "Diagnosis Puerperal Infection" [53], p. 231.

94. Jacques-René Tenon, *Mémoires sur les Hôpitaux de Paris* (Paris, 1788), pp. 222, 239–40, 269.

95. Léon LeFort, *Des Maternités* (Paris, 1866), p. 58.

96. *Aerztlicher Bericht des k.k. Gebär- und Findelhauses zu Wien . . . 1861* (Vienna, 1863), computed from cases on pp. 68–78.

97. The story is told in Sinclair, *Semmelweis* [46], pp. 48–60.

98. Douglas and McKinlay, *Maternal Mortality Scotland* [83], pp. 193–95.

99. Gustav Zinke, in "Discussion," *A/O*, 77 (1918), 118.

100. Campbell, *Maternal Mortality* [91], p. 39.

101. Franz Alois Stelzig, *Versuch einer medizinischen Topographie von Prag*, 2 vols. (Prague, 1824), II, 42.

102. Campbell, *Maternal Mortality* [91], p. 108.

103. Douglas and McKinlay, *Maternal Mortality Scotland* [83], p. 70, table 24.

104. *Bericht Gebärhaus* [96], computed from cases on pp. 68–78. From the fifty-six cases studied, I have removed a "pleuritis" victim who lasted 122 days. With her included, the average is 14.2 days.

105. Hildred M. Butler, "Bacteriological Studies of Clostridium welchii Infections in Man," *Surgery, Gynecology, Obstetrics*, 81 (1945), 475–86; and Arthur Hill, "Diagnosis Puerperal Infection" [53], p. 229.

106. Grace Meigs, *Maternal Mortality . . . in the United States* (Washington: Children's Bureau, U.S. Department of Labor, pub. no. 19, 1917), p. 16n1.

107. Eardley Holland, *Lancet*, 20 April 1935, p. 936.

108. Cullingworth, "Undiminished Mortality from Puerperal Fever in England and Wales," *Obstetrical Society of London, Transactions*, 39 (1897), 93.

109. Francis B. Smith, *The People's Health, 1830–1910* (New York: Holmes and Meier, 1979), p. 56.

110. Ann Oakley, "Wisewoman and Medicine Man: Changes in the Management of Childbirth," in Juliet Mitchell and Ann Oakley, eds., *The Rights and Wrongs of Women* (Harmondsworth: Penguin, 1976), pp. 45, 47.

111. See, for example, Suzanne Arms, *Immaculate Deception: A New Look at Women and Childbirth in America* (Boston: Houghton Mifflin, 1975), pp. 17–22.

112. Hermann Fehling, *Entwicklung der Geburtshilfe und Gynäkologie im 19. Jahrhundert* (Berlin, 1925), p. 46.

113. On the increasingly septic environment of the pre-Listerian hospital, see Edward D. Churchill, "The Pandemic of Wound Infection in Hospitals," *Journal of the History of Medicine*, 20 (1965), 389–404; and John Eric Erichsen, *On Hospitalism and the Causes of Death After Operations* (London, 1874), passim.

114. The study appeared in five parts, reprinted in *Medical Classics*, 2 (1937), 28–71.

115. O'Donel T. D. Browne, *The Rotunda Hospital, 1745–1945* (Edinburgh, 1947), p. 139. Sinclair, *Semmelweis* [46], p. 365. I have omitted recounting all the dubious attempts to "disinfect" the uterus itself once infection had taken hold, as well as efforts at "prophylactic" disinfection with strong douches—all of which did more harm than good.

116. Rudolf Dohrn, *Geschichte der Geburtshülfe der Neuzeit* (Tübingen, 1904), p. 292.

117. F. Siredey, *Les Maladies puerpérales: Etude clinique* (Paris, 1884), p. 92.

118. Emma L. Call, "The Evolution of Modern Maternity Technic," *A/O*, 58 (1908), 396.

119. Robert Boxall, "Mortality in Childbed," *JOB*, 7 (1905), 317.

120. Catharine van Tussenbroek, "Kindbett-Sterblichkeit in den Niederlanden," *Archiv für Gynäkologie*, 95 (1911–12), 32.

121. Claude E. Heaton, "Control of Puerperal Infection in the United States during the Last Century," *AJO-G*, 46 (1943), 483.

122. Edmond Weber, *Beiträge zur Mortalitäts-Statistik an septischen puerperalen Prozessen* (Berne: med. diss., 1890), p. 31.

123. Catharine Macfarlane, "A Month at Bumm's Klinik, Berlin," *AJO*, 59 (1909), 463.

124. Paul Zweifel, in "Diskussion," *ZBG*, 38 (1906), 1188.

125. For a review, see Fehling, *Entwicklung* [112], pp. 185–95.

126. von Winckel, *Handbuch* [52], III, 360, 372.

127. Munro Kerr, *Maternal Mortality* [36], p. 239.

128. Alois Valenta, "Wie soll an den Hebammenschulen die Antiseptik gelehrt . . . werden?" *ZBG*, 12 (1888), 778.

129. Frank H. Jackson, "Puerperal Sepsis," *AJO*, 54 (1906), 23.

130. De la Motte, *Traité* [11], p. 584.

131. von Winckel, *Handbuch* [52], III, 315–23.

132. E. Hönck, "Ein Beitrag zur Hebammenfrage," *ZGH*, 25 (1893), 107–45.

133. Douglas and McKinlay, *Maternal Mortality Scotland* [83], p. 178.

134. Radtke, "Ursachen Kindbettfieber" [88], p. 19.

135. Ibid., pp. 20–21, 27.

136. Siegfried Rosenfeld, "Zum Schutze der Gebärenden," *ZGH*, 57 (1906), p. 165; the "average" is an average of rates for the various *Länder*.

137. Otto R. Eichel, "A Preliminary Report of a Statistical Study of Puerperal Sepsis," *AJO-G*, 7 (1924), 672.

138. Chalmers, *Health of Glasgow* [67], p. 263.

139. Francis Ramsbotham, Notice, *LMG*, 3 (1829), 285; 5 (1830), 687.

140. John Hall Davis, *Parturition and its Difficulties* (London, 1865), deaths on pp. 344–50. Of thirty-one maternal deaths, I have assumed that fourteen came from some infectious process, namely: 6 "peritonitis," 3 "phlebitis of uterus, pyemia," 2 "pyemia," 1 "fever with enlarged spleen," 1 "disease of nervous centers with hemiplegia," and 1 "acute jaundice," the onset of which was one-day postpartum.

141. Cited in Mervyn Susser and Abraham Adelstein, *Vital Statistics: A Memorial Volume of Selections from . . . William Farr* (Metuchen, N.J.: Scarecrow Press, 1975), p. 277. Farr gives no dates or sources. I assume that Rigden had five infection deaths: four from puerperal fever and one from "heart disease." He recorded in addition three more deaths from eclampsia and one, the cause of which is not stated.

142. Dr. Wengler, "Das Auftreten von Wochenbettfieber und seine Bekämpfung in zwei Landkreisen," *Zeitschrift für Medicinal-Beamte*, 30 (1917), 176.

143. Döllner, "Zur Frage des Wochenbettfiebers," *Zeitschrift für Medicinal-Beamte*, 30 (1917), 332.

Chapter 7

1. Edward Shorter, *The Making of the Modern Family* (New York: Basic Books, 1975), pp. 227–55.

2. Queirel, *Histoire de la Maternité de Marseille* (Marseille, 1889), p. 15.

3. Quoted from another study in Alain Mathiot, *Pratique obstétricale à Lyon à la fin du XVIIIe . . . siècle* (Lyon: med. diss., 1975), pp. 20–21.

4. Joseph Schneider, *Versuch einer Topographie der Residenzstadt Fulda* (Fulda, 1806), p. 205.

5. Adams Walther, "Zur Hebammenfrage," *ZBG*, 8 (1884), 308.

6. Jacques Gélis, "Sages-femmes et accoucheurs: l'obstétrique populaire aux XVIIe et XVIIIe siècles," *Annales ESC*, 32 (1977), 947.

7. Ibid., p. 948.

8. Joseph Daquin, *Topographie médicale de la ville de Chambéry* (Chambéry, 1787), p. 80.

9. F. J. Werfer, *Versuch einer medizinischen Topographie der Stadt Gmünd* (Gmünd, 1812), p. 97.

10. Friedrich Pauli, *Medicinische Statistik . . . Landau* (Landau, 1831), p. 60.

11. H. Wollheim, *Versuch einer medizinischen Topographie und Statistik von Berlin* (Berlin, 1844), p. 117.

12. C. F. Senff, *Über Vervollkommnung der Geburtshülfe* (Halle, 1812), p. 85.

13. Eduard Otto Dann, *Topographie von Danzig* (Berlin, 1835), p. 280.

14. H. B. Semmelink, "Statistisches über 600 Geburten der Privatpraxis," *ZGH*, 71 (1912), 368.

15. R. Dohrn, "Erfahrungen bei Prüfungen und dem Nachexamen der Hebammen," *ZBG*, 30 (1906), 907.

16. John Douglas, *A Short Account of the State of Midwifery in London* (London, 1736), pp. 68–70.

17. Catherine M. Scholten, " 'On the Importance of the Obstetrick Art': Changing Customs of Childbirth in America," *William and Mary Quarterly*, 3rd ser., 34 (1977), 428–45; Jane B. Donegan, *Women and Men Midwives: Medicine, Morality, and Misogyny in Early America* (Westport: Greenwood, 1978), pp. 110–35; and Jean Donnison, *Midwives and Medical Men: A History of Inter-Professional Rivalries and Women's Rights* (New York: Schocken, 1977), p. 22 and passim.

18. A. K. Chalmers, *The Health of Glasgow, 1818–1925* (Glasgow, 1930), p. 263.

19. Ibid.

20. Robert R. Rentoul, "Is It in the Best Interest of Public Health . . . Supplying Poorer Women Only with Midwives . . . ," *Lancet*, 16 January 1897, p. 155.

21. Ibid.

22. "Report of the Infant Mortality Committee," *Obstetrical Society of London. Transactions*, 11 (1869), 134.

23. Milton J. Lewis, *"Populate or Perish": Aspects of Infant and Maternal Health in Sydney, 1870–1939* (Canberra, Australian National University: diss., 1976), p. 207n38.

24. An estimate of Dr. J. H. Aveling, cited in Francis B. Smith, *The People's Health 1830–1910* (New York: Holmes & Meier, 1979), p. 55.

25. Estimate from Thomas Darlington, "The Present Status of the Midwife," *AJO*, 63 (1911), 870.

26. Helen M. Dart, *Maternity and Child Care in Selected Rural Areas of Mississippi* (Washington: U.S. Department of Labor, Children's Bureau, pub. no. 88, 1921), p. 27.

27. Frances S. Bradley and Margaretta A. Williamson, *Rural Children in Selected Counties of North Carolina* (Washington: U.S. Department of Labor, Children's Bureau, pub. no. 33, 1918), p. 30.

28. Margaret Hagood, *Mothers of the South: Portraiture of the White Tenant Farm Woman* (1939; rpt. New York: Norton, 1977), p. 113.

29. Florence B. Sherbon and Elizabeth Moore, *Maternity and Infant Care in Two Rural Counties in Wisconsin* (Washington: U.S. Department of Labor, Children's Bureau, pub. no. 46, 1919), pp. 28, 32.

30. In the discussion of F. E. Leavitt's paper, "Obstetrics as Practiced in the Country," *St. Paul Medical Journal*, 18 (1916), 372.

31. Grace Abbott, "The Midwife in Chicago," *American Journal of Sociology*, 20 (1914–15), 684.

32. J. Clifton Edgar, "The Education, Licensing and Supervision of the Midwife," *AJO*, 73 (1916), 388.

33. Midwife statistics on Britain from 1919 to 1922 are in Janet Campbell, *Maternal Mortality* (London: Ministry of Health, Reports on Public Health no. 25, 1924), p. 31 and for 1946 and 1970 in National Birthday Trust Fund, *British Births, 1970*, vol. 1: *The First Week of Life* (London: Heinemann, 1975), p. 27 (the "midwife" figure includes student midwives). American midwife statistics for 1935 and 1946 may be found in Paul H. Jacobson, "Hospital Care and the Vanishing Midwife," *Milbank Memorial Fund Quarterly*, 34 (1956), 254; for 1970 and 1977 in *Statistical Abstract of the United States, 1979*, p. 63. "Midwife" births include as well "attendant not specified."

34. *Statistical Yearbook of the Netherlands, 1978*, p. 48.

35. Comparative data on the mid-1970s from the *Statistisches Jahrbuch für die Bundesrepublik Deutschland, 1980*, p. 671.

36. Letter of R. W. Burslem, *BMJ*, 1 December, 1979, pp. 1442–43.

37. Doreen Garside, "Midwifery in Scandinavia," *Nursing Times*, 6 May 1976, pp. 702–04.

38. Jacqueline Gottely, "Premiers résultats d'une enquête nationale sur les sages-femmes," *Cahiers de sociologie et de démographie médicales*, 16 (1976), 156; 1973 data.

39. For some medically-inspired birthing chairs, see Harold Speert, *Iconographia Gynia-*

trica: A Pictorial History of Gynecology and Obstetrics (Philadelphia: Davis, 1973), pp. 268–69.

40. All of the preceding quotations from Jean Paul Stucky, *Der Gebärstuhl: Die Gründe für sein Verschwinden im deutschen Sprachbereich* (Zurich: Juris, 1965), pp. 33, 34, 37.

41. Friedrich Julius Morgen, *Beiträge zu einer medicinischen Topographie . . . der Stadt Memel* (Memel, 1843), p. 144.

42. Harvey Graham, *Eternal Eve: The Mysteries of Birth and the Customs That Surround It*, rev. ed. (London: Hutchinson, 1960), p. 189.

43. Quoted in William Leishman, *A System of Midwifery*, 3rd ed. (Philadelphia, 1879), p. 263n1.

44. For one point of view, see chapter 8, "Pain and Childbirth: The Doctor's Fallacy," in Suzanne Arms, *Immaculate Deception: A New Look at Women and Childbirth in America* (Boston: Houghton Mifflin, 1975), p. 115ff.

45. See, for example, E. Pelkonen, *Über volkstümliche Geburtshilfe in Finnland* (Helsinki, 1931), p. 143 ("Strafe für den Sündenfall den Frauen").

46. Yvonne Verdier, *Façons de dire, façons de faire* (Paris: Gallimard, 1979), p. 93.

47. Hagood, *Mothers of South* [28], pp. 115–16.

48. Flora Thompson, *Lark Rise to Candleford* (1939; rpt. Penguin, 1973), p. 50.

49. Otto Spiegelberg, *A Text Book of Midwifery*, Eng. trans., 2 vols. (London, 1887), I, 257.

50. On women's and doctors' efforts to cope with pain before the anesthetic era, see Claire Elizabeth Fox, *Pregnancy, Childbirth and Early Infancy in Anglo-American Culture: 1675–1830* (University of Pennsylvania: diss., 1966), pp. 144–47.

51. Carl Müller, *Volksmedizinisch-geburtshilfliche Aufzeichnungen aus dem Lötschental* (Berne: Huber, 1969), p. 83; see also Pelkonen, *Finnland* [45], pp. 154, 175f.

52. For a recent account, see A. J. Youngson, *The Scientific Revolution in Victorian Medicine* (London: Croom Helm, 1979), pp. 42–72.

53. Ibid., p. 112.

54. Ibid.

55. James W. Duncan, "The 'Radical' in Obstetrics," *AJO-G*, 20 (1930), 226.

56. Eardley Holland, "Birth Injury in Relation to Labor," *AJO-G*, 33 (1937), 18.

57. Ransom S. Hooker, ed., *Maternal Mortality in New York City: A Study of All Puerperal Deaths, 1930–1932* (New York: New York Academy of Medicine, Committee on Public Health Relations, 1933), p. 113.

58. Great Britain, Ministry of Health, *Report on an Investigation into Maternal Mortality* (London, 1937; Cmd. 5422), p. 117.

59. Harry E. Beard, "Home Obstetrics," *West Virginia Medical Journal* (January, 1940), p. 19.

60. Campbell, *Maternal Mortality* [33], p. 48.

61. Leavitt, "Obstetrics in the Country" [30], p. 370.

62. Carl Joseph Gauss, "Geburten im künstlichen Dämmerschlaf," *Archiv für Gynäkologie*, 78 (1906), 579–631. For a brief outline of the history of "twilight sleep," see J. M. Munro Kerr et al., eds., *Historical Review of British Obstetrics and Gynecology, 1800–1950* (Edinburgh: Livingstone, 1954), pp. 231–34. Judith Walzer Leavitt analyzes the potentiality of the technique for enhancing women's control of delivery. "Birthing and Anesthesia: The Debate Over Twilight Sleep," *Signs*, 6 (1980), 147–64.

63. All these techniques described in Munro Kerr, ibid., pp. 231–36.

64. Youngson, *Scientific Revolution* [52], pp. 101 ff.

65. Charles Waller, *Elements of Practical Midwifery*, 4th ed. (London, 1858), pp. 151–52.

66. The phrase is W. C. Danforth's, "Is Conservative Obstetrics to be Abandoned"? *AJO-G*, 3 (1922), 610.

67. James Young, "Maternal Mortality and Maternal Mortality Rates," *AJO-G*, 31 (1936), 210.

68. George Kosmak, in a discussion following William F. Mengert's paper, "Fetal and Neonatal Mortality: Causes and Prevention," *AJO-G*, 55 (1948), 666.

69. O'Donel T. D. Browne, *The Rotunda Hospital, 1745–1945* (Edinburgh: Livingstone, 1947), p. 230.

70. Richard W. Wertz and Dorothy C. Wertz, *Lying-In: A History of Childbirth in America* (New York: Free Press, 1977), pp. 178–98.

71. The preceding facts are from Francis B. Smith, *The People's Health, 1830–1910* (New York: Holmes & Meier, 1979), p. 23.

72. Ibid., p. 24.

73. John W. Williams, "Medical Education and the Midwife Problem in the United States," *JAMA*, 58 (1912), 1–5.

74. Rudolph Holmes, "The Fads and Fancies of Obstetrics: A Comment on the Pseudo-scientific Trend of Modern Obstetrics," *AJO-G*, 2 (1921), 231.

75. Mabel Dobbin Crawford, "The Obstetric Forceps and Its Use," *Lancet*, 11 June 1932, p. 1242.

76. Stanley P. Warren, "The Prevalence of Puerperal Septicemia in Private Practice . . . ," *AJO*, 51 (1905), 302.

77. J. S. Templeton, "Obstetrics in Country Practice," *Illinois Medical Journal*, 33 (1918), 92.

78. Andrew Topping, "Prevention of Maternal Mortality," *Lancet*, 7 March 1936, p. 546.

79. R. Veitch Clark, discussing Manchester, at a meeting of the Royal Sanitary Institute, *Lancet*, 20 April 1935, p. 937.

80. Great Britain, Ministry of Health, *Report on Maternal Mortality in Wales* (London, Cmd. 5423, 1937), p. 105.

81. See Munro Kerr, *Historical Review* [62], p. 113.

82. J. Hofbauer, "Hypophysenextrakt als Wehenmittel," *ZBG*, 35 (1911), 137–41.

83. For the reader's convenience, let me list here the various editions of *Williams Obstetrics*, along with their authors, that will be cited in this chapter: 1st (1906), 2nd (1908), 5th (1926), 6th (1930) by John Whitridge Williams himself; 7th (1936) and 9th (1945) by Henricus J. Stander; 10th (1950), 11th (1956), 12th (1961), and 13th (1966) by Nicholson J. Eastman; 14th (1971) by Louis M. Hellman and Jack A. Pritchard; and 16th (1980) by Jack A. Pritchard and Paul E. MacDonald. Called simply *Obstetrics: A Textbook*, until the 10th edition, all were published in New York by Appleton-Century-Crofts.

84. Joseph B. DeLee, quoted in Morris Fishbein, *Joseph Bolivar DeLee: Crusading Obstetrician* (New York: Dutton, 1949), p. 248.

85. Hermann Fehling, *Entwicklung der Geburtshilfe und Gynäkologie im 19. Jahrhundert* (Berlin, 1925), pp. 58–59.

86. G. H. Luedtke, in the discussion of Leavitt, "Obstetrics in the Country" [30], p. 373.

87. Great Britain, *Maternal Mortality Wales* [80], p. 108.

88. Ibid.

89. Alexander Miller, "Twenty Years' Obstetric Practice," *Glasgow Medical Journal*, ser. 5,.51 (1899), 225.

90. H. E. Collier, "A Study of the Influence of Certain Social Changes Upon Maternal Mortality and Obstetrical Problems, 1834–1927," *JOB*, 37 (1930), 41n1.

91. Henry Jellett, *Causes and Prevention of Maternal Mortality* (London, 1929), p. 207.

92. Th. Heynemann, "Ergebnisse und Lehren der erweiterten geburtshilflichen Landesstatistik Hamburgs (1932–1935)," *ZGH*, 114 (1937), 252.

93. Elizabeth Moore, *Maternity and Infant Care in a Rural County in Kansas* (Washington: U.S. Department of Labor, Children's Bureau, pub. no. 26, 1917), pp. 23–24, and E. D. Plass, "A Statistical Study of 129,539 Births in Iowa," *AJO-G*, 28 (1934), computed from data in tables on pp. 298–99.

94. Henry Buxbaum, "Obstetrics in the Home," *Surgical Clinics of North America*, February, 1943, p. 57.

95. Jellett, *Causes and Prevention* [91] p. 200.

96. Douglas Miller, "Observations on Unsuccessful Forceps Cases," *BMJ*, 4 August 1928, p. 183.

97. Crawford, "Obstetric Forceps" [75], p. 1241.

98. Ibid., p. 1242.

99. James Hendry, "Unsuccessful Forceps Cases," *BMJ*, 4 Aug. 1928, p. 187.

100. Campbell, *Maternal Mortality* [33], p. 52.

101. Crawford, "Obstetric Forceps" [75], p. 1241.

102. Ibid., pp. 1241–42, and Miller, "Observations" [96], p. 184.

103. J. M. Munro Kerr, *Maternal Mortality and Morbidity* (Edinburgh, 1933), p. 51.

104. Hendry, "Unsuccessful Forceps" [99], pp. 185–86. He was quoting Lady Selborne.

105. W. Japp Sinclair, "The Injuries of Parturition: The Old and the New," *BMJ*, 4 September 1897, p. 595.

106. Jellett, *Causes and Prevention* [91], p. 238.

107. The phrase is from Dr. Dilys Jones in Janet Campbell et al., *High Maternal Mortality in Certain Areas* (London: Ministry of Health, Reports on Public Health, no. 68, 1932), p. 80.

108. Quoted in Crawford, "Obstetric Forceps" [75], p. 1243.

109. Victor Bonney, "The Continued High Maternal Mortality of Child-bearing," *Proceedings of the Royal Society of Medicine*, 12 (1918–19), 96.

110. Lapthorn Smith, in the discussion of the Bonney paper, ibid., p. 104.

111. Maurice Mottram, "The Rural Practitioner and Maternity," *BMJ*, 3 January 1925, p. 42.

112. William F. Shaw, "Unsuccessful Forceps Cases," *BMJ*, 4 August 1928, p. 189.

113. Great Britain, *Maternal Mortality Wales* [80], p. 106.

114. Excerpts in response to Leavitt's questionnaire, "Obstetrics in the Country" [30], p. 371.

115. Ernst Zürcher, *Die geburtshülfliche Landpraxis* (Trogen, 1887), pp. 4, 13.

116. Sinclair, "Injuries of Parturition" [105], pp. 592, 595.

117. Campbell, *Maternal Mortality* [33], p. 56.

118. Shaw, "Unsuccessful Forceps Cases" [112], p. 190.

119. Munro Kerr, *Maternal Mortality* [62], pp. 113–14.

120. Templeton, "Obstetrics in Country Practice" [75] p. 92.

121. Of Franklin, Tennessee, K. S. Howlett, "Country Obstetrics," *Tennessee State Medical Association Journal*, 16 (1923–24), 176.

122. Moore, *Maternity and Infant Care* [93], p. 25.

123. Sherbon, *Maternity Care Wisconsin* [29], p. 29.

124. C. Henry Davis, "Maternal Mortality: A Crime of Today," *Surgery, Gynecology and Obstetrics*, 30 (1920), 289.

125. 1908 Detroit data from Clara M. Davis, "Obstetrical Service for the Laboring Classes," *Journal of the Michigan State Medical Society*, 7 (1908), 214. 1925 to 1945 Detroit data from Harold C. Mack and R. S. Sidall, "Cesarean Section in Detroit During 1945," *AJO-G*, 56 (1948), 60. British data from National Birthday Trust Fund, *British Births 1970*, p. 25. Dutch data from Netherlands. *Statistical Yearbook of the Netherlands, 1978*, p. 48.

126. Robert Anderson letter, *BMJ*, 2 July 1921, p. 28.

127. Adolf Weber, *Bericht über Hundert in der Landpraxis operative behandelte Geburten*, (Munich, 1901) p. 4.

128. Eneas K. MacKenzie, "Rural Midwifery Practice," *Practitioner*, 115 (1925), 269.

129. Bonney, "Continued High Maternal Mortality" [109], pp. 87–89, 96.

130. Zürcher, *Geburtshülfliche Landpraxis* [115], pp. 2, 8.

131. Quoted in Leavitt, "Obstetrics in the Country" [30], p. 371.

132. Bonney, "Continued High Maternal Mortality" [109], p. 104.

133. Great Britain, *Investigation Maternal Mortality* [58], p. 23. At that point the authors were summarizing earlier reports, but controlling the local GP is clearly the intent of this report as well.

134. Edwin Daily, "Maternity Care in the United States: Planning for the Future," *AJO-G*, 49 (1945), 129.

135. Egbert Morland, *Alice and the Stork, Or the Rise in the Status of the Midwife as Exemplified in the Life of Alice Gregory* (London: Hodder & Stoughton, 1951), pp. 38, 49–50.

136. Lisbeth Burger, *Vierzig Jahre Storchentante: Aus dem Tagebuch einer Hebamme* (Breslau, 1936), pp. 166–67.

137. Julius Beer, ed., *Memoiren einer Berliner Wickelfrau* (Berlin, 1872), p. 58.

138. The preceding evidence from Morris Vogel, *The Invention of the Modern Hospital: Boston, 1870–1930* (Chicago: University of Chicago Press, 1980), pp. 117–19.

139. Emma L. Call, "The Evolution of Modern Maternity Technic," *AJO*, 58 (1908), 403.

140. Wertz and Wertz, *Lying-In* [70], p. 168.

141. On these factors in Düsseldorf and other German cities, see the debate between

Else Theisen and a group of Berlin obstetricians: Theisen, "Betrachtungen über Anstalts-
und Hausgeburten," *ZBG,* 64 (1940), 307–11; and Rott et al., "Betrachtungen über Anstalts-
und Hausgeburten," *ZBG,* 64 (1940), 1442–54.

142. Jacques Gélis, *Accoucheur de campagne sous le roi soleil* (Toulouse: Privat, 1979),
p. 45n55.

143. Alois Nöth, *Die Hebammenordnungen des XVIII. Jahrhunderts* (Würzburg:
med. diss., 1931), p. 84 (midwife ordinance of the Burggrafschaft Nürnberg). See also Max
Runge, "Über die Berechtigung des Kaiserschnittes an der Sterbenden," *ZGH,* 9 (1883),
260–62.

144. G. Lammert, *Volksmedizin und medizinischer Aberglaube in Bayern* (Würzburg,
1869), pp. 12–13.

145. Mary Donally's text is reprinted in a note in *Pediatrics,* 54 (1974), 460. The original
publication was Duncan Stewart's article "The Cesarean Operation Done with Success by
a Midwife," in *Medical Essays and Observations,* 5 (1752), 360–362, which I have not
seen. On the famous story of Jacob Nufer, the sow gelder who performed caesarean section
successfully on his wife in 1500, see Theodore Cianfrani, *A Short History of Obstetrics
and Gynecology* (Springfield, Ill.: Charles C Thomas, 1960), pp. 125, 131–32.

146. On their remote history, see Heinrich Fasbender, *Geschichte der Geburtshilfe* (Jena,
1906), pp. 136–39, 221–22.

147. Mireille Laget, "La Césarienne ou la tentation de l'impossible: XVIIᵉ et XVIIIᵉ siècle,"
Annales de Bretagne, 86 (1979), 183.

148. Jacques-René Tenon, *Mémoires sur les hôpitaux de Paris* (Paris, 1788), p. 251n33.

149. On Britain, see Fleetwood Churchill, *On the Theory and Practice of Midwifery,*
6th ed. (London, 1872), pp. 406–08. On the United States, see Robert P. Harris, "Special
Statistics of the Cesarean Operation in the United States," *AJO,* 14 (1881), 347.

150. According to M. P. Rucker, "A Brief History of Obstetrics and Gynecology in Virginia," *AJO-G,* 31 (1936), 190.

151. Harris, "Special Statistics" [149], p. 343.

152. A history of the modern caesarean remains to be written; but for basic events, see
Owen H. Wangensteen and Sarah D. Wangensteen, *The Rise of Surgery from Empiric
Craft to Scientific Discipline* (Minneapolis: Univ. of Minnesota Press, 1978), pp. 200–
13; and Harold Speert, *Essays in Eponymy: Obstetric and Gynecologic Milestones* (New
York: Macmillan, 1958), pp. 594–603.

153. Robert P. Harris, "Remarks on the Cesarean Operation," *AJO,* 11 (1878), 621.

154. Browne, *Rotunda Hospital* [69], p. 183; Vogel, *Modern Hospital* [138], p. 117;
Paul Bar, *La Maternité de l'Hôpital St. Antoine* (Paris, 1900), p. 156; and Georges Duval,
De la morbidité et de la mortalité . . . Hôpital de la Charité (Lille, 1899), p. 55.

155. Browne, ibid., p. 206.

156. J. H. Carstens, "Cesarean Section," *AJO,* 29 (1894), 776; if the pelvic antero-posterior
diameter was less than three inches.

157. Max Hirsch, "Der Weg der operativen Geburtshilfe in bevölkerungs-politischer Beleuchtung," *Archiv für Frauenkunde,* 13 (1927), 207. In the 1920s, however, four times
as many versions as caesareans continued to be done. The overall level of obstetric operations
in Baden increased rapidly from 1871 to 1910, rising thereafter scarcely at all.

158. Fehling, *Entwicklung Geburtshilfe* [85], p. 56.

159. Richard C. Norris, "The Indications and Limitations of the Induction of Labor,"
AJO, 78 (1918), 510.

160. James D. Voorhees, "Can the Frequency of Some Obstetrical Operations Be Diminished?" *AJO,* 77 (1918), 10.

161. Joseph Baer, et al., "The Present Position of Version and Extraction," *AJO-G,* 24
(1932), 600.

162. D. Anthony D'Esopo, "Trends in the Use of the Cesarean Section Operation,"
AJO-G, 58 (1949), 1122.

163. Browne, *Rotunda Hospital* [69], p. 197; only one was actually done, however.

164. Jellett, *Causes and Prevention* [91], pp. 222–23.

165. *Williams Obstetrics* [83], 2nd ed. (1908), pp. 463–64.

166. *Williams Obstetrics* [83], 6th ed. (1930), p. 568.

167. *Williams Obstetrics* [83], 10th ed. (1950), p. 1126.

168. Queen Charlotte's *Text-Book of Obstetrics,* 4th ed. (London, 1936), pp. 526–27.

169. Gilbert I. Strachan's *Textbook of Obstetrics* (London: Lewis, 1947), p. 682.

170. Plass, "Statistical Study" [93], pp. 298–99.

171. Hugo Sellheim, writing in Josef Halban and Ludwig Seitz, eds., *Biologie und Pathologie des Weibes* (Berlin, 1927), 7(1), 267–68.

172. The paper was published in 1918; Voorhees, "Frequency Obstetrical Operations" [160], pp. 5, 9.

173. Thomas E. Cone, Jr., *History of American Pediatrics* (Boston: Little, Brown, 1979), p. 151.

174. MacKenzie, "Rural Midwifery" [128], pp. 269–70.

175. Jellett, *Causes and Prevention* [91], p. 220.

176. Stephen K. Westman, *A Surgeon's Story* (London: Kimber, 1962), p. 150.

177. Frank Meriwether, "Cesarean Section Versus Craniotomy," *AJO*, 44 (1901), 207.

178. Joseph DeLee, in discussion, *AJO-G*, 2 (1921), 299.

179. See the clash between the "conservative" Englishman Eardley Holland and the "radical" Canadian James Goodall at the 1936 meeting of the American Gynecological Society, after Holland's paper deprecating "prophylactic forceps": "Birth Injury in Relation to Labor," *AJO-G*, 33 (1937), 3–13, discussion 13–18.

180. Albert H. Aldridge and Richard S. Meredith, "Obstetric Responsibility for the Prevention of Fetal Deaths," *AJO-G*, 42 (1941), 388.

181. City of Toronto, Department of Public Health, *Annual Statement*, 1979 (Toronto: Department of Public Health, 1980), p. 146 (results for 1979).

182. Calculated from data in *Annuaire Statistique de la France*, 1979, pp. 40–41, and from the *Statistical Abstract of the United States*, 1979, p. 75.

183. Spiegelberg, *Midwifery* [49], I, 253–54.

184. D. Lloyd Roberts, *The Practice of Midwifery* (London, 1896), pp. 263–64.

185. Charles Jewett, ed., *The Practice of Obstetrics*, 3rd ed. (London, 1907), p. 242.

186. J. W. Markoe, "Asepsis in Obstetrics in the Tenements," *Bulletin of the Lying-In Hospital in the City of New York*, 11 (1916–18) 171.

187. James D. Voorhees, "The Etiology of Puerperal Sepsis," *AJO*, 53 (1906), 762.

188. Thomas Watts Eden, *A Manual of Midwifery*, 3rd ed. (London, 1911), p. 277. See also J. H. E. Brock, "The Conduct of Labour and Puerperal Sepsis," *Lancet*, 16 August 1919, p. 279. ("The vulva should be shaved as for any other surgical operation. No doubt it would be a good deal opposed by patients.")

189. Fehling, *Entwicklung Geburtshilfe* [85], p. 47.

190. Leonard W. Bickle, letter, *BMJ*, 20 November 1920, p. 803, and Ploeger, "Statisticher Bericht über die Geburten der königlichen Universitäts-Frauenklinik in Berlin," *ZGH*, 53 1905), 242.

191. *Williams Obstetrics* [83], 7th ed. (1936), p. 394.

192. *Williams Obstetrics* [83], 2nd ed. (1908), p. 304; 5th ed. (1926), p. 349; and 7th ed. (1936), p. 394, respectively.

193. *Williams Obstetrics* [83], 5th ed. (1926), p. 349. This finding was first reported in R. A. Johnston and R. S. Sidall, "Is the Usual Method of Preparing Patients for Delivery Beneficial or Necessary?" *AJO-G*, 4 (1922), 645–50; the study was of "preparation" as a whole, not just shaving.

194. Summary of a paper by Le Lorier on "La Morbidité et la mortalité maternelles à la Maternité de l'Hôpital Boucicaut de 1924 à 1928," *Gynécologie et Obstétrique*, 20 (1929), 595; Florence E. Barrett, "The Prophylactic Treatment of Puerperal Sepsis," *Lancet*, 23 June 1923, p. 1280; Manuel S. Tansinsin, "A Statistical Study of Puerperal Morbidity in Hospital Practice," *AJO-G*, 18 (1929), 99; and Joseph B. DeLee, *The Principles and Practice of Obstetrics*, 6th ed. (Philadelphia, 1933), p. 297.

195. *Williams Obstetrics* [83], 16th ed., p. 408.

196. *Williams Obstetrics* [83] 12th ed., p. 436.

197. Leishman, *System of Midwifery* [43], pp. 265–66.

198. W. S. Playfair, *A Treatise on the Science and Practice of Midwifery*, 3rd ed. (Philadelphia, 1880), p. 279.

199. Charles D. Meigs, *Obstetrics*, 5th ed. (Philadelphia, 1867), p. 329.

200. Richard C. Norris, ed., *An American Text-Book of Obstetrics* (Philadelphia, 1905), p. 369.

201. DeLee, *Principles and Practice* [194], pp. 297–98.

202. Ibid., 5th ed., p. 320.

203. *Williams Obstetrics* [83], 7th ed., pp. 407–8.

348 Notes for pages 169–72

204. P. Cazeaux, *Obstetrics: The Theory and Practice,* 7th U.S. ed. (Philadelphia, 1884), p. 394; Spiegelberg, *Midwifery* [49], I, 256; W. F. T. Haultain, *Practical Handbook of Midwifery and Gynaecology,* 5th ed. (Edinburgh: Livingstone, 1957), p. 67; and Matthew M. Garrey, et al., *Obstetrics Illustrated,* 2nd ed. (Edinburgh: Churchill-Livingstone, 1974), p. 209 ("Delivery of the baby may be conducted in the left lateral or in the dorsal position").

205. Robert Percival, *Holland and Brews Manual of Obstetrics,* 14th ed. (Edinburgh: Churchill-Livingstone, 1980), p. 385.

206. See the 16th ed. of *Williams Obstetrics* [83], p. 416.

207. For a brief history of inducing labor, see Hugo Ehrenfest, *Fetal, Newborn, and Maternal Morbidity and Mortality* (New York: White House Conference on Child Health, Report of the Subcommittee on Factors and Causes of Fetal . . . Mortality 1933), pp. 184–88.

208. On Bellevue Hospital, see remarks by Harold C. Bailey in the discussion of various papers, *AJO-G,* 1 (1920–21), 74–75; on Evanston Hospital, Robert M. Grier, "Maternal Morbidity," *AJO-G,* 34 (1937), 302; and on the United States as a whole in 1967, American College of Obstetricians and Gynecologists, *National Study of Maternity Care: Survey of Obstetric Practice and Associated Services in Hospitals in the United States* (Chicago: ACOG, 1970), p. 16.

209. James Walker, "Fetal Anoxia," *JOB,* 61 (1954), 166, 168.

210. *Williams Obstetrics* [83], 16th ed. pp. 414, 683, 937, 950–51.

211. On British rates for 1965 and 1972, see the essay by Peter Howie, "The Induction of Labor," in Tim Chard and Martin Richards, eds., *Benefits and Hazards of the New Obstetrics* (London: Heinemann, 1977), p. 93. For 1970, National Birthday Trust Fund, *British Births,* p. 79. For mid-1970s data, see Ian Donald, *Practical Obstetric Problems,* 5th ed. (London: Lloyd-Luke, 1979), p. 512 ("over 40 percent" for Glasgow). The Watford Maternity Unit had in 1974 a 55-percent rate (see Richard H. Tipton and B. V. Lewis, Letter, *BMJ,* 15 February 1975, p. 391). Oxford, too, had a 55-percent rate in 1974 (John Bonnar, Letter, *BMJ,* 13 March 1976, p. 652).

212. Margaret F. Myles, *Textbook for Midwives,* 8th ed. (Edinburgh: Churchill-Livingstone, 1975), p. 549; note that the 1st edition of this book in 1953 was much more conservative (p. 585). Among the British literature emphasizing the dangers of prolonging pregnancy, see Neville R. Butler and Eva D. Alberman, *Perinatal Problems: The Second Report of the 1958 British Perinatal Mortality Survey* (Edinburgh: Livingstone-Churchill, 1969), pp. 268–72; R. A. Cole et al., "Elective Induction of Labour," *Lancet,* 5 April 1975, p. 768; and K. O'Driscoll et al., "Selective Induction of Labour," *BMJ,* 27 December 1975, p. 728.

213. Fasbender, *Geschichte Geburtshilfe* [146], p. 595. Fielding Ould, *A Treatise of Midwifery* (Dublin, 1742), pp. 145–46.

214. Rudolf Beck, *Geburten und Geburtshilfe in ländlichen Verhältnissen: eine statistische Studie aus den Geburtstabellen des Amtes Sursee über die letzten 39 Jahre* (Basel: med. diss., 1930), p. 47.

215. Erwin Zweifel, "Erfahrungen an den letzten 10,000 Geburten," *Archiv für Gynäkologie,* 101 (1913–14), 681.

216. Henry Buxbaum, "Out-Patient Obstetrics," *AJO-G,* 31 (1936), 413.

217. DeLee, *Principles and Practice* [194], p. 322

218. See the discussion of Anna Broomall's paper in *AJO,* 11 (1878), 605–6.

219. Jewett, *Practice of Obstetrics* [185], p. 253.

220. Alfred L. Galabin, *Practice of Midwifery,* 7th ed. (London, 1910), p. 648.

221. Robert W. Johnstone, *Text-book of Midwifery,* 7th ed. (London, 1934), p. 157.

222. Eastman, *Williams Obstetrics* [83], p. 412.

223. Howard C. Taylor, "Indications and Technique of Episiotomy," *American Journal of Surgery,* NS, 35 (1937), 403.

224. DeLee, *Principles and Practice* [194], pp. 322, 331; Eastman, *Williams Obstetrics* [83], p. 410.

225. Norman R. Kretzschmar, "A Study of 2987 Consecutive Episiotomies," *AJO-G,* 35 (1938), 621–22.

226. H. Bristol Nelson and Daniel Abramson, "The Advantages of Conservative Obstetrics," *AJO-G,* 41 (1941), 802.

227. Ontario, Ministry of Health, *Hospital Statistics,* 1978/79, p. 92; and H. Glosemeyer and H. Stockhausen, "Mediolaterale Episiotomie oder mediane Episiotomie?" *Geburtshilfe*

und Frauenheilkunde, 38 (1978), 34–37. On Brighton, see Constance L. Beynon, "Midline Episiotomy as a Routine Procedure," *JOB,* 81 (1974), 128.

228. Juliet Willmott, "Too Many Episiotomies," *Midwives Chronicle,* February 1980, p. 46.

229. Ibid., p. 46.

230. United States data for 1975 from Chard and Richards, *Benefits and Hazards,* p. 39, citing unpublished data from the American Hospital Record Study of the Commission on Professional and Hospital Activities.

231. Tenon, *Mémoires sur les hôpitaux* [148], p. 252.

232. M. Semon, "Über die in dem Provinzial-Hebammeninstitut zu Danzig in den Jahren 1887–1897 ausgeführten Zangenentbindungen," *ZGH,* 39 (1898), 139, reporting data from twelve other lying-in hospitals.

233. Browne, *Rotunda Hospital* [69], p. 206.

234. Ehrenfest, *Fetal Morbidity* [207], p. 224.

235. Ibid., pp. 221–22.

236. Joseph DeLee, "The Prophylactic Forceps Operation," *AJO-G,* 1 (1920–21), 34–44, quote from p. 43.

237. Report on the 1921 meeting of the American Gynecological Society, *AJO-G,* 2 (1921), 298–300 and 306–07.

238. Williams, *Williams Obstetrics* [83], 6th ed., p. 481.

239. Chard and Richards, *Benefits and Hazards* [211], p. 39.

240. Browne, *Rotunda Hospital* [69], p. 206. 1974 data on the National Maternity Hospital in Dublin from John Bonnar, Letter, *BMJ,* 13 March 1976, p. 652. In selected British hospitals in the 1970s, 17.8 percent. See Iain Chalmers et al., "Obstetric Practice and Outcome of Pregnancy in Cardiff Residents, 1965–73," *BMJ,* 27 March 1976, p. 736; and Jean Fedrick and Patricia Yudkin, "Obstetric Practice in the Oxford Record Linkage Study Area, 1965–72," *BMJ,* p. 739. Average of the two studies.

241. Ehrenfest, *Fetal Morbidity* [207], p. 220. Ehrenfest opposed the obstetric "radicals."

242. Eastman, *Williams Obstetrics* [83], 10th ed., p. 1058.

243. The current (16th ed.) of *Williams Obstetrics,* 16th ed. [83], p. 1044; Ontario, *Hospital Statistics,* annual volumes, 1975 to 1977/78.

244. Ontario, *Hospital Statistics* [227], 1978/79, p. 92.

245. Bonnar, Letter, *BMJ,* 13 March 1976, p. 652.

246. Eastman, *Williams Obstetrics* [83], 11th ed., p. 1135; 13th ed., p. 1126.

247. O. Hunter Jones, "Cesarean Section in Present-Day Obstetrics," *AJO-G,* 126 (1976), 527. The increase in caesareans is not due to a rising percentage of repeat sections on mothers who have already had a section once. In two series the share of first-time ("primary") sections has risen since the 1940s. See Jones's data on Charlotte, N.C., from 1940 to 1975, "Caesarean Section," p. 522, and Lester T. Hibbard, "Changing Trends in Cesarean Section," *AJO-G,* 125 (1976), 799, on the USC Medical Center.

248. The 1941 quote is from the discussion of George H. Ryder, "A Comparison of the Classical and Lower Segment Cesarean Section," *AJO-G,* 41 (1941), 1037.

249. American College of Obstetricians and Gynecologists, *National Study* [208], p. 10.

250. National Birthday Trust Fund, *British Births* [33], p. 27.

251. William C. Keettel, "An Appraisal of Maternity Care in Iowa," *JAMA,* 27 January 1969, pp. 721, 724.

252. Ehrenfest's phrase, *Fetal Morbidity* [207], p. 220.

Chapter 8

1. A. Guisan, "La Médecine judiciare au XVIIIᵉ siècle, d'après les procédures criminelles vaudoises," *Revue suisse de médecine,* 13 (1912–13), 674.

2. Egon Weinzierl, *Die uneheliche Mutterschaft* (Berlin, 1925), pp. 39–41.

3. Quoted in Helmuth Jahns, *Das Delikt der Abtreibung im Landgerichtsbezirk Duisburg in der Zeit von 1910 bis 1935* (Bonn: staatswiss. diss., 1938), p. 36.

4. Emma Goldman, *Living My Life*, 2 vols. (1931; rpt. New York: Dover, 1970), I, 185–86.

5. See, for example, Franz Xaver Güntner, *Kindesmord und Fruchtabtreibung in gerichtsärztlicher Beziehung* (Prague, 1845), p. 71.

6. Johann Storch, *Unterricht vor Heb-Ammen*, vol. I of *Von Kranckheiten der Weiber*, 8 vols. (Gotha, 1746–53), p. 162.

7. Cited in Alan Macfarlane, "Illegitimacy and Illegitimates in English History," in Peter Laslett et al., eds., *Bastardy and Its Comparative History* (Cambridge: Harvard Univ. Press, 1980), p. 77.

8. E. Pelkonen, *Über volkstümliche Geburtshilfe in Finnland* (Helsinki, 1931), p. 60.

9. Ambroise Tardieu, *Étude médico-légale sur l'avortement* (Paris, 1868), p. 28.

10. Carl Heinrich Stratz, *Die Frauen auf Java: eine gynäkologische Studie* (Stuttgart, 1897), pp. 47–48, describes the technique; see more recently Josefina R. Reynes, "The Significance of Abortion in Bohol," mimeograph of the Bohol Province MCH/FP Project, Tagbilaran City, Philippines, October, 1979, pp. 18–19; and Tongplaew Narkavonnakit, "Abortion in Rural Thailand: A Survey of Practitioners," *Studies in Family Planning*, 10 (1979), 226.

11. P. Fraenkel, "Über den Tod beim Abort," *ZBG*, 50 (1926), 2217; see also G. Leubuscher, "Krimineller Abort in Thüringen," *Vierteljahrsschrift für gerichtliche Medizin*, ser. 3, 50 (1915), 9, who says that massage was used *mehrfach* [numerous times].

12. See Wolfgang Jöchle, "Menses-Inducing Drugs: Their Role in Antique, Medieval and Renaissance Gynecology and Birth Control," *Contraception*, 10 (1974), 425–39; and Ruth Hähnel, "Der künstliche Abortus im Altertum," [*Sudhoff's*] *Archiv für die Geschichte der Medizin*, 29 (1936), 224–55.

13. Christian Gottlieb Troppanneger, *Decisiones Medico-Forenses . . . de Lethalitate Vulnerum* (Dresden, 1733), pp. 225–26.

14. See the list in Jules Massé, *Botanique médicale*, 11th ed. (Paris, 1867), pp. 281–86.

15. Alexander Berg, *Der Krankheitskomplex der Kolik-und Gebärmutterleiden in Volksmedizin und Medizingeschichte* (Berlin, 1935), p. 57 on East Prussia.

16. The most important contribution to this somewhat romanticized historiographic trend is Muriel Joy Hughes, *Women Healers in Medieval Life and Literature* (Freeport, N.Y., 1943), esp. pp. 22–36.

17. J. Thomsen, "Ein Fall von Abtreibung der Leibesfrucht," *Vierteljahrsschrift für gerichtliche und öffentliche Medicin*, NF, 1 (1864), 316.

18. Dr. Flügel, *Volksmedizin und Aberglaube im Frankenwalde*, (Munich, 1863), p. 47.

19. See L. Schenkel-Hulliger et al., "Experimental Models in the Search for Antigestagenic Compounds with Menses-Inducing Activity," *Journal of Steroid Biochemistry*, 11 (1979), 757.

20. F. J. McCann, quoted in summary in *BMJ*, 2 February 1929, p. 203.

21. Otto Kostenzer, "Das Arzneibuch 'der alten Frau Taentzlin' zu Schwaz," *Veröffentlichungen des Tiroler Landesmuseum Ferdinandeum*, 55 (1975); see, for example, the recipe "Zu fürkhommen ainer yeden frawen ir krannckhait" (p. 38).

22. J. B. Chomel, *Abregé de l'histoire des plantes usuelles*, 2 vols. (Paris, 1739), I, 149–50.

23. Storch, *Kranckheiten der Weiber* [6], III, 199–200.

24. Otto Stoll, *Die Erhebungen über Volksmedizin in der Schweiz* (Zurich, 1901), p. 24; offprint from the *Schweiz. Archiv für Volkskunde*, 5 (1901).

25. Coralie W. Rendle Short, "Causes of Maternal Death Among Africans in Kampala, Uganda," *JOB*, 68 (1961), 45.

26. Harvey Graham, *Eternal Eve: The Mysteries of Birth and the Customs That Surround It*, rev. ed. (London: Hutchinson, 1960), p. 17.

27. Warren R. Dawson, *A Leechbook or Collection of Medical Recipes of the Fifteenth Century* (London, 1934), p. 97.

28. Percivall Willughby, *Observations in Midwifery* (1863; rpt. East Ardsley: S. R. Publishers, 1972), p. 59.

29. Among innumerable examples, see R. de Westphalen, *Petit dictionnaire des traditions populaires messines* (Metz, 1934), pp. 4–6; Eugène Olivier, *Médecine et santé dans le*

pays de Vaud au XVIIIe siècle (Lausanne, 1939), I, 273, 277; and Moritz Gerhard Thilenius, *Kurzer Unterricht für die Hebammen und Wöchnerinnen auf dem Lande* (Cassell, 1769), p. 50.

30. B. D. H. Miller, " 'She Who Hath Drunk Any Potion' . . . . , " *Medium Aevum,* 31 (1962), 191.

31. Guillaume Mauquest de la Motte, *Traité complet des acouchemens,* rev. ed. (1715; rpt. Leiden, 1729), p. 68.

32. Edward Moore, letter on midwifery cases, *Lancet,* 22 March 1862, p. 307.

33. On these Third World countries see, for example, J. C. Saha et al., "Ecbolic Properties of Indian Medicinal Plants," *Indian Journal of Medical Research,* 49 (1961), 130–51; R. Moreno Azorero and B. Schvartzman, "268 plantas medicinales utilizadas para regular !a fecundidad en algunos paises de Sudamérica," *Reproducción,* 2 (1975), 163–83; and Yun Cheung Kong, "Potential Anti-fertility Plants from Chinese Medicine," *American Journal of Chinese Medicine,* 4 (1976), 105–28.

34. See World Health Organization, *Ninth Annual Report, Special Programme of Research . . . in Human Reproduction* (Geneva: World Health Organization, 1980), pp. 84–85. For a substantive report on the progress of this research, see Norman S. Farnsworth et al., "Potential Value of Plants as Sources of New Antifertility Agents," *Journal of Pharmaceutical Sciences,* 64 (1975), 535–98 and 717–54.

35. J. R. Spinner, "Zur Toxikologie des Eukalyptusöls und anderer ätherischer Oele, mit besonderer Berücksichtigung ihrer fruchtabtreibenden Wirkung," *Deutsche medizinische Wochenschrift,* 8 April 1920, p. 389.

36. Felix von Oefele, "Anticonceptionelle Arzneistoffe," *Heilkunde,* 2 (1897–98), 494.

37. Cited in Wolfgang Schneider, *Lexikon zur Arzneimittelgeschichte,* 7 vols. (Frankfurt a/M.: Govi Verlag, 1968–75), V/1, 335 ("Aufsteigen und Wehetum der Mutter").

38. Gerhard Madaus, *Lehrbuch der biologischen Heilmittel* (1938; rpt. Hildesheim: Georg Olms, 1976), III, 2504.

39. H. H. Ploss, *Zur Geschichte, Verbreitung und Methode der Frucht-Abtreibung* (Leipzig, 1883), p. 47.

40. Dawson, *Leechbook* [27], p. 125.

41. Béla Issekutz, *Die Geschichte der Arzneimittelforschung* (Budapest: Akadémiai Kiadó, 1971), p. 330.

42. J. Alksnis, "Materialien zur lettischen Volksmedizin," in Rudolf Kobert, ed. *Historische Studien aus dem Pharmakologischen Institute . . . Dorpat,* IV (Halle, 1894), p. 226.

43. E. Ferdut, *De l'avortement* (Paris, 1865), p. 83; Madaus, *Lehrbuch,* p. 2503.

44. Dr. Weihe, "Use of Ergot in Inducing Abortion," *LMG,* 18 (1836), 543.

45. James Whitehead, *On the Causes and Treatment of Abortion and Sterility* (London, 1847), p. 254.

46. John H. Morgan, "An Essay on the Causes of the Production of Abortion among Our Negro Population," *Nashville Journal of Medicine and Surgery,* 19 (1860), 120.

47. O. Vago, "Toxische und kaustische Komplikationen durch Gebrauch sogenannter fruchtabtreibender Arzneimittel," *ZGH,* 170 (1969), 273.

48. Louis S. Goodman and Alfred Gilman, *The Pharmacological Basis of Therapeutics,* 5th ed. (New York: Macmillan, 1975), p. 874.

49. Lafeuille, *La Vérité sur l'avortement* (Paris, n.d.), p. 100.

50. Dr. Moïssidés, "Contribution à l'étude de l'avortement dans l'antiquité grecque," *Janus,* 26 (1922), 143; Madaus, *Lehrbuch,* [38], 2373–76; P. Fournier, *Le livre des plantes médicinales et vénéneuses de France,* 3 vols. (Paris, 1947–48), III, 357–58; and Elseluise Haberling, *Beiträge zur Geschichte des Hebammenstandes, I: Der Hebammenstand in Deutschland von seinen Anfängen bis zum Dreissigjährigen Krieg* (Berlin, 1940), p. 71.

51. Ernest Guenther, *Essential Oils,* 6 vols. (New York: Van Nostrand, 1948–52), III, 383–84 and, Otto Gessner, *Gift- und Arzneipflanzen von Mitteleuropa,* 3rd ed. (Heidelberg: Winter, 1974), pp. 311–12.

52. Jean Renaux, "A Propos des propriétés abortives des essences de rue et de sabine," *Archives internationales de pharmacodynamie,* 66 (1941), 472.

53. André Patoir et al., "Etude expérimentale comparative de quelques abortifs," *Gynécologie et obstétrique,* 39 (1939), p. 201.

54. T. Hélie, "De l'action vénéneuse de la rue et de son influence sur la grossesse,"

Annales d'hygiène et de médecine légales, 20 (1838), 181–82. For the view that rue acted through its general toxicity, see T. Gallard, *De l'avortement au point de vue médico-légal* (Paris, 1878), p. 20.

55. Saha, "Indian Medicinal Plants" [33], p. 140; Andrée Levesque, "Grandmother Took Ergot," *Broadsheet*, November 1976, p. 30; Rudolf Temesváry, *Volksbräuche und Aberglaube in der Geburtshilfe und der Pflege des Neugebornen in Ungarn* (Leipzig, 1900) p. 18; and Morgan, "Abortion" [46], p. 118.

56. Louis Caradec, *Topographie médico-hygiènique du département du Finistère* (Brest, 1860), p. 337.

57. Heinrich Marzell, *Volksbotanik: Die Pflanze im deutschen Brauchtum* (Berlin, 1935), p. 106 (*Verwendung nur für Liebhaber*).

58. Torald Sollmann, *A Manual of Pharmacology*, 6th ed. (Philadelphia, 1942), p. 168.

59. Morgan, "Abortion" [46], pp. 117–18.

60. R. Frank Chandler et al., "Herbal Remedies of the Maritime Indians," *Journal of Ethnopharmacology*, 1 (1979), 62, and George A. Conway and John C. Slocumb, "Plants used as Abortifacients and Emmenagogues by Spanish New Mexicans," *Journal of Ethnopharmacology*, 1 (1979), 62, 253.

61. John Metcalf, "Statistics in Midwifery," *American Journal of the Medical Sciences*, NS, 6 (Oct. 1843), 339.

62. Ely van de Warker, *The Detection of Criminal Abortion* (1872; rpt. New York: Arno Press, 1974), p. 73.

63. Frederick Taussig, *Abortion, Spontaneous and Induced: Medical and Social Aspects* (St. Louis, 1936), p. 353.

64. Saha, "Indian Medicinal Plants" [33], p. 141.

65. Saint Hildegarde reference in Fournier, *Plantes médicinales*, [50], I, 394.

66. Renaux, "Propriétés abortives" [52], 472; Lucy Prochnow, "Experimentelle Beiträge zur Kenntnis der Wirkung der Volksabortiva," *Archives internationales de pharmacodynamie*, 12 (1911), p. 317.

67. Patoir et al. "Etude expérimentale" [53], pp. 204–5.

68. Quoted in Heinrich Lehmann, *Beiträge zur Geschichte von . . . Juniperus Sabina* (Basel: phil. diss., 1935), pp. 132–33. The German: "Zuletst so verfüren die jüngen huren/ geben jnen Seuen-palmen gepulvert/oder darüber zu trincken/dardurch vil kinder verderbt werd. Zu solchem handel gehört ein scharpffer Inquisitor und meyster."

69. Quoted in Louis Lewin, *Die Fruchtabtreibung durch Gifte und andere Mittel*, 3rd ed. (Berlin, 1922), p. 328.

70. von Oefele, "Antikonceptionelle Arzneistoffe" [36], p. 490.

71. Marzell, *Volksbotanik* [57], p. 180.

72. G. Lammert, *Volksmedizin und medizinischer Aberglaube in Bayern* (Würzburg, 1869), p. 162; and Lewin, *Fruchtabtreibung* [69], p. 328.

73. Augustus Granville, *A Report of the Practice of Midwifery at the Westminster General Dispensary during 1818* (London, 1819), p. 148.

74. Raimund Werb, *Die Wandlung der Abtreibungsmethoden und ihre forensische Bedeutung* (Marburg: med. diss., 1936), p. 17.

75. Jonas Frykman, "Sexual Intercourse and Social Norms: A Study of Illegitimate Births in Sweden, 1831–1933," *Ethnologia Scandinavica*, 1975, p. 135.

76. Lewin, *Fruchtabtreibung* [69], pp. 333–35.

77. Rudolph Lex, "Die Abtreibung der Leibesfrucht," *Vierteljahrsschrift für gerichtliche und öffentliche Medicin*, NF, 4 (1866), 239–40.

78. M. Kronfeld, "Volksthümliche Abortiva und Aphrodisiaca in Oesterreich," *Wiener medizinische Wochenschrift*, 2 November 1889, p. 1699. "So geläufig wie das Einmaleins."

79. See Guenther, *Essential Oils* [51], I, 68–77.

80. G. Marczal et al., "Phenol-Ether Components of Diuretic Effect in Parsley," *Acta Agronomica Academiae Scientiarum Hungaricae*, 26 (1977), 7–13, especially the graph on p. 12.

81. Madaus, *Lehrbuch* [38], I, 319.

82. Thomsen, "Abtreibung" [17], p. 325.

83. Roger Goulard, "Avorteurs et avorteuses à la Bastille," *Bulletin de la société française d'histoire de la médecine*, 15 (1921), 267–82.

84. Hermann W. Freund, "Das Hebammenwesen," in Joseph Krieger, ed., *Topographie der Stadt Strassburg* (Strasbourg, 1889), p. 303.

85. Dr. Coutèle, *Observations sur la constitution médicale de l'année 1808 à Albi* (Albi, 1809), p. 101.

86. Jean-Marie Munaret, *Le Médecin des villes et des campagnes* (Paris, 1862), pp. 458–59.

87. Johann Ludwig Casper, *Practisches Handbuch der gerichtlichen Medicin*, 4th ed., 2 vols. (Berlin, 1864), I, 236.

88. Stoll, *Erhebungen* [24] p. 13.

89. de la Motte, *Traité* [31], pp. 285–86.

90. Keith L. Moore, *The Developing Human: Clinically Oriented Embryology* (Philadelphia: Saunders, 1974), pp. 63, 73.

91. Joseph Capuron, *La Médecine légale relative à l'art des accouchemens* (Paris, 1821), p. 314.

92. Henry Oldham, "Clinical Lecture on the Induction of Abortion in a Case of Contracted Vagina from Cicatrization," *LMG*, NS, 9 (1849), 45–46.

93. Tardieu, *L'Avortement* [10], p. 118.

94. Dr. Martin, *Mémoires de médecine* (Paris, 1835), pp. 288–89.

95. Joubert, "Fausse couche," in Denis Diderot, ed., *Encyclopédie*, vol. 6 (1766), p. 452.

96. Sir Bernard Spilsbury speaking at Medico-Legal Society, *BMJ*, 2 February 1929, p. 203.

97. James C. Mohr, *Abortion in America* (New York: Oxford Univ. Press, 1978), pp. 30–31.

98. Great Britain, Ministry of Health, *Report on Maternal Mortality in Wales* (London, cmd. 5423, 1937), p. 70.

99. Leopold Kohn, *Beitrag zum suspeketen und kriminellen Abort an Hand von 76 Fällen der Zürcher Frauenklinik* (Zurich: med. diss., 1917), p. 14.

100. A. Haberda, "Gerichtsärztliche Erfahrungen über die Fruchtabtreibung in Wien," *Vierteljahrsschrift für gerichtliche Medizin*, 3F, 56 (1918) suppl., 56–57.

101. Atle Berg, "Statistiche Untersuchungen der von 1920 bis 1929 im Städtischen Krankenhaus Ulleваal in Oslo behandelten Aborte," *Acta Obstetricia et Gynecologica Scandinavica*, 11 (1931), 69–70.

102. Thomas V. Pearce, "Three Hundred Cases of Abortion," *JOB*, 37 (1930), 797 (overall admissions measured by the number of admissions for ectopic pregnancy).

103. Janet Campbell et al., eds., *High Maternal Mortality in Certain Areas* (London: Great Britain, Ministry of Health; Reports on Public Health, no. 68, 1932), p. 42.

104. P. Balard, note in *Presse médicale*, 9 January 1937, p. 49.

105. On the Kiel area, see Elisabeth Baldauf, *Die Frauenarbeit in der Landwirtschaft* (Kiel: staatswiss. diss., 1932), p. 57 (on Landbezirk Kiel).

106. See Friedrich Prinzing, *Handbuch der medizinischen Statistik*, 2nd ed. (Jena, 1931), p. 44 ("Fehlgeburten per 100 Entbindungen in öffentlichen Universitäts- und Privatanstalten").

107. E. Bonnaire, "Du travail de l'avortement," *Presse médicale*, 3 May 1905, p. 274.

108. H. Rothe, "Die Einschränkung des künstlichen Aborts," *ZBG*, 41 (1917), 179 ("Und wie oft hören wir in der Sprechstunde, dann fahre ich eben nach Berlin").

109. Ralph Benson, *Handbook of Obstetrics and Gynecology*, 6th ed. (Los Altos, Cal.: Lange, 1977), p. 260.

110. C. J. Roberts and C. R. Lowe, "Where Have All the Conceptions Gone?" *Lancet*, 1 March 1975, pp. 498–99.

111. Cited in Erik Lindqvist, *Über die Aborte in Malmö, 1897–1928* (Helsinki, 1931), p. 241.

112. Cited in Emil Bovin, "Die Resultate exspektativer Behandlung . . . , " *Acta Gynecologica Scandinavica*, 3 (1924–25), 107 (citing "Richter's" results).

113. Dr. Blondel, paper given to the Société d'obstétrique de Paris, *Presse médicale*, 26 March 1902, p. 296.

114. E. Roesle, "Die Ergebnisse der Magdeburger Fehlgeburtenstatistik," *Statistisches Jahrbuch der Stadt Magdeburg*, 1927, p. 135.

115. Philipp Ehlers, *Die Sterblichkeit "im Kindbett"* (Stuttgart, 1900), p. 40; F. Strassmann, *Lehrbuch der gerichtlichen Medizin*, 2nd ed. (Stuttgart, 1931), p. 107 ("Über 90 per Hundert aller Fälle von Sepsis oder Bauchfellentzündung nach Abort durch einen krimi-

nellen Eingriff hervorgerufen [sind]''); and George Gellhorn, "The Treatment of Septic Abortion," *Transactions. American Gynecological Society,* 53 (1928), p. 21, ("Ninety percent or more of all abortions are criminal abortions").

116. H. Fr. Harbitz, "Aetiologische und klinische Untersuchungen von Aborten," *Acta Obstetricia et Gynecologica Scandinavica,* 11 (1931), 51.

117. Josef Krug, "Die Fehlgeburten im Deutschen Reich," *Münchener medizinische Wochenschrift,* 15 November 1940, p. 1277.

118. Roesle, "Fehlgeburtensstatistik" [114], p. 137.

119. Lindqvist, *Aborte Malmö* [111], p. 243.

120. E. Philipp, "Der heutige Stand der Bekämpfung der Fehlgeburt," *ZBG,* 64 (1940), 248.

121. Cited in W. Latzko, "Die Behandlung des fieberhaften Abortus," *ZBG,* 45 (1921), 426.

122. Ehlers, *Sterblichkeit* [115], pp. 30, 33.

123. Karl Freudenberg, "Berechnungen zur Abtreibungsstatistik," *Zeitschrift für Hygiene und Infektionskrankheiten,* 104 (1925), 545.

124. Karl Freudenberg, "Berechnungen über die Häufigkeit der tödlichen Fehlgeburten in Deutschland," *Münchener medizinische Wochenschrift,* 6 May 1932, p. 759. Other authors offered less credible estimates many thousands higher. See L. Bouchacourt, "A Propos de quelques cas récents de poursuites judiciares pour avortement clandestin," *Journal des praticiens,* 44 suppl. (1930), 1884; and O. Pankow, "Strafbare und straflose Schwangerschaftsunterbrechungen," *Deutsche medizinische Wochenschrift,* 12 October 1928, p. 1713.

125. These examples are from Sigismund Peller, *Fehlgeburt und Bevölkerungsfrage* (Stuttgart, 1930), p. 141; Wilhelm Liepmann, "Die Gefahren des Aborts," *Deutsche medizinische Wochenschrift,* 1 March 1929, p. 351; and Bouchacourt, ibid., p. 1884n1.

126. Dunstan Brewer, discussion after a paper by Andrew Topping on "Prevention of Maternal Mortality: The Rochdale Experiment," *Lancet,* 7 March 1936, p. 547.

127. F. Pietrusky, "Zur Frage der kriminellen Fruchtabtreibung," *Deutsche Zeitschrift für die gesamte gerichtliche Medizin,* 14 (1929), 54–55.

128. Great Britain, Ministry of Health, *Maternal Mortality Wales,* p. 74.

129. Friedrich Moser, *Über Morbidität und Mortalität bei Abortus* (Berne: med. diss., 1900), p. 23; J. M. Munro Kerr, *Maternal Mortality and Morbidity* (Edinburgh, 1933), p. 46; and Taussig, *Abortion* [63], p. 382.

130. Campbell, *High Maternal Mortality* [103], p. 42.

131. Autopsy findings in Breslau and Halle, Pietrusky, "Kriminelle Fruchtabtreibung" [127], pp. 60–61.

132. See the statistics in Wilhelm Liepmann, *Die Abtreibung* (Berlin, 1927), p. 6. Hugo Lappin presents a range of studies in *Statistik der Aborte in den Jahren 1925–26* (Munich: med. diss., 1927), pp. 15–16.

133. Roesle, "Fehlgeburtenstatistik" [114], p. 137; and Ernst Brezina and Valerie Reuterer, "Über den Abortus in Österreich," *Archiv für Hygiene,* 14 (1935), 335.

134. Taussig, *Abortion* [63], pp. 386–87; Hans Nevermann, "Zur Frage der Mortalität durch Schwangerschaft, Geburt und Wochenbett," *ZBG,* 52 (1928), 2357; and Great Britain, Ministry of Health, Home Office, *Report of the Interdepartmental Committee on Abortion* (London, 1939), p. 15, on sulfa drugs.

135. Dr. Fuchs, "Wandlungen des Abortusproblems," *ZBG,* 55 (1931), 1921.

136. John A. Lyons, "Premature Interruption of Pregnancy," *AJO,* 56 (1907), 682.

137. Frank H. Jackson, "Criminal Abortion," *AJO,* 58 (1909), 663.

138. H. Wellington Yates, "Treatment of Abortion," *AJO-G,* 3 (1922), 43–45.

139. Edward Weiss, *AJO-G,* 3 (1922), 82.

140. Max Nassauer, *Der moderne Kindermord* (Leipzig, 1919), 18.

141. Adolphe Pinard, *Revue pénitentiaire et de droit pénal,* 41–42 (1917), 186.

142. See the estimates in Max Hirsch, *Fruchtabtreibung* (Stuttgart, 1921), pp. 2–8.

143. Ibid., p. 8.

144. Data on Berlin, 1882–1915, presented in Karl Hartmann, *Die Häufigkeit des Abortes: Ein statistischer Beitrag aus der Universitätsfrauenklinik in Marburg* (Marburg: med. diss., 1919), pp. 13–14 (studies of patients in gynecologic clinics, who were either forty-five at the time of the interview or had had over three births). 1915–1916 from Agnes Bluhm, "Zur Kenntnis der Gattungsleistungen der Industriearbeiterinnen im Kriege," *Archiv für*

Rassen- und Gesellschaftsbiologie, 13 (1921), 76 (married women in a factory social-insurance plan).

145. Bleichröder, "Ueber die Zunahme der Fehlgeburten in den Berliner städtischen Krankenhäusern," *Berliner klinische Wochenschrift*, 9 March 1914, p. 452.

146. C. Hamburger, *Berliner klinische Wochenschrift*, 20 November 1916, p. 1269.

147. Freudenberg, "Berechnungen" [123].

148. Sigismund Peller, "Studien zur Statistik des Abortus," *ZBG*, 53 (1929), 2221 (married women giving birth for the second time in Vienna's Piskacek Clinic).

149. P. E. Treffers, "Abortion in Amsterdam," *Population Studies*, 20 (1966–67), 300 (taken from pregnancy histories of obstetric patients in an Amsterdam hospital).

150. On Munich, see Hartmann, *Aborte* [144], pp. 13–14 (patients in gynecological clinics).

151. Virginia Clay Hamilton, "Some Sociologic and Psychologic Observations on Abortion: A Study of 537 Cases," *AJO-G*, 39 (1940), 920 (the final diagnosis in sixty-seven cases was "not pregnant").

152. Lisbeth Burger, *Vierzig Jahre Storchentante: Aus dem Tagebuch einer Hebamme* (Breslau, 1936), p. 227.

153. Quoted in Madeleine Simms, "Midwives and Abortion in the 1930's," *Midwife and Health Visitor*, 10 (1974), 115.

154. See, for example, Linda Gordon, *Woman's Body, Woman's Right: A Social History of Birth Control in America* (New York: Viking/Grossman, 1976), pp. 35–45.

155. Heinrich Fasbender, *Geschichte der Geburtshilfe* (Jena, 1906), p. 859.

156. W. Schütte, "Die Fruchtabtreibung durch innerlich gereichte Abortivmittel und durch den Einhautstich," *Zeitschrift für die staatliche Arzneikunde*, 46 Ergänzungsheft (1855), 107.

157. Ibid., p. 106.

158. James F. Scott, "Criminal Abortion," *AJO*, 33 (1896), 84; and a paper presented in 1895 at the Washington Obstetrical and Gynecological Society.

159. Ferdut, *De l'avortement* [43], p. 86.

160. Frederic Griffith, "Instruments for the Production of Abortion Sold in the Market Places of Paris, *Medical Record*, 30 January 1904, pp. 171–72.

161. Franz Maria Feldhaus, *Die Technik der Vorzeit, der geschichtlichen Zeit und der Naturvölker* (Munich: Moos, 1965), p. 1074 (entry "Spritze").

162. Reproduced in C. J. S. Thompson, *The History and Evolution of Surgical Instruments* (New York, 1942), p. 103.

163. Depicted, for example, in Elisabeth Bennion, *Antique Medical Instruments* (London: Sotheby, 1979), pp. 169–75.

164. The remote history in Fasbender, *Geschichte Geburtshilfe* [155], pp. 858–62.

165. J. Lazarewitch, "Induction of Premature Labour by Injection to the Fundus of the Uterus," *Transactions. Obstetrical Society of London*, 9 (1867), 161–202. I am obliged to Susan Lawrence for this reference.

166. Ferdut, *De l'avortement* [43], p. 86.

167. Tardieu, *L'avortement* [9], pp. 66–67.

168. See, for example, M. Mourral, testifying about objects seized in a raid on an abortionist's home, in *Revue pénitentiaire*, 173.

169. Ernst Puppel, "Der kriminelle Abort in Thüringen, 1915–1926," *Deutsche Zeitschrift für die gesamte gerichtliche Medizin*, 12 (1928), 579.

170. Ibid., p. 579.

171. According to Dr. Vibert, note in *Semaine médicale*, 1892, p. 458.

172. W. Benthin, "Ueber kriminelle Fruchtabtreibung," *ZGH*, 77 (1915), 597.

173. Artur Horvat, "Beitrag zur Statistik krimineller Aborte," *MGH*, 59 (1922), 281.

174. Haberda, "Gerichtsärztliche Erfahrungen" [100], p. 82 ("Die jetzt häufig genannten 'Mutterspritzen,' deren Verkauf . . . im Strafgesetz verboten und mit Strafe bedroht sein sollte, kennen wir in Wien seit etwa 10 Jahren").

175. Hans Schneickert, "Die gewerbsmässige Abtreibung und deren Bekämpfung," *Monatsschrift für Kriminalpsychologie*, 2 (1905–06), pp. 630–31 ("Neuerdings kommen auch Gummispritzen in den Handel").

176. Konstantin Inderheggen, *Das Delikt der Abtreibung im Landgerichtsbezirk M.-Gladbach in der Zeit von 1908 bis 1938* (Bonn: staatswiss. diss., 1939), p. 42. "Mechanical

procedures" meant mainly syringe. I am grateful for this reference to my student Mr. James Woycke, who is currently preparing a doctoral dissertation on changes in German birth control practices.

177. Pierre-Louis Duclerget, *Contribution à l'étude de l'avortement criminellement provoqué* (Nancy: med. diss., 1922), p. 57; not all the cases reported were from his hospital.

178. Quoted in ibid., p. 21.

179. See, for example, Adolphe Pinard's comment in *Presse médicale*, 18 March 1905, p. 175; Max Gerstmann, "Statistisches über Aborte," *MGH*, 68 (1925), 221 ("Weniger die geschulte Abtreiberin, als die ihren Beruf wenigstens meistens sauber und steril ausübt, als die Patienten selbst, die beim Abtreibungsgeschäft sich pathogene Keime in den Uterus bringen, verschlechtern in dieser Weise die Statistik").

180. See Jahns, *Delikt Abtreibung Duisburg* [3], p. 53, for example.

181. For details, see Hans-Georg Heinemann, *An der Rostocker Universitäts-Frauenklinik beobachtete Perforationen des graviden Uterus bei Abortusausräumung (1920–30)* (Rostock: med. diss., 1931); Erich Münchmeyer, Über die pathologisch-anatomischen Befunde der im Gerichtlich-medizinischen Institut zu München vorliegenden Fälle von tödlich verlaufener Fruchtabtreibung (Munich: med. diss., 1927); and Judith Traube, *Ueber die Perforation des Uterus mit der Kornzange bei Aborten* (Berlin: med. diss., 1912).

182. See Alfred Percheval, *Des manoeuvres abortives chez les femmes qui ne sont pas enceintes* (Paris: med. diss., 1911), p. 45; and Arthur Schönbek, "Ein Fall von kriminellem Abortus," *ZBG*, 29 (1905), 1497–98.

183. For examples, see Münchmeyer, *Befunde* [181], passim; and Weissenrieder, "Fruchtabtreibung Tod durch Luftembolie," *Zeitschrift für Medizinalbeamte*, 23 (1910), 585–93.

184. Jahns, *Delikt Abtreibung Duisburg* [3], p. 61 ("Das ist das verfluchte Weib, das mich halbtot gemacht hat. Das kennt man in Oesterreich nicht. Das kann man hier alles lernen").

185. Fr. Thomä, "Abtreibungsversuch bei fehlender Schwangerschaft," *ZGB*, 36 (1912), 1429–31.

186. Dr. Schnell, "Die beim weiblichen Geschlecht gebräuchlichen Gummiartikel zur Verhütung und Unterbrechung der Schwangerschaft," *Zeitschrift für Medizinalbeamte*, 30 (1917), 568.

187. See Doléris note, *Presse médicale*, 18 February 1905, p. 111; Griffith, "Instruments Market Places Paris" [160], p. 172; and W. Benthin, "Uber kriminelle Fruchtabtreibung," *ZGH*, 77 (1915), 626 ("Leider sind die Spritzen in den Drogerien, bei Bandagisten, selbst in den Friseurgeschäften gegen ein geringes Entgelt erhältlich").

188. Pinard, *Revue pénitentiaire* [141], p. 174.

189. Petzsch, *Abtreibung und Findelhäuser* (Greifswald, 1929), p. 16; A. Grotjahn, *Geburten-Rückgang und Geburten-Regelung* (Berlin, 1921), pp. 72–73; and quote from Benthin, "Kriminelle Fruchtabtreibung" [187], p. 609.

190. Kohn, *Beitrag Zürcher Frauenklinik* [99], p. 13; Duclerget, *Avortement Nancy* [177], p. 60; on Königsberg, Walter Offermann, "Beitrag zur Behandlung des fieberhaften Abortes und einiges über die kriminellen Aborte überhaupt," *ZGH*, 84 (1921), 382; and Hans Reichling, *Abortivmittel und Methoden des kriminellen Aborts im Landgerichtsbezirk Essen* (Münster: med. diss., 1939), pp. 19–20. I have this reference thanks to James Woycke.

191. Harbitz, "Untersuchungen von Aborten" [116], p. 51; and H. S. Pasmore, "A Clinical and Sociological Study of Abortion," *JOB*, 44 (1937), 459.

192. The references to syringes in Gordon, *Woman's Body* [154], do not distinguish between vaginal and uterine douching (pp. 64–66).

193. Mohr, *Abortion in America* [96], p. 70.

194. Hunter Robb, "The Induction of Abortion," in Charles Jewett, ed., *Practice of Obstetrics*, 3rd ed. (London, 1907), p. 696.

195. This procedure described in Haberda, "Gerichtsärztliche Erfahrungen" [100], pp. 83–86.

196. Quoted in J. Milton Mabbott, "The Regulation of Midwives in New York," *AJO*, 55 (1907), 520. On Portland, see Raymond E. Watkins, "A Five-Year Study of Abortion," *AJO-G*, 26 (1933), 162.

197. See Horatio R. Storer, "The Use and Abuse of Uterine Tents," *American Journal of the Medical Sciences*, NS, 37 (1859), 59; and J. M. Munro Kerr, *Operative Midwifery*,

2nd ed. (London, 1911), p. 449. I am grateful to Susan Lawrence for these references, and for the following one as well.

198. W. Edward Pritchard, "Abortion Procured by Tents of Common Sea Tangle," *Transactions. Obstetrical Society of London,* 5 (1863), 198–99.

199. T. Gallard, *L'Avortement au point de vue médico-legal* (Paris, 1878), p. 29.

200. Dr. Kiefer speaking in a discussion period, *ZBG,* 50 (1926), 2216.

201. Campbell, *High Maternal Mortality* [103], p. 82. The author was evidently unaware of the true application of the bark, believing it to be taken as a drug.

202. Pasmore, "Study of Abortion" [191], p. 459.

203. Great Britain, Committee on Abortion [134], p. 62.

204. One is depicted in Harold Speert, *Iconographia Gyniatrica: A Pictorial History of Gynecology and Obstetrics* (Philadelphia: Davis, 1973), p. 463.

205. For a detailed history of the uterine curette, I am indebted to Susan Lawrence's unpublished paper "Instrumental Therapeutic Abortion and Induction of Premature Labor in the Nineteenth Century" (1978).

206. The earliest reference to appear in the *Surgeon General's Index,* vol. 19, 1914, is V.-L.-S. Candelier, *Du Curettage total de l'uterus comme méthode d'avortement provoqué* (Lille, 1896). Paul F. Mundé, in his important 1878 paper on the subject, makes no reference to curettage for abortion ("The Dull Wire Curette in Gynecological Practice," *Transactions. Edinburgh Obstetrical Society,* 5 [1877–80], 48–64).

207. See Davis B. Hart, *Guide to Midwifery* (London, 1912), p. 415.

208. Nicolson J. Eastman, *Williams Obstetrics,* 10th ed. (New York: Appleton-Century-Crofts, 1950), p. 1045.

209. Cited in Roger Darquenne, "L'Obstétrique aux XVIIIᵉ et XIXᵉ siècles," in *Ecoles et livres d'école en Hainaut du XVIᵉ au XIXᵉ siécle* (Mons: Ed. universitaires, 1971), p. 306.

210. Rothe, "Einschränkung des künstlichen Aborts" [108], 179 ("Sie haben gewiss Husten").

211. Grotjahn, *Geburten-Rückgang* [189], p. 58.

212. R. Hoffstätter, "Tentamen abortus provocandi deficiente graviditate," *Beiträge zur gerichtlichen Medizin,* 5 (1922), 36–37.

213. Gallard, *L'Avortement* [199], p. 29. It is clear from the text that the *hystéromètre* is, in fact, a uterine curette.

214. Reichling, *Abortivmittel Essen* [190], p. 23.

215. Jack A. Pritchard and Paul C. MacDonald, *Williams Obstetrics,* 16th ed. (New York: Appleton-Century-Crofts, 1980), p. 528.

216. M. Magid and N. Pantschenko, "Versuche der Fruchtabtreibung und intrauterine Eingriffe bei ektopischer Schwangerschaft," *ZBG,* 57 (1933), 706.

217. In the considerable literature, see, for example, Arthur Stein, "Attempted Abortion in the Absence of Uterine Pregnancy," *AJO,* 75 (1917), 644–51; and Hans Hermann Schmid, "Tentamen abortus provocandi deficiente graviditate," *ZBG,* 36 (1912), 1457–61.

218. Said Dr. Hammerschlag in a discussion, *ZBG,* 50 (1926), 2216 ("Die Abtreiber infizieren, die Ärzte verletzen").

219. Arthur M. Hill, "Post-Abortal and Puerperal Gas Gangrene," *JOB,* NS, 43 (1936), table II after p. 249.

220. On the increase generally, see Werb, *Wandlung Abtreibungsmethoden* [74], p. 44.

221. See Liepmann, *Abtreibung* [132], pp. 10–11; and Heinemann, *Rostocker Perforationen* [181], p. 2.

222. Sigismund Peller, *Fehlgeburt und Bevölkerungsfrage* [125], p. 142.

223. See Jalmar H. Simons on Minneapolis, "Statistical Analysis of One Thousand Abortions," *AJO-G,* 37 (1939), 843 (33 percent of the abortions with drugs, mainly ergot and quinine).

224. Virginia Clay Hamilton, "The Clinical and Laboratory Differentiation of Spontaneous and Induced Abortion," *AJO-G,* 41 (1941), 62.

225. Ibid., pp. 64–65.

226. Ibid., p. 65.

227. The relevant studies are: Kohn, *Beitrag zum suspekten Abort* [99], p. 13 (24 percent). On Königsberg, Benthin, "Kriminelle Fruchtabtreibung" [172], pp. 595–96 (120 cases). Hellmuth Hahn, *Gerichtärztliche Erfahrungen über den kriminellen Abort am Land-*

gericht Göttingen in den Jahren 1909-1919 (Göttingen: med. diss., 1920), p. 18 (98 cases). Puppel, "Krimineller Abort in Thüringen" [169], p. 578 ("Very rare"). Inderheggen, *Abtreibung im Landgericht M.-Gladbach* [176], p. 38 (12 percent). Reichling, *Abortivmittel Essen* [190], pp. 19–20 (219 cases; 11 percent). On Elisabethgrad (later Kirovgrad), S. Weissenberg, "Hundert Fehlgeburten, ihre Ursachen und Folgen," *Archiv für Rassen- und Gesellschafts-Biologie*, 7 (1910), 609–10. 49 cases (45 percent). Harbitz, "Untersuchungen von Aborten" [116], p. 51 (among the 159 who confessed, 19 percent).

228. Quoted in Ethel M. Elderton, *Report on the English Birthrate* (London, 1914), p. 137.

229. Simms, "Midwives and Abortion" [153], p. 114.

230. Great Britain, *Committe on Abortion* [134], p. 41.

231. Hans Zahler, *Die Krankheit im Volksglauben des Simmenthals* (Berne, 1898), p. 56.

232. Margarete Möckli von Seggern, *Arbeiter und Medizin: Die Einstellung des Zürcher Industriearbeiters zur wissenschaftlichen und volkstümlichen Heilkunde* (Basel: Krebs, 1965), p. 148.

233. Rudolf Kobert, *Lehrbuch der Intoxikationen*, 2 vols. (Stuttgart, 1902–06), II, 598–99.

234. On the counterfeiting of saffron, see Madaus, *Lehrbuch* [38], II, 1124. On saffron's ineffectiveness in Thuringia, possibly linked to adulteration, see Leubuscher, "Krimineller Abort" [11], p. 11.

235. Ant. Joseph Scholz, *Pharmazeutisch-gebräuchliche Coniferen-Blattdrogen insbesondere Juniperus Sabina und seine Verfälschungen* (Basel: phil. diss., 1923), p. 55.

236. André Patoir et al., "Sur l'emploi fréquent des toxiques végétaux dits abortifs," *Presse médicale*, 3–6 December 1941, p. 1292.

237. Among various investigations, see "Quacks and Abortion: A Critical and Analytical Inquiry," *Lancet*, 10 December 1898, pp. 1570–71, 17 December, pp. 1652–53, 24 December, pp. 1723–25, 31 December, pp. 1807–09; "The Composition of Certain Secret Remedies," *BMJ*, 7 December 1907, pp. 1653–58; British Medical Association, *More Secret Remedies: What They Cost and What They Contain* (London, 1912), pp. 184–209; G. Roche Lynch's comments in *BMJ*, 2 February 1929, p. 204; Martin Cole and A. F. M. Brierley, "Abortifacient Drugs," *Journal of Sex Research*, 4 (1968), 16–25; P. S. Brown, "Female Pills and the Reputation of Iron as an Abortifacient," *Medical History*, 21 (1977), 291–304; Arthur J. Cramp, *Nostrums and Quackery* (Chicago, 1921), II, 160–82, and *Nostrums and Quackery and Pseudo-Medicine* (1936), III, 64–66; and A. Beythien and H. Hempel, "Über die Tätigkeit des Chemischen Untersuchungsamtes der Stadt Dresden im Jahre 1914," *Pharmazeutische Zentralhalle*, 56 (1915), 372.

238. See Bernard Spilsbury's remarks in *BMJ*, 2 February 1929, p. 203.

239. Letter from around 1914. The Women's Co-operative Guild, *Maternity: Letters from Working-Women* (1915; rpt. New York: Garland, 1980), p. 45.

240. On Sweden, see G. Hedrén, "Zur Statistik und Kasuistik der Fruchtabtreibung," *Vierteljahrsschrift für gerichtliche Medizin*, 3rd ser., 29 (1905), 55.

241. Kobert, *Lehrbuch* [233], II, 283.

242. Hedrén, "Fruchtabtreibung" [240], pp. 50–55; Lewin, *Fruchtabtreibung* [69] pp. 248–56; and Werb, *Wandlung Abtreibungsmethoden* [74], pp. 7–8.

243. Hedrén, ibid., p. 52. Kobert believed that fifty matches would yield a fatal dose (*Lehrbuch* [233], II, 285).

244. Lewin, *Fruchtabtreibung* [69], p. 276.

245. Dawson, *Leechbook*, [27], p. 99.

246. Lewin, *Fruchtabtreibung* [69], p. 281.

247. Arthur Hall and W. B. Ransom, "Plumbism from the Ingestion of Diachylon as an Abortifacient," *BMJ*, 24 February 1906, p. 428.

248. G. Schwarzwaeller, "Zur Fruchtabtreibung durch Gifte," *Berliner klinische Wochenschrift*, 18 February 1901, p. 194.

249. Morris M. Datnow, "An Experimental Investigation Concerning Toxic Abortion Produced by Chemical Agents," *JOG*, 35 (1928), p. 710 and passim.

250. Ibid., p. 710.

251. *Forty-Third Annual Report of the Local Government Board, 1913–14. Supplement in Continuation of the Report of the Medical Officer . . . Containing a Third Report on Infant Mortality* (London, Cd. 7511, 1914), pp. 67–70.

252. *Pharmaceutical Journal*, 17 March 1906, p. 337.

253. Ibid., 10 March 1906, p. 305.

254. Great Britain, *Committee on Abortion* [134], pp. 56–57.

255. Said Lynch [237], p. 204.

256. Pearce, "Three Hundred Cases Abortion" [102], p. 782.

257. The basic story is told in Issekutz, *Arzneimittelforschung* [41], pp. 45–53; for a brief English account, see Goodman and Gilman, *Pharmacological Basis* [46], p. 1062.

258. Cited in Madaus, *Lehrbuch* [38], I, 950.

259. Issekutz, *Arzneimittelforschung* [41], pp. 46–47.

260. Lewin, *Fruchtabtreibung* [69] p. 364, citing French experiments from the 1870s.

261. *Sixth Report of the Medical Officer of the Privy Council, 1863* (London, 1864), p. 457, citing a "Report by Dr. Henry J. Hunter on the Excessive Mortality of Infants in Some Rural Districts of England."

262. Oefele, "Anticonceptionelle Arzneistoffe" [36], p. 493 (under discussion of "Salix").

263. National Birth Rate Commission, *The Declining Birth-Rate. Its Causes and Effects*, 2nd ed. (London, 1917), p. 274.

264. R. M. Mayer, "Tod nach Fruchtabtreibung mit Chinin," *Archiv für Toxikologie*, 6 (1935), 37.

265. Harbitz, "Untersuchungen von Aborten" [116], p. 51.

266. Simons, "Statistical Analysis of One Thousand Abortions" [223], p. 843.

267. Simms, "Midwives and Abortion" [153], p. 114.

268. Great Britain, *Committee on Abortion* [134], p. 42.

269. Summarized in *Presse médicale*, 7 January 1903, p. 28.

270. See K. Hofbauer, "Betrachtungen zur Chininwirkung am Herzen bei einer Chinintoxikation nach Abortversuch," *Wiener medizinische Wochenschrift*, 106 (1956), 377; and K. Willner and L. Heinrichs, "Subakute tödliche Chininvergiftung nach Abortversuch," *Archiv für Toxikologie*, 19 (1961), 224–25.

271. M. Canale, "Clinica degli avvelenamenti da abortivi chimici," *Minerva Ginecologica*, 21 (1969), 1184.

272. Lewin, *Fruchtabtreibung* [69], p. 364 ("Alle stimmen jedoch darin überein, dass grosse Chinindosen den Uterus ganz still legen.")

273. Edgar Rentoul and Hamilton Smith, *Glaister's Medical Jurisprudence and Toxicology*, 13th ed. (Edinburgh: Churchill, 1973), p. 386.

274. Moïssidés, "Contribution avortement grecque" [50], p. 143 (under "Selinon").

275. Daniel Fabre and Jacques Lacroix, *La Vie quotidienne des paysans du Languedoc au XIXe siècle* (Paris: Hachette, 1973), p. 190.

276. Madaus, *Lehrbuch* [38], III, 2091.

277. Quoted in Siegmar Schultze (pseud.: Dr. Aigremont), *Volkserotik und Pflanzenwelt*, 2 vols. (Halle, 1908–09), I, 139.

278. Madaus, *Lehrbuch* [38], III, 2092; Schneider, *Lexikon* [37], III, 43.

279. See A. Tschirch, *Handbuch der Pharmakognosie*, 3 vols. (Leipzig, 1907–27), II, 1260.

280. Carl Stange, "Bemerkungen über die ätherischen Oele . . . des Petersiliensamens," *Repertorium für die Pharmacie*, 15 (1823), 108–09.

281. For the story, see Joret and (Augustin?) Homolle, *Mémoire sur l'apiol* (Paris, 1855), pp. 6–7, 43–44.

282. Thomas Sanctuary, "Concerning the Action of Certain Remedies in 'Functional' Amenorrhea," *Lancet*, 10 January 1885, p. 59. Among other reports of apiol's "success" as an emmenagogue, see I. Galligo, "Studj Terapeutici Sull'Apiolo," *Imparziale*, 1 (1861–62), 7; Marotte, "De l'utilité de l'apiol dans l'aménorrhée et la dysménorrhée," *Bulletin de thérapeutique médicale*, 65 (1863), 295–349; V.-A. Fauconneau-Dufresne, *De l'emploi de l'apiol* (Paris, 1876), pp. 10–16; and A. Lamouroux, *Étude sur l'apiol* (Paris, 1881), conclusions on p. 16.

283. Roberts Bartholow, *Practical Treatise on Materia Medica and Therapeutics*, 3rd ed. (New York, 1879), p. 512.

284. "Quacks and Abortion," *Lancet*, 10 December 1898, p. 1570; 24 December 1898, p. 1725.

285. Dr. Glatard, "Un Cas d'intoxication par l'apiol," *Bulletin médicale de l'Algérie*, 2nd ser., 21 (1910), 461.

286. George B. Wood and Franklin Bache, *The Dispensatory of the United States*, 12th ed. (Philadelphia, 1868), pp. 640–41.
287. Mentioned in *Pharmazeutische Zentralhalle*, 41 (1900), 784.
288. William Martindale, *The Extra Pharmacopoeia*, 4th ed. (London, 1885), pp. 80–81.
289. Lamouroux, *L'Apiol* [282], p. 3.
290. Mentioned in *Pharmaceutical Journal*, 90 (1913), 130.
291. For its rocky history in the *Codex*, see Raymond-Jean-Paul Quilichini, *Contribution à l'étude analytique de l'apiol* (Bordeaux: med. diss., 1952), pp. 61–62.
292. *Jahresbericht über die Fortschritte der Pharmacognosie*, NF, 18–19 (1883–84), 706; this is the first reference to apiol in the *Jahresberichte*, which began publication in 1866.
293. *Merck Index of Chemicals and Drugs* (Rahway, N.J., 1889) p. 20.
294. *Pharmazeutische Zentralhalle*, 44 (1903), 8.
295. Mentioned in *Pharmazeutische Zentralhalle*, 53 (1912), 1039.
296. Spinner, "Zur Toxikologie des Eukalyptusöls," [35] p. 391.
297. Werb, *Wandlung Abtreibungsmethoden* [74], pp. 18–19.
298. A. Beythien and H. Hempel, "Über die Tätigkeit des Chemischen Untersuchungsamtes der Stadt Dresden im Jahre 1927," *Pharmazeutische Zentralhalle*, 69 (1928), 340.
299. Professor Kochmann, "Anthemis nobilis und Apiol, sind sie Abortivmittel?" *Archiv für Toxikologie*, 2 (1931), 36.
300. Walther Ripperger, *Grundlagen zur praktischen Pflanzenheilkunde* (Stuttgart, 1937), p. 297.
301. Note in *Pharmazeutische Zeitung*, 80 (1935), 227.
302. G. Joachimoglu, "Apiolum viride als Abortivum," *Deutsche medizinische Wochenschrift*, 3 December 1926, p. 2080.
303. Ph. Chapelle, "L'Apiol liquide; son long passé irréprochable et les graves accidents récents qu'on lui attribue faussement," *Journal de Pharmacie et de chimie*, ser. 8, 18 (1933), 25; the author represented a pharmaceutical company.
304. Patoir, "Emploi fréquent abortifs" [236], 1292.
305. Henri Roger and Maurice Recordier, "Les Polynévrites phosphocréosotiques," *Annales de médecine*, 35 (1934), 47.
306. Trillat et al., "Un Cas d'intoxication mortelle par l'apiol," *Bulletin de la société d'obstétrique et de gynécologie*, 1931, p. 615.
307. Étienne Chabrol et al., "A Propos des formes graves mais curables de l'intoxication par l'apiol," *Bulletins et mémoires de la société médicale des hôpitaux de Paris*, 56 (1941), 810.
308. Nicolo Candela, "Sull'aborto criminoso con mezzi chimici," *Annali di Ostetricia e Ginecologia*, 50 (1928), 1519.
309. Francesco D'Aprile, "Sull'aborto criminoso," *Annali di Ostetricia e Ginecologia*, 50 (1928), 1226.
310. See, for example, the entries in Jacob Gutman, *Modern Drug Encyclopedia* (New York, 1934), p. 443.
311. *Physicians Desk Reference*, 1971, p. 1248.
312. E. Schifferli, "Einige Fälle von Abtreibung durch 'Apiol'-Präparate," *Deutsche Zeitschrift für die gesamte gerichtliche Medizin*, 30 (1938), 55–58.
313. H. Jagdhold, "Apiol als Abortivum," *Archiv für Toxikologie*, 4 (1933), 126–27.
314. The deaths were reported as follows: Brenot, "Intoxication mortelle par l'apiol," *Journal suisse de pharmacie*, 3 January 1914, pp. 6–7, a summary of the original report, which appeared in *Bourgogne médicale*, 15 July 1913. D'Aprile, "Sull'aborto criminoso" [309], reporting three deaths in Italy in the 1920s; Trillat, "Cas d'intoxication" [306], pp. 615–16; L. Laederich et al., "Intoxication mortelle par l'apiol," *Bulletins et mémoires de la société médicale des hôpitaux de Paris*, 3rd ser., 48 (1932), 746–57; A. Patoir and G. Patoir, "L'Hépato-néphrite apiolique," *L'Echo médical du Nord*, 3rd ser., 4 (1935), 319; Pietro Piccioli, "Avvelenamento da apiolo ingerito a scopo abortivo," *Giornale del Medico Practico*, 19 (1937), 22–23 (they considered it an apiol death, yet they found traces of parsley in the victim's intestine at autopsy, so it could have been poisoning from decoction of parsley); Adrien Debuirre, *Étude clinique et expérimentale des quelques produits abortifs d'origine végétale* (Lille: med. diss., 1938), pp. 20–22; Roger Papet, *A Propos de quelques cas d'intoxication grave par ingestion d'apiol dans un but abortif* (Lyon:

med. diss., 1939), pp. 32–33; Mauro Barni, "L'Intossicazione da apiolo," *Minerva Medicolegale*, 72 (1952), 6–7; Louis Lowenstein and Donald H. Ballew, "Fatal Acute Hemolytic Anemia . . . from Ingestion of a Compound Containing Apiol," *Canadian Medical Association Journal*, 1 February 1958, pp. 195–96 (given that "Apergol," the ingested substance, contained savin and ergotin as well, it is not clear that the toxic symptoms were entirely due to apiol); and Ch. Vitani, "Difficultés rencontrées à propos des avortements par toxiques," *Médecine légale et dommage corporel*, 2 (1969), 153–54.

315. Konstantin Lowenberg, "Cerebral Damage in a Case of Fatal Poisoning Due to a Compound of Ergot and Apiol (Ergoapiol)," *JAMA*, 19 February 1938, pp. 573–75.

316. In the substantial post–Second World War Italian literature on the subject, see Armando Prassoli, "Su Di un Caso di Avvelenamento Mortale da Ingestione a Scopo Abortivo di Decotto di Radici di Prezzemolo," *Folia Gynecologica*, 42 (1947), 257–78; Corrado Belvederi, "Su Quattro Casi di Anuria Postabortiva," *Rivista Italiana di Ginecologia*, 32 (1949), 349–70; Clemente Puccini, "Alcune Considerazioni sugli Avvelenamenti da Apiolo," *Minerva Medicolegale*, 81 (1961), 194–200 (apiol was found in several body organs at autopsy, yet the victim had ingested a parsley decoction; hence the apiol may not have been the cause of death); Michele Mumolo, "Su Di un Caso di Intossicazione Acuta e Mortale da Apiolo," *Recenti Progressi in Medicina*, 36 (1964), 139–51 (she drank a parsley decoction, but also had endometritis; apiol found at autopsy); and V. Mele, "Sulla Intossicazione da Prezzemolo Usato come Mezzo Abortivo," *Folia Medica*, 51 (1968), 601–13.

317. J. Chevalier, "A Propos de l'Apiol," *Bulletin général de thérapeutique médicale*, 158 (1909), 103.

318. Georg Strassmann, "Brauchbare und unbrauchbare Abtreibungsmittel," *MGH*, 75 (1926–27), 82.

319. J. W. G. ter Braak, "Polyneuritis nach Gebrauch eines Abortivums," *Deutsche Zeitschrift für Nervenheilkunde*, 125 (1932), 95.

320. F. von Neureiter et al., *Handwörterbuch der gerichtlichen Medizin* (Berlin, 1940), p. 58.

321. Gessner, *Gift- und Arzneipflanzen* [51], p. 307.

322. Candela, "Sull'aborto Criminoso" [308], cases 1–8 and obs. A and B, pp. 1208–15.

323. Rodolfo Marri, "Contributo alla farmacologia degli olii eterei: ricerche sperimentali sull'Apiolo," *Archivio italiano di scienze farmacologiche*, 8 (1939), summary of findings on p. 266.

324. For experimental evidence that placental lesions figure prominently in apiol's abortive action, see André Patoir, "Intoxication apiolique expérimentale," *L'Echo médical du Nord*, NS, 6 (1936), pp. 650–51, and Patoir et al., "Étude expérimentale," 39 (1939), 202–03; Armando Prassoli, "L'Azione dell'Apiolo sulla Cellula Coriale e sulla Placenta Della Cavia," *Folia Gynecologica*, 42 (1947), conclusions summarized on p. 307.

325. *British Pharmaceutical Codex*, 1949 ed., p. 1443.

326. *Dispensatory of the United States*, 1955 ed., p. 1796.

327. See "Trade Information Letter" no. 175, sent out by Canada's Department of National Health and Welfare on 14 August 1959. I have a copy of this thanks to W. A. Robertson, Chief of the Product Regulation Division of Canada's Bureau of Drug Surveillance.

328. Jagdhold mentioned his encounter with the *Münchener medizinische Wochenschrift* on p. 126; his defense of apiol was published in the *Archiv für Toxikologie* [313].

329. Lewin, *Fruchtabtreibung* [69], 3rd ed., p. 223. The fourth edition in 1925 does not expand this reference.

330. Editorial in *Pharmaceutical Journal*, 17 June 1939, p. 612.

331. G. R. Brown, Personal communication, 2 July 1979.

332. Arthur Osol, Personal communication, 9 July 1979.

333. The most comprehensive early report on the epidemic is J. W. G. ter Braak, "Polyneuritis nach Gebrauch eines Abortivum" [319]. A later review is Werner Naumann, "Über Polyneuritiden nach Gebrauch von Apiol," *Archiv für Toxikologie*, 8 (1937), 207–10. On the American "ginger paralysis" epidemic, see Manuel L. Weber, "A Follow-Up Study of Thirty-Five Cases of Paralysis Caused by Adulterated Jamaica-Ginger Extract," *United States Veterans' Administration Medical Bulletin*, 13 (1937), 228–42.

334. See the note in *AJO-G*, 28 (1934), 305.

335. Taussig, *Abortion* [63], p. 353.

336. See J. R. Walmsley, "Apiol," *Quarterly Journal of Pharmacy*, 1 (1928), 388–94.

337. *Dispensatory of the United States*, 1947 ed., p. 1543.

338. Note on the "Emmenagogue Oils" which mentions apiol as well, *JAMA*, 8 November 1913, p. 1725; as evidence they cited David I. Macht, "The Action of So-Called Emmenagogue Oils on the Isolated Uterus," *JAMA*, 12 July 1913, pp. 105–07.

339. *Annual Reprint of the Reports of the Council on Pharmacy and Chemistry of the American Medical Association for 1923* (Chicago, 1924), pp. 12–13. Franz Berger's review of apiol's physiological effects, *Handbuch der Drogenkunde*, 7 vols. (Vienna: Maudrich, 1949–67), V (1960), p. 330 ("Durch die Eigenschaft, die glatte Muskulatur des Uterus zu erregen und damit eine starke Durchblutung der Becken- und Bauchorgane zu verursachen, kann es als Abortivum wirken").

340. Torald Sollmann, *Manual of Pharmacology*, 6th ed. (1942), p. 168.

Chapter 9

1. U.S. Department of Health and Human Services, *Vital Statistics of the United States, 1978, vol. II, section 5: Life Tables* (Hyattsville: U.S. Department of Health and Human Services, pub. no. [PHS] 81–1104, 1980), p. 5–4.

2. Ashley Montagu, *The Natural Superiority of Women* (New York: Macmillan, 1953), p. 80.

3. On the longer life expectancy of men today in poorer countries, see G. Acsádi and J. Nemeskéri, *History of Human Life Span and Mortality* (Budapest: Akadémiai Kiadó, 1970), p. 185, table 56.

4. For data on a number of countries, see Fr. Oesterlen, *Handbuch der medicinischen Statistik* (Tübingen, 1865), pp. 170–71.

5. Ibid., p. 163.

6. Marilyn M. McMillen, "Differential Mortality by Sex in Fetal and Neonatal Deaths," *Science*, 6 April 1979, pp. 89–90. See also the references in Ingrid Waldron, "Why Do Women Live Longer Than Men?" *Journal of Human Stress*, March, 1976, p. 3.

7. See the data in Louis I. Dublin and Alfred J. Lotka, *Length of Life: A Study of the Life Table* (New York, 1936): "Indications seem to be that up to the beginning of the nineteenth century an average length of life of 35 to 40 years may have been common." (p. 56). For male-female differences, see the data in pp. 45–58.

8. See *Dodeligheten og dens Arsaker i Norge, 1856–1955* (Oslo: Statistisk Sentralbyra, 1961), p. 185, table 124.

9. Acsádi and Nemeskéri, *Human Life Span* [3], p. 184, table 55.

10. Ibid., p. 183.

11. Keith Wrightson and David Levine, *Poverty and Piety in an English Village: Terling, 1525–1700* (New York: Academic Press, 1979), p. 59 ("Life expectation at various ages").

12. Alois Bek, *Die Bevölkerungsbewegung im ländlichen Raum in den letzten 250 Jahren* (Hohenheim: landwirt. diss., n. d.), p. 120.

13. Among other studies, see Hans Christian Johansen, *Befolkningsudvikling og Familiestruktur i det 18. Arhundrede* (Odense: Odense University Press, 1976), p. 121, based on age-specific mortality rates. Jacques Dupâquier, *La Population rurale du Bassin Parisien à l'époque de Louis XIV* (Paris: Editions de l'école de H.E.S.S., 1979), p. 287, table 103 of ratios of *quotients de mortalité*, which show a female surplus mortality until age thirty. Arthur Imhof's study of marriages in four nineteenth-century German communities found that by age forty-nine, 18 percent of the husbands and 25 percent of the wives had died. "Die Übersterblichkeit verheirateter Frauen im fruchtbaren Alter," *Zeitschrift für Bevölkerungswissenschaft*, 1979, p. 497. See also the data in Nels Wayne Mogensen, *Aspects de la société augeronne aux XVIIᵉ et XVIIIᵉ siècles* (Paris-Sorbonne: thèse III cycle, 1971), p. 119. See also the burial ratios for 1700–96 in Claude Bruneel, *La Mortalité dans les campagnes: Le Duché de Brabant aux XVIIᵉ et XVIIIᵉ siècles* (Louvain: Editions Nauwelaerts, 1977), p. 422.

14. *Historisk statistik för Sverige*, del. 1: *Befolkning* (Stockholm: Statistiska Centralbyran, 1969), p. 111 (presents age-specific mortality rates by sex for Sweden from 1751 on).

15. Paul H. Jacobson, "An Estimate of the Expectation of Life in the United States in

1850," *Milbank Memorial Fund Quarterly*, 35 (1957), 198; table 1 ("Approximate life table, white population").

16. *Statistische Nachrichten über das Grossherzogthum Oldenburg*, 11 (1870), 224 (life-table mortality rates).

17. Ibid., computed from life-table mortality rates on pp. 39, 44.

18. Ibid., p. 78 for Belgium; for Norway, *Dodeligheten* [8], p. 51.

19. The most convenient compilation of age-specific English mortality statistics by age, sex, and cause-of-death is W. P. D. Logan, "Mortality in England and Wales from 1848 to 1947," *Population Studies*, 4 (1950–51), 132–78 (tables throughout).

20. English women in 1977 die slightly more often than men of digestive diseases, but this represents an exception to the international pattern. See World Health Organization, *World Health Statistics Annual 1979* (Geneva: World Health Organization, 1979), passim for the appropriate data.

21. Bud Berzing, *Sex Songs of the Ancient Letts* (New York: University Books, 1969), pp. 140–41.

22. Dr. Rame, *Essai historique et médical sur Lodève* (Lodève, 1841), p. 72.

23. For a somewhat overdrawn picture of tuberculosis in the nineteenth century as a "fashionable" middle-class disease, see Susan Sontag, *Illness as Metaphor* (New York: Farrar, Straus & Giroux, 1977).

24. See *Denmark, Its Medical Organization, Hygiene and Demography*, (Copenhagen, 1891, p. 429); *Dodeligheten* [8] p. 121; and on Stockholm, Max Mosse and Gustav Tugendreich, *Krankheit und soziale Lage* (Munich, 1913), p. 251.

25. Friedrich Prinzing, "Krankheitsstatistik (spezielle)," in A. Grotjahn and J. Kaup, eds., *Handwörterbuch der sozialen Hygiene*, 2 vols. (Leizig, 1912), I, 673 (data on the Leipziger Ortskrankenkasse).

26. Elizabeth Wicht-Candolfi, *La Mortalité à Genève, 1730–1739* (Université de Genève: mémoire de maîtrise, 1971), pp. 35–37, 64–67; data on "population résidente" for 1798 by age and sex were used as the denominator in these calculations, from Alfred Perrenoud, *La Population de Genève, XVIe–XIXe siècles* (Geneva: Lib. Jullien, 1979), p. 532.

27. *Denmark Hygiene* [24], p. 429 (data on *morbis cordis*).

28. Prinzing, "Krankheitsstatistik" [25], p. 673 (Ortskrankenkasse data).

29. Computed from data in Wicht-Candolfi, *Mortalité à Genève* [26]; included in abdominal and gastrointestinal infections were "abcès. inflammation bas ventre," "misereré, colique," "inflammation entrailles," "hydropique," "hydropsie matrice," "diarrhée," and "devoiement, vomissement."

30. Jonas Graetzer, *Edmund Halley und Caspar Neumann: Ein Beitrag zur Bevölkerungs-Statistik* (Breslau, 1883), data on pp. 66–75 ("Geschwulst und innerliche Geschwür").

31. Philipp Ehlers, *Die Sterblichkeit "im Kindbett" in Berlin und Preussen, 1877–1896* (Stuttgart, 1900), p. 39.

32. Prinzing, "Krankheitsstatistik" [25], p. 673.

33. Evelyn B. Ackerman, "Use by Patients of a French Provincial Hospital, 1895–1923," *Bulletin of the History of Medicine*, 54 (1980), 199.

34. Dublin and Lotka, *Length of Life* [7], p. 210.

35. Leslie Schoenfield, "Diseases of the Gallbladder," in Kurt J. Isselbacher et al., eds., *Harrison's Principles of Internal Medicine*, 9th ed. (New York: McGraw-Hill, 1980), p. 1490.

36. Denys Jennings, "Perforated Peptic Ulcer: Changes in Age-Incidence and Sex-Distribution in the Last 150 Years," *Lancet*, 2 March 1940, p. 396, figure 1.

37. Ibid., pp. 444–45. See also H. B. M. Murphy, "Historic Changes in the Sex Ratios for Different Disorders," *Social Science and Medicine*, 12B (1978), 143–45.

38. Jennings, "Perforated Peptic Ulcer," p. 396.

39. Hermann Fehling, *Entwicklung der Geburtshilfe und Gynäkologie im 19. Jahrhundert* (Berlin, 1925), p. 263.

40. F. Bisset Hawkins, *Elements of Medical Statistics* (London, 1829), computed from tables on pp. 87–99. Adult deaths over 15 from 1821 to 1824.

41. *Denmark Hygiene* [24], pp. 428–30 (towns only).

42. See, for example, the statistics for the United States and West Germany in *World Health Statistics Annual, 1979*, pp. 137, 305.

43. U.S. Department of Health, Education and Welfare, NCHS, *Office Visits by Women . . . 1977* (Hyattsville: Department of Health, Education and Welfare, Vital and Health Statistics Series 13, no. 45, pub. no. [PHS] 80–1796, 1980), p. 11, figure 7.

44. *Denmark Hygiene* [24], pp. 428–30; on Breslau, Graetzer, *Beitrag Bevölkerungssta-tistik* [30], pp. 66–75; on Norway, *Dodeligheten* [8], p. 151.

45. Dominique Tabutin, "La Surmortalité féminine en Europe avant 1940," *Population*, 33 (1978), 135; for 1848–72; I have also found useful two unpublished papers by Michel Poulain and Dominique Tabutin, "Mortalité aux jeunes ages en Europe et en Amérique du Nord du XIXe à nos jours," working paper no. 76 (August 1979), and "La Surmortalité des petites filles en Belgique au XIXe et au début du XXe siècle," working paper no. 77 (October 1979), Département de Démographie, Université Catholique de Louvain.

46. See, for example, David T. Purtilo and John L. Sullivan, "Immunological Bases for Superior Survival of Females," *American Journal of the Diseases of Children*, 133 (1979), 1251–52.

47. Verena Martin-Kies, *Der Alltag eines Engadiner Arztes um 1700* (Chur: Calven Kommissionsverlag, 1977), p. 88.

48. Franz Mezler, *Versuch einer medizinischen Topographie der Stadt Sigmaringen* (Freiburg, 1822), pp. 164, 346.

49. Dr. Goldschmidt, *Volksmedicin im nordwestlichen Deutschland* (Bremen, 1854), p. 39.

50. Gertrud Dyhrenfurth, *Ein schlesisches Dorf und Rittergut* (Leipzig, 1906), tabulated from pp. 104–13.

51. Marta Wohlgemuth, *Die Bäuerin in zwei badischen Gemeinden* (Karlsruhe, 1913), tabulated from pp. 118–21.

52. Mezler, *Topographie* [48], pp. 349, 351.

53. Maria Bidlingmaier, *Die Bäuerin in zwei Gemeinden Württembergs* (Tübingen: staatswiss. diss., 1918), p. 105.

54. B. Walkmeister-Dambach, *Leben und Arbeit der Bündner Bäuerin*, offprint from *Schweizerische landwirtschaftliche Monatshefte*, 1928, p. 13.

55. Dyhrenfurth, *Schlesisches Dorf* [50], tabulated from pp. 105–13, question 17.

56. Elisabeth Baldauf, *Die Frauenarbeit in der Landwirtschaft* (Kiel: staatswiss. diss., 1932), p. 119.

57. Friedrich Prinzing, "Die kleine Sterblichkeit des weiblichen Geschlechts in den Kulturstaaten und ihre Ursachen," *Archiv für Rassen- und Gesellschafts-Biologie*, 2 (1905), 378.

58. *Dodeligheten* [8], p. 123.

59. Robert E. Kennedy, Jr., *The Irish: Emigration, Marriage and Fertility* (Berkeley: University of California Press, 1973), pp. 59–60.

60. F. A. M. Kerckhaert and F. W. A. Van Poppel, *Tables de mortalité abrégées par sexe et état matrimonial pour les Pays-Bas, période 1850–1970* (Tilburg: Instituut voor Social Wetenschappelijk, 1974), computed from tables passim.

61. *Dodeligheten* [8], p. 188.

62. Cited in Oesterlen, *Handbuch* [4], p. 190 (data for 1855–57).

63. Friedrich Prinzing, "Sterblichkeitsstatistik (spezielle)," in Grotjahn and Kaup, *Handwörterbuch Hygiene*, II, 545–46; data for 1896–1905.

64. Bernard Christian Faust, *Gedanken über Hebammen . . . auf dem Lande* (Frankfurt, 1784), p. 11.

65. Wilhelm Brenner-Schaeffer, *Darstellung der sanitätlichen Volks-Sitten und des medizinischen Volks-Aberglaubens im . . . Oberpfalz* (Amberg, 1861), p. 11.

66. Joseph Wolfsteiner, in *Bavaria: Landes- und Volkskunde des Königreichs Bayern, vol. 2: Oberpfalz und Regensburg* (Munich, 1863), p. 329.

67. Imhof, "Übersterblichkeit verheirateter Frauen," p. 497, table 2.

68. Logan, "Mortality in England and Wales" [19], pp. 158–59, table 7A; *Denmark Hygiene* [24], p. 428; and Georg Wilhelm Consbruch, *Medicinische Ephemeriden nebst einer medicinischen Topographie der Grafschaft Ravensberg* (Chemnitz, 1793), end table, for 1782–84.

69. Bettie Freeman, "Fertility and Longevity in Married Women Dying after the End of the Reproductive Period," *Human Biology*, 7 (1935), 407, table 6.

70. *Dodeligheten* [8], p. 188.

71. U.S. Department of Health, Education and Welfare, National Cancer Institute, *SEER*

Program: Cancer Incidence and Mortality in the United States, 1973–1976 (Bethesda: Department of Health, Education and Welfare, pub. no. [NIH] 78–1837), pp. 2, 4, 66.

72. H. Oeser et al., "Die Konstanz der Krebsgefährdung des Menschen," *Deutsche medizinische Wochenschrift,* 15 February 1974, pp. 273–77.

73. In addition to Oeser, see W. Lock, note, *ibid.,* 24 May 1974, p. 1157; and a response in that issue by Oeser, pp. 1158–59. See also O. Gsell, "Trend der Carcinomsterblichkeit der letzten 50–60 Jahre, dargestellt am Beispiel der Schweiz," *Zeitschrift für Krebsforschung,* 72 (1969), 199, figure 2, for women.

74. Edwin Silverberg, *Gynecologic Cancer: Statistical and Epidemiological Information* (n.p.: American Cancer Society, 1975), p. 23, figure 2.

75. Dr. Rigoni-Stern, "Fatti statistici relativi alle malattie cancerose . . . ," *Giornale per servire al progressi della patologia,* ser. 2, 2 (1842), 509.

76. Hubert Walter, *Bevölkerungsgeschichte der Stadt Einbeck* (Hildesheim: Lax, 1960), p. 116.

77. Friedrich Pauli, *Medicinische Statistik der Stadt . . . Landau* (Landau, 1831), pp. 101–02 (causes of death assigned by a doctor).

78. Ernst Julius Meyer, *Versuch einer medicinischen Topographie und Statistik . . . Dresden* (Stolberg am Harz, 1840), p. 333.

79. Franz Alois Stelzig, *Versuch einer medizinischen Topographie von Prag,* 2 vols. (Prague, 1824), II, 87, table 4.

80. H. J. G. Bloom et al., "Natural History of Untreated Breast Cancer (1805–1933)," *BMJ,* 28 July 1962, p. 217.

81. On England-Wales, see Logan, "Mortality in England and Wales" [19], pp. 158–59, table 7A; on Denmark, *Denmark Hygiene* [24], p. 429 (towns only); on Norway, *Dodeligheten* [8], p. 150 (ages 30–39); and for the United States, World Health Organization, *Statistics Annual* [20], p. 135 (ages 35–44).

82. Robert Hamilton, *Observations on Scrophulous Affections with Remarks on Schirrus, Cancer, and Rachitis* (London, 1791), pp. 67–71.

83. Bloom, "Natural History" [80], p. 215.

84. John Macfarlane, "Remarks on Carcinoma of the Mamma," *LMG,* NS, 2 (1838), 378.

85. Franz Strohmayr, *Versuch einer physisch-medicinischen Topographie von . . . St. Pölten* (Vienna, 1813), p. 262.

86. Johann Ebel, *Schilderung des Gebirgsvolkes vom Kanton Appenzell* (Leipzig, 1798), p. 400.

87. Hamilton, *Observations* [82], p. 70.

88. Béla Issekutz, *Die Geschichte der Arzneimittelforschung* (Budapest: Akadémiai Kiadó, 1971), p. 33.

89. For example, Lawson Tait, *Diseases of Women,* 2nd ed. (New York, 1879), p. 62, on uterine cancer.

90. For illustrations, see Harold Speert, *Iconographia Gyniatrica: A Pictorial History of Gynecology and Obstetrics* (Philadelphia: Davis, 1973), pp. 29–30.

91. On Halsted, see William A. Cooper, "The History of the Radical Mastectomy," *Annals of Medical History,* ser. 3, 3 (1941), 48–50; and Edward L. Lewison, *Breast Cancer and Its Diagnosis* (Baltimore: Williams and Wilkins, 1955), pp. 19–21.

92. Raymond M. Cunningham, "Management of Breast Cancer," *Southern Medical Journal,* 69 (1976), 261 (a regionary recurrence rate of only 20 percent).

93. Bloom, "Natural History" [80], p. 218, table 11.

94. Silverberg, *Gynecologic Cancer* [74], pp. 24–25, figures 3–4 (age distribution, United States).

95. Paul Diepgen, *Frau und Frauenheilkunde in der Kultur des Mittelalters* (Stuttgart: Thieme, 1963), p. 170 (quoting Serapion of Alexandria, an ancient Greek physician).

96. François Mauriceau, *Observations sur la grossesse et l'accouchement des femmes* (Paris, 1694), pp. 9–10.

97. Robert Semple, "Menstruation at Advanced Periods of Life," *LMG,* 15 (1835), 467–68.

98. Joseph Adams, *Observations on Morbid Poisons, Phagedena, and Cancer* (London, 1795), p. 176.

99. John Leake, *Medical Instructions Towards the Prevention and Cure of Chronic Diseases Peculiar to Women,* 5th ed. (London, 1781), pp. 116, 117.

100. Ibid., pp. 114–16.
101. Tait, *Diseases of Women* [89], p. 62.
102. F. J. Beyerlé, *Über den Krebs der Gebärmutter* (n.p., 1818), p. 71, referring to "der gemeine Mann hier zu Land."
103. Hans Zahler, *Die Krankheit im Volksglauben des Simmenthals: Ein Beitrag zur Ethnographie des Berner Oberlandes* (Berne, 1898), p. 82 ("Für Die fystlen und Kräbs").
104. Percivall Willughby, *Observations in Midwifery* (1863; rpt. East Ardsley: S. R. Publishers, 1972), pp. 227–30.
105. Harold Speert, *Essays in Eponymy: Obstetric and Gynecologic Milestones* (New York: Macmillan, 1958), p. 673. On radium, see Robert Abbe, "Radium in Surgery," *JAMA,* 21 July 1906, pp. 183–85. See also Joseph Stallworthy, "Progress in Gynecologic Oncology: A Personal Retrospective View," *Gynecologic Oncology,* 8 (1979), 259.
106. O'Donel T. D. Browne, *Rotunda Hospital, 1745–1945* (Edinburgh: Livingstone, 1947), p. 227.
107. Charles C. Norris and F. Sidney Dunne, "Carcinoma of the Body of the Uterus," *AJO-G,* 32 (1936), 988.
108. Silverberg, *Gynecologic Cancer* [74], p. 46; figures for "all stages," treated with surgery, radiation, chemotherapy, and hormonal therapy; fifteen-year survival figures available only for 1950–59.
109. Ibid., p. 35.
110. See Eugene D. Weinberg, "Iron and Infection," *Microbiological Reviews,* 42 (1978), 45–66.
111. Prinzing, "Krankheitsstatistik" [25], p. 673.
112. Innes H. Pearse and Lucy H. Crocker, *The Peckham Experiment: A Study in the Living Structure of Society* (London, 1943), p. 315.
113. Margery Spring Rice, *Working-Class Wives: Their Health and Conditions,* 2nd ed. (London: Virago, 1981), pp. 37–38.
114. On the role of soil, see Leslie J. Witts, *Hypochromic Anemia* (London: Heinemann, 1969), p. 14.
115. Magnus Huss, *Über die endemischen Krankheiten Schwedens,* German trans. (Bremen, 1854), p. 132n62.
116. Witts, *Hypochromic Anemia* [114], p. 106.
117. William Crosby, "Who Needs Iron?" *NEJM,* 8 September 1977, p. 544.
118. Quoted in Dr. Ashwell, "Observations on Chlorosis," *Guy's Hospital Reports,* 1 (1836), 560–61.
119. Quoted in Virgil F. Fairbanks, *Clinical Disorders of Iron Metabolism,* 2nd ed. (New York: Grune & Stratton, 1971), p. 9.
120. Johannes Lange, quoted in Ralph H. Major, *Classic Descriptions of Disease,* 2nd ed. (New York, 1939), pp. 528–29.
121. Johann Storch, *Von Kranckheiten der Weiber,* 8 vols. (Gotha, 1746–53), II, 64–67.
122. Zahler, *Krankheit Simmenthal* [103], pp. 94–95 (for "Bleichsucht des Frauenzimmers").
123. Heinrich Höhn, "Volksheilkunde (I)," *Württembergische Jahrbücher,* 1917–18, p. 138; Höhn supplied the word "chlorosis."
124. Fairbanks, *Disorders of Iron Metabolism* [119], p. 18.
125. Dr. Douvillé, *Topographie physique et médicale de Compiègne* (Anvers, 1881), p. 196.
126. Witts, *Hypochromic Anemia* [114], p. 33.
127. Axel Hansen, "Die Chlorose im Altertum." [*Sudhoff's*] *Archiv für die Geschichte der Medizin,* 24 (1931), 176.
128. H. St. H. Vertue, "Chlorosis and Stenosis," *Guy's Hospital Reports,* 104 (1955), 334 ("chlorosis . . . in reality has a separate nature" from "chronic microcytic anemia").
129. Bartholomäus von Battisti, *Abhandlungen von den Krankheiten des schönen Geschlechts* (Vienna, 1784), p. 38.
130. See the brilliant but unpersuasive essay by Karl Figlio, "Chlorosis and Chronic Disease in Nineteenth-Century Britain: The Social Constitution of Somatic Illness in a Capitalist Society," *Social History,* 3 (1978), 167–97.
131. Th. Deneke, "Über die auffallende Abnahme der Chlorose," *Deutsche medizinische Wochenschrift,* 4 July 1924, p. 902.

132. J. M. H. Campbell, "Chlorosis: A Study of the Guy's Hospital Cases During the Last Thirty Years," *Guy's Hospital Reports*, 73 (1923), 253.

133. Ibid., p. 253.

134. Richard Cabot, "The General Pathology of the Blood-Forming Organs," in William Osler, ed., *Modern Medicine: Its Theory and Practice* (Philadelphia, 1909), pp. 639–640.

135. R. J. Weissenbach, "La Chlorose est-elle en voie de disparition? Et pourquoi?" *Progrès médical*, 3 May 1924, p. 271.

136. Hansen, "Chlorose Altertum" [127], p. 176.

137. H. Sellheim, *ZBG*, 50 (1926), 2069–70.

138. Storch, *Weiberkranckheiten* [121], II, 72.

139. Dr. Ashwell, "Observations on Chlorosis" [118], p. 530.

140. Cited in Eugene Stransky, "On the History of Chlorosis," *Episteme*, 8 (1974), 37.

141. Campbell, "Chlorosis" [132], pp. 255–56; see also Cabot, "Blood-Forming Organs" [134], p. 642.

142. Vertue, "Chlorosis and Stenosis" [128], pp. 341–43.

143. Robert P. Hudson, "The Biography of Disease: Lessons from Chlorosis," *Bulletin of the History of Medicine*, 51 (1977), 457–61.

144. H. Boëns-Boissau, *Traité pratique des maladies, des accidents . . . des houilleurs* (Brussels, 1862), pp. 73–77 on "les jeunes filles employées aux travaux des charbonnages." On Zola's use of this work, see Richard H. Zakarian, *Zola's "Germinal": A Critical Study of its Primary Sources* (Geneva: Droz, 1972), pp. 104–5.

145. Huss, *Krankheiten Schwedens* [115], pp. 119–30; in summarizing these reports, however, Huss does mention corsets among the *Bauermädchen* [daughters of the landholding peasants], p. 129.

146. *Bavaria: Landes-und Volkskunde des Königreichs Bayern. vol. IV: Unterfranken* (Munich, 1866), p. 215 ("Bleichsucht"); and Jean-Auguste Crouzet, *Topographie médical . . . de Lodève* (Montpellier, 1912 written in 1898), p. 167.

147. Campbell, "Chlorosis" [132], p. 281; and Cabot, "Blood-Forming Organs" [134], p. 641.

148. Sarah Stage, *Female Complaints: Lydia Pinkham and the Business of Women's Medicine* (New York: Norton, 1979), p. 85.

149. Vincent Harris, "Observations on Anemia," *Saint Bartholomew's Hospital Reports*, 20 (1884), 87.

150. From the English translation, *Joyfull Newes Out of the Newe Founde Worlde*, which appeared in 1577, as quoted in Fairbanks, *Disorders Iron Metabolism* [119], p. 5.

151. R. G. Latham, ed., *The Works of Thomas Sydenham*, 2 vols. (London, 1848–50), II, 103, 232.

152. See Russell L. Haden, "Historical Aspects of Iron Therapy in Anemia," *JAMA*, 17 September 1938, p. 1060; and Fairbanks, *Disorders Iron Metabolism* [119], pp. 14–15.

153. On this mini fall-and-rise, see ibid., pp. 15–16, 29–30.

Chapter 10

1. Robert W. Kistner, *Gynecology*, 3rd ed. (Chicago: Year Book, 1979), p. 80.

2. Warren R. Dawson, ed., *A Leechbook of the Fifteenth Century* (London, 1934), p. 189.

3. Anton Elsener, *Medizinisch-topographische Bemerkungen über einen Theil des Urnerlandes* (Altdorf, 1811), p. 84.

4. This account is from Kistner, *Gynecology* [1], p. 80.

5. "Office Visits for Male Genitourinary Conditions: National Ambulatory Medical Care Survey: United States, 1977–78," *Advance Data from Vital and Health Statistics of the National Center for Health Statistics*, no. 63 (3 Nov. 1980), p. 4.

6. Cited in Leslie T. Morton, *A Medical Bibliography*, 3rd ed. (London: Deutsch, 1970), p. 600, entry 5207.

7. C. P. Anyon et al., "A Study of Candida in One Thousand and Seven Women," *New Zealand Medical Journal*, 73 (1971), 10.

8. William Smellie, *A Treatise on the Theory and Practice of Midwifery* (London, 1752), p. 163.

9. Among the many doctors who wondered that their "whites" patients sometimes later found themselves sterile, see Joseph Schneider, *Versuch einer Topographie der Residenzstadt Fulda* (Fulda, 1806), p. 191.

10. Percivall Willughby, *Observations in Midwifery* (1863; rpt. East Ardsley: S. R. Publishers, 1972), pp. 241–42.

11. Friederich Colland, *Untersuchung der gewöhnlichen Ursachen so vieler frühzeitig-todtgebohrner . . . Kinder* (Vienna, 1800), pp. 71–72.

12. William Black, *An Arithmetical and Medical Analysis of the Diseases and Mortality of the Human Species*, 2nd ed. (London, 1789), p. 194.

13. Eduard Otto Dann, *Topographie von Danzig* (Berlin, 1835), p. 249.

14. Ely van de Warker, "A Gynecological Study of the Oneida Community," *AJO*, 17 (1884), 805, table 5.

15. Marie C. Stopes, *"The First Five Thousand": Being the First Report of the First Birth Control Clinic in the British Empire* (London, 1925), p. 53.

16. J.-B. Denis Bucquet, *Topographie médicale de la ville de Laval, manuscrit inédit de 1808* (Angers, 1894; ms written in 1808), pp. 70–71.

17. Dr. Rame, *Essai historique et médical sur Lodève* (Lodève, 1841), p. 75.

18. F. J. Werfer, *Versuch einer medizinischen Topographie . . . Gmünd* (Gmünd, 1813), p. 138.

19. Johann Rambach, *Versuch einer physisch-medizinischen Beschreibung von Hamburg* (Hamburg, 1801), p. 335.

20. Dr. Ludwig Mauthner in an 1841 report; quoted in Gustav Otruba, "Lebenserwartung und Todesursachen der Wiener," *Jahrbuch des Vereines für Geschichte der Stadt Wien*, 15/16 (1959–60), 214 ("Steckermädel").

21. Dr. Zengerle, "Auszug . . . medicinischen Topographie des Oberamtsbezirks Wangen," *Medicinisches Correspondenz-Blatt des württembergischen ärztlichen Vereins*, 18 (1848), 255.

22. F. Schuler, "Die glarnerische Baumwollindustrie und ihr Einfluss auf die Gesundheit der Arbeiter," *Vierteljahrsschrift für Gesundheitspflege*, 4 (1972), 110, 132.

23. Jean-Baptiste-Marin Lesaas, *Essai sur la topographie médicale de la ville d'Elbeuf* (Rouen, 1874), p. 26.

24. See Langdon Parsons and Sheldon C. Sommers, *Gynecology*, 2nd ed. (Philadelphia: Saunders, 1978), pp. 109–10; and Gilles R. G. Monif, *Infectious Diseases in Obstetrics and Gynecology* (New York: Harper & Row, 1974), p. 107.

25. Although I do not wholly subscribe to his views on this, see Jean-Pierre Peter, "Entre femmes et médecins: Violence et singularités dans les discours du corps . . . fin du XVIIIe siècle," *Ethnologie française*, 6 (1976), 341–48.

26. Quoted in Josef Werlin, "Rezepte zur Frauenheilkunde aus dem 16. Jahrhundert," *Medizinische Monatsschrift*, 20 (1966), 266.

27. G. Lammert, *Volksmedizin und medizinischer Aberglaube in Bayern* (Würzburg, 1869), pp. 149–50.

28. Hans Zahler, *Die Krankheit im Volksglauben des Simmenthals* (Berne, 1898), p. 71.

29. Jacques Idoux, *Exploration des traditions thérapeutiques des guérisseurs . . . du Département de la Moselle* (Metz: pharm. diss., 1975), p. 92.

30. James Whitehead, *On the Causes and Treatment of Abortion and Sterility* (London, 1847), p. 255.

31. E. Pelkonen, *Über volkstümliche Geburtshilfe in Finnland* (Helsinki, 1931), p. 30.

32. Francis Ramsbotham, note, *LMG*, NS, 6 (1848), 910.

33. Bud Berzing, ed., *Sex Songs of the Ancient Letts* (New York: University Books, 1969), p. 39.

34. K. H. Lübben, *Beiträge zur Kenntnis der Rhön* (Weimar, 1881), p. 76.

35. Rudolf Temesváry, *Volksbräuche und Aberglauben in der Geburtshilfe . . . in Ungarn* (Leipzig, 1900), p. 98.

36. Maria Bidlingmaier, *Die Bäuerin in zwei Gemeinden Württembergs* (Tübingen: staatswiss. diss., 1918), p. 147.

37. Dr. Märkel, "Medicinisch-topographische und ethnographische Beschreibung . . . Roding, 1860," manuscript in the Staatsarchiv Amberg, Landgerichtsarzt Roding, no. 2.

38. Paul Diepgen, *Frau und Frauenheilkunde in der Kultur des Mittelalters* (Stuttgart: Thieme, 1963), p. 174.

39. Pelkonen, *Geburtshilfe Finnland* [31], pp. 17–18.

40. Margarete Möckli von Seggern, *Arbeiter und Medizin: Die Einstellung des Zürcher Industriearbeiters zur wissenschaftlichen und volkstümlichen Heilkunde* (Basel: Krebs, 1965), p. 40.

41. See, for example, Bucquet, *Topographie médicale* [16], p. 71. Many manuscript reports on *muguet* are to be found in the SRM series, nos. 175–82, of the Académie de Médecine in Paris.

42. Johann Osiander, *Volksarzneymittel*, 3rd ed. (Tübingen, 1838), p. 417; on the procystocide effect of *Salvia officinalis* (sage), among other volatile oils, see N. Jankov et al., "Action of Some Essential Oils on *Trichomonas Vaginalis*," *Folia Medica*, 10 (1968), 309.

43. See, for example, Richard Quain, *Dictionary of Medicine*, 6 vols. (London, 1886), III, 826.

44. *Merck's Manual of the Materia Medica*, 5th ed. (New York, 1923), p. 325.

45. Kistner, *Gynecology* [1], p. 86.

46. *Merck Manual* [44], pp. 174–75.

47. Ibid., pp. 324–26.

48. Arthur Curtis, *A Text-Book of Gynecology* (Philadelphia, 1930), p. 269.

49. See the references in E. D. Plass et al., "Monilia Vulvovaginitis," *AJO-G*, 21 (1931), 320–34.

50. Louis S. Goodman and Alfred Gilman, *The Pharmacological Basis of Therapeutics*, 5th ed. (New York: Macmillan, 1975), p. 1086.

51. Graz data from Otto Burkard, "Erhebungen über Tripperverbreitung und Tripperfolgen in Arbeiterkreisen," *Zeitschrift für Bekämpfung der Geschlechtskrankheiten*, 12 (1911–12), 248, 253.

52. Monif, *Infectious Diseases* [24], p. 179.

53. Parsons and Sommers, *Gynecology* [24], p. 833.

54. Eugène Olivier, *Médecine et santé dans le pays de Vaud au XVIIIᵉ siècle, 1675–1798*, 2 vols. (Lausanne, 1939), II, 696.

55. J. B. Kyll, "Über syphilitische Ansteckung von Wöchnerinnen durch Milchaussaugerinnen," *Zeitschrift für die Staatsarzneikunde*, 17 (1837), 454.

56. H. J. Källmark, *Eine statistische Untersuchung über Syphilis* (Uppsala: med. diss., 1931), p. 35.

57. Johann Storch, *Von Weiberkranckheiten*, 8 vols. (Gotha, 1746–53), VIII, 243–44.

58. Guillaume de la Motte, *Traité complet des accouchemens*, rev. ed. (Leiden, 1729), pp. 663–64.

59. J.-B. F. Descuret, *La Médecine des passions* (Paris, 1841), p. 488.

60. Bertel von Bonsdorff, *The History of Medicine in Finland, 1828–1918* (Helsinki: Finnish Society of Sciences, 1975), p. 66.

61. Morton, *Bibliography* [6], p. 599, for dates.

62. See, for example, the citations in Alain Corbin, *Les Filles de noce: misère sexuelle et prostitution (19ᵉ et 20ᵉ siècles)* (Paris: Montaigne, 1978), pp. 362–90.

63. Edward Shorter, *The Making of the Modern Family* (New York: Basic Books, 1975), ch. 3.

64. Källmark, *Syphilis* [56], p. 71.

65. Lisbeth Burger, *40 Jahre Storchentante: Aus dem Tagebuch einer Hebamme* (Breslau, 1936), p. 133.

66. U.S. Bureau of the Census, *Historical Statistics of the United States*, 2 vols. (Washington, D.C.: Government Printing Office, 1975), I, 77.

67. Friedrich Prinzing, "Krankheitsstatistik (spezielle)," in A. Grotjahn and J. Kaup, eds., *Handwörterbuch der sozialen Hygiene*, 2 vols. (Leipzig, 1912), I, 673.

68. A. Blaschko, "Geschlechtskrankheiten," in Grotjahn and Kaup, *Handwörterbuch*, I, 400.

69. Lida J. Usilton, "Prevalence of Venereal Disease in the United States," *Venereal Disease Information*, 11 (1930), 556.

70. Max Mosse and Gustav Tugendreich, *Krankheit und soziale Lage* (Munich, 1913), p. 510.

71. Emil Noeggerath, *Die latente Gonorrhoe im weiblichen Geschlecht* (Bonn, 1872), p. 65.

72. Statistic based on Finish data from about 1924 to 1936, cited in Elisabeth Rees and E. H. Annels, "Gonococcal Salpingitis," *British Journal of Venereal Disease*, 45 (1969), 206.

73. Ibid., p. 205.

74. Arthur H. Curtis, "Bacteriology and Pathology of Fallopian Tubes Removed at Operation," *Surgery, Gynecology and Obstetrics*, 33 (1921), 625.

75. Howard C. Taylor, "Notes on Fifty Years of Progress in Gynecology," *American Journal of Surgery*, NS, 51 (1941), 99.

76. Phillips Cutright and Edward Shorter, "The Effects of Health on the Completed Fertility of Nonwhite and White U.S. Women Born Between 1867 and 1935," *Journal of Social History*, 13 (1979), 192–217.

77. Alma Thomas (pseudonym, "Anneliese Bergsteiger"), *Erinnerungen einer Hebamme* (Osterwieck, 1941), p. 42 (*Typische Tripper-Einkind-Ehe*).

78. Noeggerath, *Latente Gonorrhoe* [71], p. 81.

79. On V.D.'s antifertility effects as a whole, see Anne Retel-Laurentin, "Evaluation du rôle de certaines maladies dans l'infécondité," *Population*, 33 (1978), 117, graph 2.

80. Massimo Livi-Bacci, *A History of Italian Fertility During the Last Two Centuries* (Princeton: Princeton Univ. Press, 1977), p. 263, table 7.6.

81. Paul Ehrlich and S. Hata, *Die experimentelle Chemotherapie der Spirillosen* (Berlin, 1910), p. 136.

82. Harry F. Dowling, *Fighting Infection: Conquests of the Twentieth Century* (Cambridge: Harvard Univ. Press, 1977), p. 146.

83. Richard H. Schwarz, "Acute Pelvic Inflammatory Disease," in Monif, ed., *Infectious Diseases* [24], p. 381.

84. Lennart Jacobson and Lars Weström, "Objectivized Diagnosis of Acute Pelvic Inflammatory Disease," *AJO-G*, 105 (1969), 1092. On the role of tubal infections in infertility as a whole, see *Merck Manual* [44], 13th ed., p. 933.

85. W. J. Sinclair "The Injuries of Parturition: the Old and the New," *BMJ*, 4 September 1897, pp. 589–90.

86. Thomas A. Emmet, "The Necessity for Early Delivery, as Demonstrated by the Analysis of 161 Cases of Vesico-Vaginal Fistula," *American Gynecological Society. Transactions*, 3 (1878), 116–17 table; appropriate statistics available for only 73 cases.

87. Willughby, *Observations* [10], p. 54.

88. De la Motte, *Traité* [58], pp. 513–14.

89. George Fielding, "Case of Recto-Vaginal Fistula Successfully Treated," *LMG*, 18 (1836), 49.

90. Paul A. Janssens, *Paleopathology: Diseases and Injuries of Prehistoric Man* (London: Baker, 1970), p. 118.

91. Both quotes from Henry C. Falk and M. Leon Tancer, "Vesicovaginal Fistula: An Historical Survey," *Obstetrics and Gynecology*, 3 (1954), 338–39.

92. Harold Speert, *Essays in Eponymy: Obstetric and Gynecologic Milestones* (New York: Macmillan, 1958), pp. 442–43.

93. "Summarische Auszüge aus den Tagebüchern des königlichen clinischen Institut's (Göttingen, 1787)," printed text with handwritten entries about patients, in Göttingen Staats-und Universitätsbibliothek: entry for October, 1786.

94. MaryRose MacDonald, seminar paper, University of Toronto, 1980.

95. Robert Bland, *Some Calculations of the Number of Accidents or Deaths Which Happen in Consequence of Parturition* (London, 1781), p. 7.

96. Paul Portal, *La Pratique des accouchemens* (Paris, 1685), p. 10.

97. Cited in Franz von Winckel, *Allgemeine Gynäkologie* (Wiesbaden, 1909), p. 157.

98. Fleetwood Churchill, *On the Theory and Practice of Midwifery*, 3d U.S. ed. (Philadelphia, 1848), p. 467.

99. Douglas Miller, "Observations on Unsuccessful Forceps Cases," *BMJ*, 4 August 1928, p. 185.

100. Sinclair, "Injuries of Parturition" [85], p. 594; see also Emmet ("Vesico-vaginal Fistula" [86], p. 124), who attributed the decline to greater forceps use.

101. See John R. Kight, "John Peter Mettauer and the First Successful Closure of Vesico-vaginal Fistula in the United States," A/O-G, 99 (1967), 885–92.

102. The story is told in Seale Harris, Women's Surgeon: The Life Story of J. Marion Sims (New York: Macmillan, 1950), pp. 82–102.

103. Barbara Ehrenreich and Deirdre English, For Her Own Good: 150 Years of the Experts' Advice to Women (New York: Doubleday Anchor, 1979), pp. 124–25.

104. This was Sinclair's opinion, at least. "Injuries of Parturition" [85], pp. 589–92.

105. Nicolas Puzos, Traité des accouchemens (Paris, 1759), p. 133.

106. De la Motte, Traité [58], pp. 617–18.

107. Women's Co-operative Guild, Maternity: Letters from Working-Women (London, 1915), p. 70.

108. According to Elseluise Haberling, Beiträge zur Geschichte des Hebammenstandes, I: Der Hebammenstand in Deutschland von seinen Anfängen bis zum Dreissigjährigen Krieg (Berlin, 1940), p. 72.

109. Jacques Mesnard, Le Guide des accoucheurs, 2nd ed. (Paris, 1753), pp. 333–34.

110. Adams Walther, "Zur Hebammenfrage," ZBG, 8 (1884), 306.

111. Stopes, First Five Thousand [15], pp. 32–33.

112. De la Motte, Traité [58], p. 638.

113. See J. Matthews Duncan, Clinical Lectures on the Diseases of Women (London, 1889), p. 423. This condition is called "rectocele."

114. Gertrud Dyhrenfurth, Ein schlesisches Dorf und Rittergut (Leipzig, 1906), pp. 104–13.

115. Mme. Rondet, Guide des sages-femmes (Paris, 1836), pp. 5–6.

116. George Van S. Smith et al., "Procidentia," A/O—G, 17 (1929), 669–70; the average number of children per patient was 3.9.

117. John Duffy, ed., The Rudolph Matas History of Medicine in Louisiana, 2 vols. (Baton Rouge: Louisiana State Univ. Press, 1962), II, 65–66.

118. Ilza Veith, Hysteria: The History of a Disease (Chicago: University of Chicago Press, 1965), p. 23.

119. Rondet, Guide des sages-femmes [115], pp. 15, 30.

120. Quoted in Marcelle Bouteiller, Médecine populaire d'hier et d'aujourd'hui (Paris: Maisonneuve, 1966), pp. 68–70.

121. Beryl Rowland, ed., Medieval Woman's Guide to Health: The First English Gyneco-logical Handbook (Kent: Kent State Univ. Press, 1981), p. 103.

122. See, for example, Zahler, Simmenthal [28], pp. 68, 89; and Werlin, "Rezcpte zur Frauenheilkunde" [26], p. 266.

123. See Mosse and Tugendreich, Soziale Hygiene [70], p. 248; John Roberton, Essays and Notes on the Physiology and Diseases of Women (London, 1851), p. 406; and John Leake, Medical Instructions Towards the Prevention and Cure of Chronic Diseases Peculiar to Women, 5th ed. (London, 1781), I, 129.

124. Thomas Madden, A/O, 5 (1872–73), 53.

125. Rondet, Guide des sages-femmes [115], p. 20.

126. "Gutachten eine Ehescheidungsklage, wegen angeblich relativer Unmöglichkeit der ehelichen Beiwohnung, betreffend," Zeitschrift für die Staatsarzneikunde, 25 Ergänzungs-heft (1838), 99.

127. [Jean-Marie] Munaret, Le Médecin des villes et des campagnes, 3rd ed. (Paris, 1862), p. 422.

128. Bernhard Christian Faust, Gedanken über Hebammen . . . auf dem Lande (Frank-furt/M., 1784), p. 20.

129. Quoted in Elaine Tyler May, Great Expectations: Marriage and Divorce in Post-Victorian America (Chicago: University of Chicago Press, 1980), p. 36.

130. See Speert, Essays in Eponymy [92], pp. 108–115. On the history of repairs for prolapse, see also, "History and Review of the Literature on Prolapse of the Uterus and Vagina," Acta Obstetricia et Gynecologica Scandinavica, 36 supp. 1 (1957), 18–26; and Ludwig A. Emge and R. B. Durfee, "Pelvic Organ Prolapse: Four Thousand Years of Treat-ment," Clinical Obstetrics and Gynecology, 9 (1966), 997–1032.

131. U.S. Department of Health, Education and Welfare, Office Visits by Women: The

National Ambulatory Medical Care Survey, United States, 1977 (Hyattsville: National Center for Health Statistics, DHEW Pub. No. [PHS] 80–1796, 1980), pp. 26–27.
132. U.S. Department of Health, Education and Welfare, *Acute Conditions, Incidence and Associated Disability, United States, July 1977–June 1978* (Hyattsville: National Center for Health Statistics, DHEW Pub. No. [PHS] 79–1560, 1979), p. 10.
133. Ibid., p. 11.
134. Louise Bourgeois, *Observations diverses sur la stérilité* (Paris, 1626), p. 37.
135. Catharine Beecher, *Letters to the People on Health and Happiness* (New York, 1855), pp. 121, 122, 125, 129.
136. Paul Mundé, "A Report of the Gynecological Service of Mount Sinai Hospital," *AJO,* 32 (1895), 466.
137. James N. West, "When Shall We Perform Myomectomy," *AJO,* 56 (1907), 701–02.
138. Ibid.
139. Cesar Hawkins, note, *LMG,* 12 (1833), 459.
140. See Lawrence D. Longo, "The Rise and Fall of Battey's Operation: A Fashion in Surgery," *Bulletin of the History of Medicine,* 53 (1979), 244–67.
141. Ibid., p. 253.
142. Mundé, "Report Gynecological Service" [136], p. 679.
143. John A. Sampson *Archives of Surgery,* 3 (1921), 245–323. See also Magnus Haines, "The Emergence of Pathology in Gynecology," *Journal of Clinical Pathology,* 24 (1971), 378–79.
144. See C. Frederic Fluhmann, "The Rise and Fall of Suspension Operations for Uterine Retrodisplacement," *Johns Hopkins Medical Journal,* 96 (1955), 59–70.
145. Ibid., p. 67.
146. Sarah Stage, *Female Complaints: Lydia Pinkham and the Business of Women's Medicine* (New York: Norton, 1979), ch. 3.
147. Stopes, *First Five Thousand* [15], p. 34.
148. Margery Spring Rice, *Working-Class Wives: Their Health and Conditions,* 2nd ed. (London: Virago, 1981), p. 45.
149. Hunter Robb, "The Use of Morphine and other Strong Sedatives in Gynecological Practice," *Maryland Medical Journal,* 14 May 1892, pp. 617–18.
150. Françoise Loux and Philippe Richard, *Sagesses du corps: La Santé et la maladie dans les proverbes français* (Paris: Maisonneuve, 1978), p. 133 ("A larmes de femme et boiterie de chien il ne faut pas se fier"; "maux de femmes, comme l'aurore, vers midi déjà s'évaporent").
151. G. Himmelfarb, "Zur Kasuistik der Scheidenverletzungen durch den Coitus," *ZBG,* 14 (1890), 395–98.
152. Shorter, *Modern Family* [63].
153. Ehrenreich and English, *For Her Own Good* [103], pp. 104–05.
154. Ben Barker-Benfield, "Sexual Surgery in Late-Nineteenth-Century America," *International Journal of Health Services,* 5 (1975), 287.
155. Barbara J. Berg, *The Remembered Gate: Origins of American Feminism* (Oxford: Oxford Univ. Press, 1978), pp. 121–22.
156. Berzing, *Sex Songs* [33], p. 63.
157. James Hingeston, "Remarks on Enlargement of the Prostate," *LMG,* 11 (1833), 75.
158. Thomas Shapter, *The Climate of the South of Devon,* 2nd ed. (London, 1862), p. 260.
159. Elizabeth Wicht-Candolfi, *La Mortalité à Genève, 1730–1739* (Univ. de Genève: Mémoire de maîtrise, 1971), pp. 64–67. One woman died of "rétention d'urine" too.
160. W. P. D. Logan, "Mortality in England and Wales from 1848 to 1947," *Population Studies,* 4 (1950–51), table 2 on pp. 138–39, table 7 on pp. 158–59.
161. On the composition of stone in nineteenth-century Europe, see Edwin L. Prien, "The Riddle of Urinary Stone Disease," *JAMA,* 19 April 1971, p. 504. On Napoleon III, see Harold Ellis, *A History of Bladder Stone* (Oxford: Blackwell, 1969), pp. 50–56.
162. From tabulations in Jonas Graetzer, *Edmund Halley und Caspar Neumann. Ein Beitrag zur Geschichte der Bevölkerungs-Statistik* (Breslau, 1883), pp. 66–75; Protestants only.

163. Benjamin C. Brodie, *Lectures on the Diseases of the Urinary Organs*, 3d ed. (London, 1842), p. 273.

164. Quoted in Owen H. Wangensteen and Sarah D. Wangensteen, *The Rise of Surgery from Empiric Craft to Scientific Discipline* (Minneapolis: University of Minnesota Press, 1978), p. 85.

165. Ellis, *Bladder Stone* [161], p. 16.

166. John Forbes, "Sketch of the Medical Topography of the Hundred of Penwith," *Transactions of the Provincial Medical and Surgical Association*, 2 (1834), p. 198.

167. Thomas Shapter, "On the Medical Topography of Exeter," *Transactions of the Provincial Medical and Surgical Association*, 10 (1842), 163.

168. J. Hartwell Harrison et al., eds., *Campbell's Urology*, 4th ed. (Philadelphia: Saunders, 1978), I, 781.

169. A. Batty Shaw, "East Anglian Bladder Stone," *Journal of the Royal Society of Medicine*, 72 (1979), 226, figure 5. On the frequency of urinary-tract stones in the United States from 1977 to 1978 see National Center for Health Statistics, "Office Visits" [5], p. 4.

170. Harrison, *Campbell's Urology* [168], II, 950.

171. Ibid., II, 1085.

172. National Center for Health Statistics, "Office Visits" [5], pp. 2–4.

173. Wangensteen and Wangensteen, *Rise of Surgery* [164], p. 103.

Chapter 11

1. Martine Segalen, *Mari et femme dans la société paysanne* (Paris: Flammarion, 1980), pp. 136, 138.

2. For a résumé, see Ilza Veith, *Hysteria: The History of a Disease* (Chicago: University of Chicago Press, 1965), ch. 2.

3. The standard work is Alexander Berg, *Der Krankheitskomplex der Kolik—und Gebärmutterleiden in Volksmedizin* (Berlin, 1935), quote from p. 50.

4. Ibid., p. 52.

5. Ibid., p. 53.

6. G. Lammert, *Volksmedizin und medizinischer Aberglaube in Bayern* (Würzburg, 1869), p. 252.

7. Carly Seyfarth, *Aberglaube und Zauberei in der Volksmedizin Sachsens* (Leipzig, 1913), p. 89 ("Mutter, du Luder, packe dich nach deinem Hause").

8. For recent summaries of the vast menstrual taboo literature, see Penelope Shuttle and Peter Redgrove, *The Wise Wound: Menstruation and Everywoman* (London: Gollancz, 1978); and Paula Weideger, *Menstruation and Menopause: The Physiology and Psychology, the Myth and the Reality* (New York: Alfred A. Knopf, 1976).

9. Quoted in Heinrich Fasbender, *Geschichte der Geburtshilfe* (1906; rpt. Hildesheim: Olms, 1964), p. 89.

10. Guillaume de la Motte, *Traité complet des acouchemens*, rev. ed. (Leiden, 1729), p. 57.

11. Lucienne Roubin, *Chambrettes des Provençaux* (Paris: Plon, 1970), p. 157.

12. Bernard Edeine, *La Sologne: Contribution aux études d'technologie métropolitaine*, 2 vols. (Paris: Mouton, 1974), II, 658.

13. Rudolf Temesváry, *Volksbräuche und Aberglauben in der Geburtshilfe und der Pflege des Neugebornen in Ungarn* (Leipzig, 1900), p. 3.

14. Yvonne Verdier, *Façons de dire, façons de faire* (Paris: Gallimard, 1979), p. 43.

15. See Weideger, *Menstruation* [8], p. 91, for a woodcut of ritual bathing among the Jewish women of Fürth; on Hildegard of Bingen, see Esther Fischer-Homberger, *Krankheit Frau* (Berne: Huber, 1979), p. 54.

16. See Hans Fehr, *Die Rechtstellung der Frau und der Kinder in den Weistümern* (Jena, 1912), pp. 4–10.

17. E. Pelkonen, *Über volkstümliche Geburtshilfe in Finnland* (Helsinki, 1931), p. 117.

18. Temesváry, *Geburtshilfe Ungarn* [13], pp. 89–90.

19. Max Hippe, "Die Gräber der Wöchnerinnen," *Mitteilungen der schlesischen Gesellschaft für Volkskunde,* 7 (1905), 102.

20. Temesváry, *Geburtshilfe Ungarn* [13], p. 100.

21. Ludwig Strackerjan, *Aberglaube und Sagen aus dem Herzogtum Oldenburg,* 2 vols. (Oldenburg, 1909), II, 204.

22. Freddy Sarg, *La Naissance en Alsace* (Strasbourg: Oberlin, 1974), p. 57.

23. Jacques Toussaert, *Le Sentiment religieux en Flandre à la fin du Moyen-Age* (Paris: Plon, 1963), pp. 100–01.

24. J. E. Vaux, *Church Folk Lore* (London, 1902), p. 112. I am grateful to Alwyne Graham for this reference.

25. Franz Hempler, *Psychologie des Volksglaubens . . . des Weichsellandes* (Königsberg, 1930), p. 89 ("das Gesicht der gestorbenen Wöchnerin ganz 'zerspickt vom Bart der Unterirdischen' '").

26. Arnold Van Gennep, *Manuel de folklore français contemporain,* 7 vols. (Paris: Picard, 1943–58), I (i), 120.

27. Sarg, *Naissance en Alsace* [22], p. 43.

28. Lammert, *Volksmedizin Bayern* [6], p. 177.

29. L.-J.-B. Bérenger-Féraud, *Réminiscences populaires de la Provence* (Paris, 1885), pp. 176–77.

30. Christian Jensen, *Die nordfriesischen Inseln* (Hamburg, 1891), pp. 344–45.

31. Seyfarth, *Aberglaube Sachsens* [7], p. 27.

32. On Luther, see Reinhard Worschech, *Frauenfeste und Frauenbräuche in vergleichender Betrachtung mit besonderer Berücksichtigung Frankens* (Würzburg: phil. diss., 1971), p. 218; on Breslau, see Hippe, "Gräber der Wöchnerinnen" [19], p. 102.

33. Hippe, ibid. p. 103.

34. Ibid., p. 103.

35. B. Kahle, "Noch einmal die 'Gräber der Wöchnerinnen,' " *Mitteilungen der schlesischen Gesellschaft für Volkskunde,* 8 (1906), 60.

36. Th. Imme, "Geburt und Kindheit in Sitte und Volksglauben Altessens und seiner Umgebung," *Zeitschift des Vereins für rheinische und westfälische Volkskunde,* 10 (1913), 170.

37. Kahle, "Noch einmal" [35], p. 60.

38. See World Health Organization, Eastern Mediterranean Regional Office, *Traditional Practices Affecting the Health of Women and Children* (Alexandria: World Health Organization, 1979), passim.

39. See, for example, Georg Burckhard, *Die deutschen Hebammenordnungen von ihren ersten Anfängen bis auf die Neuzeit* (Leipzig, 1912), p. 22.

40. See Edward Shorter, "The 'Veillée' and the Great Transformation," in Jacques Beauroy et al., eds., *The Wolf and the Lamb: Popular Culture in France* (Saratoga: Anma Libri, 1977), pp. 127–40.

41. Segalen, *Mari et femme* [1], p. 151.

42. Roderick Phillips, "Gender Solidarities in Eighteenth-Century Urban France: the Example of Rouen," *Histoire sociale/Social History,* 13 (1980), 332.

43. See André Varagnac, *Civilisation traditionnelle et genres de vie* (Paris: Albin Michel, 1948), pp. 182–212.

44. Worschech, *Frauenfeste* [32], pp. 184–85.

45. Ibid., p. 108.

46. Ibid., p. 111.

47. Alois Nöth, *Die Hebammenordnungen des XVIII. Jahrhunderts* (Würzburg: med. diss., 1931), p. 156.

48. Walter Diener, *Hunsrücker Volkskunde* (Bonn, 1925), pp. 146–47.

49. Ruth-E. Mohrmann, *Volksleben in Wilster im 16. und 17. Jahrhundert* (Neumünster: Wachholtz, 1977), p. 304.

50. For example, for France, see G. Michel Coissac, *Mon Limousin* (Paris, 1913), p. 260; and Van Gennep, *Manuel folklore,* I (i), 120–21. I have cited here only a portion of the numerous references.

51. Worschech, *Frauenfeste* [32], p. 223.

52. Ibid., p. 218.

53. See Van Gennep, *Manuel folklore* [26], I (ii), 743, 751; The reference by Van Gennep is to all female deaths, not just puerperas.

54. Quoted in an unsigned note in *Mein Elsassland*, 1 (1920), 106 ("Morjerot un Wiwerweh esch am Metäuj nix meh").

55. I have attempted to document the rise of the companionate marriage in Edward Shorter, *The Making of the Modern Family* (New York: Basic Books, 1975).

56. See most recently Carl N. Degler, *At Odds: Women and the Family in America from the Revolution to the Present* (New York: Oxford, 1980), ch. 7 and passim.

57. Verdier, *Façons de dire* [14], pp. 97–98; different women are speaking.

58. See, in particular, Carroll Smith-Rosenberg, "The Female World of Love and Ritual: Relations between Women in Nineteenth-Century America," *Signs*, 1 (1975), 1–29; and Nancy F. Cott, *The Bonds of Womanhood: 'Women's Sphere' in New England, 1780–1835* (New Haven: Yale Univ. Press, 1977), passim.

59. J. Jill Suitor, "Husbands' Participation in Childbirth: A Nineteenth-Century Phenomenon," *Journal of Family History*, 6 (1981), 278–93.

60. H. Höhn, "Sitte und Brauch bei Tod und Begräbnis," *Württembergische Jahrbücher*, 1913, p. 356.

61. H. Höhn, "Sitte und Brauch bei Geburt, Taufe und in der Kindheit," *Württembergische Jahrbücher*, 1909, p. 263.

62. Johann Rehli, "Tod and Sterben im Vorderprättigau," *Schweizerisches Archiv für Volkskunde*, 36 (1937–38), 159.

NOTES TO TABLES

Table 5.1 (page 72)

Marie Kopp, *Birth Control in Practice* (1934; rpt. New York: Arno Press, 1972), pp. 127–128. Based on interviews with 10,000 mothers in Margaret Sanger's Birth Control Clinical Research Bureau from 1923 to 1929. Kopp's data indicate that each woman had been pregnant an average of four times. On the assumption that around a quarter of those pregnancies ended in miscarriage or induced abortion, I give an average of three full-term births per woman at the time of interview.

Table 5.2 (page 89)

Emile Rigaud, *Examen clinique de 396 cas de rétrécissements du bassin observés à la Maternité de Paris de 1860 à 1870* (Paris, 1870), pp. 131–34. Pages 134–36 summarize the results of some additional cases observed by G.-C. Stanesco over a sixteen-year period in the Clinique d'Accouchements of Paris.

Table 5.3 (page 94)

ALL HEMORRHAGES

—Rotunda Hospital, Dublin (1770s). Cited in Fleetwood Churchill, *On the Theory and Practice of Midwifery*, 3rd ed. (Philadelphia, 1848), p. 431 (2.3 per 1,000).
—Rotunda Hospital, Dublin (1826–31). Robert Collins, *A Practical Treatise of Midwifery* (Boston, 1841), pp. 59f (half of the 131 hemorrhages in 16,000 deliveries were judged "severe") (8.0 per 1,000).
—London (1820–28). See Francis Ramsbotham, *The Principles and Practice of Obstetric Medicine and Surgery* (London, 1841) (9.2 per 1,000).
—Royal Maternity Charity, western district London (1842–64). See John Hall Davis, *Parturition and Its Difficulties, with Clinical Illustrations and Statistics of 13,783 Deliveries* (London, 1865) (12.0 per 1,000).
—Munich Lying-In Hospital. Carl von Hecker, *Beobachtungen und Untersuchungen aus der Gebäranstalt zu München, 1859–1879* (Munich, 1881), p. 10 (based on 17,000 deliveries, among which were more multiparous than primiparous mothers; 24.8 per 1,000).
—Cincinnati hospital (1894–1913). Magnus A. Tate, "Maternal Obstetrical Records in the Cincinnati Hospital for a Period of Twenty Years," *Lancet-Clinic*, 9 May 1914, p. 558 (based on 4,300 deliveries; 1.9 per 1,000).

—Sursee (1891–1929). See Rudolf Beck, *Geburten und Geburtshilfe in ländlichen Verhältnissen: eine statistische Studie aus den Geburtstabellen des Amtes Sursee über die letzten 39 Jahre* (Basel: med. diss., 1930) (54.5 per 1,000).

—New York City (1920). See Kopp note above (13.3 per 1,000).

—Chicago Lying-In (1931–45). M. Edward Davis, "A Review of the Maternal Mortality at the Chicago Lying-In Hospital," *AJO-G*, 51 (1946), 499–500 (about 20 per 1,000).

PLACENTA PREVIA

—Rotunda Hospital, Dublin, (1770s and 1826–31). See Churchill, *Theory and Practice;* and Collins, *Practical Treatise* (rates are .4 and .7 per 1,000).

—London (1820–28). See Ramsbotham, *Obstetric Medicine* (1.5 per 1,000).

—London (1842–64). See Davis, (1.9).

—Munich Lying-In Hospital (1859–79). See Hecker, *Beobachtungen* (2.4).

—Late nineteenth century rates for Bavaria, Kurhessen, and Sachsen, and for Berlin in 1895. Erwin Zweifel, "Erfahrungen an den letzten 10,000 Geburten mit besonderer Berücksichtigung des Altersbildes," *Archiv für Gynäkologie,* 101 (1913–14), 689–90 (rates 1.5, .6, .6, and 1.3, respectively).

—Rates are presented for a number of lying-in hospitals late in the nineteenth century, Wilhelm Bokelmann, "Die Mortalität der königl. Universitätsfrauenklinik zu Berlin," *ZGH,* 12 (1886), 147; and Ploeger, "Statistischer Bericht über die Geburten der . . . Frauenklinik in Berlin während 15 Jahren," *ZGH,* 53 (1905), 237 (These rates average to 4.2 per 1,000).

—Adolphe Pinard, *Du Fonctionnement de la Maternité de Lariboisière* (Paris, 1889), passim (5.8 per 1,000).

—Sources for the following will be found in preceding notes and in notes to chapter 5: Mecklenburg (1904), (2.6 per 1,000) Büttner, "Mecklenburg-Schwerins Geburtshilfe"; Cincinnati (1894–1913), (.9) Tate, "Obstetrical Records"; Sursee (1891–1935), (4) Beck, *Geburten und Geburtshilfe;* Chicago (1931–45), (.6) Davis, *Parturition.*

—Cleveland Maternity Hospital (1922–30). Arthur H. Bill, "Placenta Previa," *AJO-G,* 21 (1931), 104 (3.0 per 1,000 in 34,000 deliveries).

—Helsinki Maternity Hospital (1910–24). Sally Hjelt, "Placenta previa," *Finska Läk-Sällsk Handlungen,* 67 (March, 1925), 254–55, 3.2 per 1,000; (German summary at end).

—Hamburg (1932–35). Th. Heynemann, "Ergebnisse und Lehren der erweiterten geburtshilflichen Landesstatistik Hamburgs," *ZGH,* 114 (1937), 262 (based on 69,000 deliveries; 4.8 per 1,000; half were treated through caesarean).

—Current. Jack A. Pritchard and Paul C. MacDonald estimate placenta previa at about .5 per 100 deliveries and postpartum hemorrhage (with the loss of more than 1,000 milliliters of blood) at about 5 percent. But because earlier, definitions of a major hemorrhage were probably restricted to even greater blood losses, putting "6 percent" in the table would have given rise to misleading impressions. Pritchard and MacDonald, *Williams Obstetrics,* 16th ed. (New York: Appleton-Century-Crofts, 1980), p. 508 for placenta previa, and p. 877 for postpartum hemorrhage.

Table 5.4 (page 97)

MAINLY FIRST MOTHERS (PRIMIPARAS)

—Paris Maternité (1804–11). Marie-Louise Lachapelle, *Pratique des accouchemens,* (Paris, 1825), III, 3 (for 16,000 deliveries, 2.3 per 1,000).

—Bourg Hospital (1823–29). Cited in Alfred Velpeau, *Traité complet de l'art des accouchemens,* 2nd ed. (Paris, 1834), II, 121 (for 11,000 deliveries, 4.2 per 1,000).

—Rotunda Hospital, Dublin (1826–31). See Collins, *Practical Treatise,* reference p. 123 (among 30 cases, 29 were to primiparous women; 5.8 per 1,000).

—*Aerztlicher Bericht des k. k. Gebär- und Findelhauses zu Wien, 1861* (Vienna, 1863), p. 4 (among 8,700 deliveries, 2.4 per 1,000).

—Data for German maternity hospitals late in the nineteenth century, Bokelmann, "Mor-

talität," and Ploeger, "Statistischer Bericht"—For the Munich Gebäranstalt, see Hecker, *Beobachtungen* (3.9 per 1,000).
—Munich (1909–13). See Zweifel, "Erfahrungen" (12.1 per 1,000).
—Sursee (1891–1929). See Beck, *Geburten und Geburtshilfe* (4.7 per 1,000).

MAINLY MOTHERS OF ESTABLISHED FAMILIES (MULTIPARAS)

—For Dublin's Rotunda Hospital and London (1820–28 and 1842–64), see preceding tables (the respective rates are: 1.2 and .6 per 1,000).
—Lewes (1813–28). Gideon Mantell, "On the Secale Cornutum," *LMG,* 2 (1828), 782 (in 2,400 deliveries, 6 eclamptics).
—Paris. See Pinard, *Du Fonctionnement* (table 5.3) (rates for multiparas only is 4.7 per 1,000).
—Munich Lying-In Hospital. See Hecker, *Beobachtungen* (table 5.3) (rate for multiparas only is .5 per 1,000).
—Baden (1886–1900). Max Hirsch, "Der Weg der operativen Geburtshilfe," *Archiv für Frauenkunde,* 13 (1927), 211 (1.0 per 1,000).
—Cette (ca. 1855–70). Adolphe Dumas, *Quelques faits d'éclampsie puerpérale* (Montpellier, 1871), p. 21 (for 12,000 births 1.6 per 1,000).
—For Sursee (1.0 per 1,000, multiparas only), Munich Uni-Klinik (2.9 per 1,000, multiparas only), Mecklenburg (2.7), and Baden (1901–25) (1.6), see previous references in this table and preceding tables.
—Kansas (ca. 1916). Elizabeth Moore, *Maternity and Infant Care in a Rural County in Kansas* (1917; rpt. New York: Arno Press, 1972), p. 30 (in 1,269 pregnancies of 330 mothers interviewed in 1916, 3 cases of eclampsia; 2.4 per 1,000).
—For Hamburg (2.9 per 1,000) and Cincinnati (2.8), see preceding notes.
—New Zealand (1928–33). J. M. Munro Kerr, et al., eds., *Historical Review of British Obstetrics and Gynaecology, 1800–1950* (Edinburgh: Livingstone, 1954), p. 155 (3.1 per 1,000).
—Sloane Hospital, New York City (1901–23). James D. Voorhees, "Can the Frequency of Some Obstetrical Operations be Diminished?" *AJO,* 77 (1918), 4. The average of the rates for 1901–5, 1911–15 and 1919–23 is 10.4 per 1,000, but the rate declines considerably over that time. Of the 54 cases in the latter period, 29 were emergency admissions from outside—a fact suggesting that the incidence among the hospital's booked cases was much lower.

Table 5.5 (page 99)

GERMAN VILLAGES

—Data on 140 *altmärkische Dörfer* (1766–74), Salzwedel and Arendsee (1766–74), Kurmark and Neumark Brandenburg (1789–98), and Ravensberg (1782–92), from Boris Schaefer, *Die Wöchnerinnensterblichkeit im 18ten Jahrhundert* (Berlin: med. diss., 1923), pp. 47, 55, 56. Data for Apolda (1768–74 and 1784–86) from Schulze, "Anhang zu den Auszügen aus den Kirchenbüchern im Weimarischen besonders die Wöchnerinnen betreffend," *Johann Christ. Starks Archiv für die Geburtshülfe,* 1(ii) (1787), 95–96. Data for Herzogthum Eisenach (1783–86) from Heusinger, "Geburts—und Sterbelisten," *Johann Christ. Starks Archiv für die Geburtshülfe,* 1(ii) (1787), pp. 96–97. Data for the Calvörde district (1688–1790) from August Hinze, "Tabellarische Verzeichnisse der Getauften, Getrauten . . . nach den Kirchenbüchern des calvördischen Physicats-Districts," *Johann Christ. Starks Archiv für die Geburtshülfe,* 4 (1792), 289–95 (these data supply, moreover, the only values for the 1650–99 period). Data for Mecklenburg-Schwerin (1789–1849) from Masius, "Die 30-jährigen Bevölkerungs . . . listen," *Zeitschrift für die Staatsarzneikunde,* 3 (1823), 27. Data for Ostfriesland (1765–1807) from Toel, "Bevölkerungs . . . Listen Osnabrück," *Zeitschrift für die Staatsarzneikunde,* 10 (1825), table 5 following p. 92. Data for Querfurt (1841–50) from Schraube, "Medicinisch-topographische Skizze des Kreises Querfurt," *Monatsblatt für medicinische Statistik,* nos. 8–10 (1864), births on p. 59, maternal deaths on p. 69. Data on two groups of villages in Austria from Franz Fliri, *Bevölkerungsgeographische Untersuchungen im Unterinntal* (Innsbruck: Universitäts-Verlag Wagner, 1948), p. 56, and Gisela Winkler, *Bevölkerungsgeographische Untersuchungen im Martelltal* (Innsbruck: Verlag Wagner, 1973), pp. 70–71 (the time span for both is 1700 on). Data for Zillhausen (1755–1854) from Elisabeth Eckle, *Über die Gesundheitsverhältnisse in Zillhausen von der Mitte des 18. bis zum Beginn des 20. Jahrhunderts* (Freie Universität Berlin: med. diss., n.d.), pp. 25–26. Data for Württemberg (1821–25), from a work by "Riecke" cited in Alfred Velpeau, *Traité complet de l'art des accouchemens*, 2nd ed. (Paris, 1835), I, 131.

BRABANT VILLAGES

—Claude Bruneel, *La Mortalité dans les campagnes: Le Duché de Brabant aux XVIe et XVIIIe siècles* (Louvain: Nauwelaerts, 1977), p. 455 (3 villages for 1624–40, 6 for 1701–56, 5 for 1750–91).

LONDON

—1583–99. From Thomas R. Forbes, *Chronicle from Aldgate: Life and Death in Shakespeare's London* (New Haven: Yale University Press, 1971), p. 106 (St. Botolph's parish).
—1629–36. Data on "christenings" from John Graunt, *Natural and Political Observations Made Upon the Bills of Mortality* (rpt. Baltimore: Johns Hopkins, 1939), pp. 80–81. Added to "christenings" in order to complete the denominator were numbers of "abortives" and stillborn taken from J. Marshall, *Mortality of the Metropolis* (London, 1832), end table for "period I." Data on number of deaths in childbirth are from Marshall as well.
—1670–99 (with many gaps). Data on number baptized, abortives, stillborn, and maternal deaths, all from Thomas Short, *New Observations on . . . Bills of Mortality* (1750; rpt. London: Gregg International, 1973), pp. 188–89.
—1701–46. Data on number of christenings from W. Heberden, *Observations on the Increase and Decrease of Different Diseases* (1801; rpt. Gregg International, 1973), pp. 2–5. Data on abortives, stillbirths, and maternal deaths from William Black, *An Arithmetical and Medical Analysis of the Diseases and Mortality of the Human Species* (1789; rpt. London: Gregg International, 1973), table following p. 42.
—1747–95 (represents 1747–77 and 1795). Taken from Black, ibid., and Heberden, ibid.
—1828–50. From the outpatient service of the eastern district of the Royal Maternity Charity, based on 49,000 domestic deliveries by "well-educated midwives," cited in J. M. Munro Kerr et al., eds., *Historical Review of British Obstetrics and Gynaecology, 1800–1950* (Edinburgh: Livingstone, 1954), p. 263.

EDINBURGH

—I took the lower of two sets of estimates of maternal mortality for the three decades, given in Michael Flinn, et al., eds., *Scottish Population History from the 17th Century to the 1930s* (Cambridge: Cambridge University Press, 1977), p. 296.

KÖNIGSBERG (1769–1814)

—From Schaefer, *Wöchnerinnensterblichkeit*, pp. 40–41.

BERLIN

—1720–1822. Ibid., pp. 15–28.
—1835–41. From H. Wollheim, *Versuch einer medicinischen Topographie und Statistik von Berlin* (Berlin, 1844), pp. 362–85.

Table 5.6 (page 102)

BADEN (1864–66)

—Alfred Hegar, *Die Sterblichkeit während Schwangerschaft, Geburt und Wochenbett* (Freiburg, 1868), pp. 7–16 (187 maternal deaths in 34,600 home deliveries in the Oberrhein-kreis, 1864–66, primarily midwife-assisted). Among the 107 "infection" deaths I included 24 from "peritonitis," 2 from "albuminuria-hydrops," and 80 from various other conditions in which some infective process was evidently at work. Among the related "medical" deaths are 11 from tuberculosis, 3 from typhus, and 7 owing to various conditions. Almost all deaths occurred in pregnancies at term.

NEW YORK CITY (1930–32)

—Ransom S. Hooker, *Maternal Mortality in New York City: A Study of All Puerperal Deaths, 1930–1932* (New York, 1933), table on pp. 232–33 (1,564 maternal deaths in 348,000 home and hospital deliveries, 1930–32). Of the 510 sepsis deaths, 148 followed caesarean delivery; 8 of the 14 "miscellaneous" deaths were owing to pernicious vomiting. Chief among the 344 deaths from related "medical" diseases were "chronic heart disease," 99; lobar pneumonia, 52; influenza, 21; and chronic nephritis, 18. There were 357 additional deaths from abortion, 262 of them septic; and 120 deaths from ectopic gestation.

UNITED STATES (1976)

—*Vital Statistics of the United States, 1976*, vol. II: *Mortality* (Hyattsville, Md.: U.S. National Center for Health Statistics, 1980), 134–39 (335 maternal deaths in 3,168,000 deliveries). Of the "phlebitis-embolism" deaths, only 3 occurred from phlebitis, 54 from embolus. I included 5 deaths from "retained placenta" in the category "shock-traumatic delivery." There were no deaths from pernicious vomiting. Among the 45 "medical" deaths were 20 from cerebral hemorrhage, 8 from "liver necrosis" (once called "yellow liver of pregnancy"), 6 from renal disease, 8 from blood dyscrasias, and 2 from urinary tract infection. Excluded were 39 ectopic pregnancy deaths and 16 abortion deaths. Heart-disease deaths related to pregnancy or delivery are not classified separately. In the 1950s they ranked fourth among the causes of maternal death. K. Ueland, "Cardiac Surgery and Pregnancy," *AJO-G*, 92 (1965), 150.

Table 7.1 (page 157)

GERMANY

—1877 and 1891. From Philipp Ehlers, *Die Sterblichkeit "Im Kindbett"* (Stuttgart, 1900), p. 1 (for Prussia).
—1924 and 1936. From W. Bickenbach, "Über die Müttersterblichkeit bei klinischer Geburtshilfe," *ZBG*, 64 (1940), 818 (German Reich).
—1952 and 1962. H. Rummel, "Die Entwicklung der Anstaltsgeburtshilfe in der Bundesre-publik," *Medizinische Welt*, December, 1966, p. 2538. By 1962, 93 percent of all births in East Germany occurred in hospital, (p. 2539).
—1970 and 1973. K.-H. Wulf, "Panoramawandel in der Geburtshilfe," *Geburtshilfe und Frauenheilkunde*, 35 (1975), 395 (presumably for West Germany).

UNITED STATES (1935–50)

—Cited in Neal Devitt, "The Transition from Home to Hospital Birth in the United States, 1930–1960," *Birth and the Family Journal*, 4 (1977), 5. 1977 from *U.S. Statistical Abstract, 1979*, p. 63.

Table 7.2 (page 162)

—On the 1890s–1900s mortality in general, see Rudolph W. Holmes' summary of case reports, "Cesarean Section for Placenta Previa: An Improper Procedure," *JAMA*, 44 (1905), 1594. The mortality rate of sections for placenta previa was 20 percent.

1900–1909

—C. P. Monahan, et al., "The Experience of the Johns Hopkins Hospital with Cesarean Section," *AJO-G*, 44 (1942), 1001 (whites only); James D. Voorhees, "Can the Frequency of Some Obstetrical Operations Be Diminished?" *AJO*, 77 (1918), 10.

1910–19

—Monahan, et al. and Voorhees, see 1900–1909; Morris Courtiss, "Analytic Study of 1000 Cases of Cesarean Section," *AJO-G*, 32 (1932), 680–81 (for the Massachusetts Memorial Hospital); Isadore Daichman, "Review of Cesarean Section," *AJO-G*, 37 (1939), 138 (for the Jewish Hospital of New York City); J. P. Greenhill, "Analysis of 874 Cervical Cesarean Sections Performed at the Chicago Lying-In Hospital," *AJO-G*, 19 (1930), 615 (includes both outpatient and ward services); E. M. Hawks, "Maternal Mortality in 582 Abdominal Cesarean Sections," *AJO-G*, 18 (1929), 396 (for the New York Nursery and Child's Hospital); and E. D. Plass, "The Relation of Forceps and Cesarean Section to Maternal and Infant Morbidity and Mortality," *AJO-G*, 22 (1931), 190 (on the Hartford General Hospital).

1920–29

—See all the studies cited for 1900–09 and 1910–19; in addition, Ralph L. Barrett, "A Fifteen-Year Study of Cesarean Section in the Woman's Hospital in the State of New York' " *AJO-G*, 37 (1939), 436; William J. Dieckmann, "Cesarean Section Mortality," *AJO-G*, 50 (1945), 32 (citing data for New Orleans' hospitals and the Boston Lying-In Hospital); and E. D. Plass, "A Statistical Study of 129,539 births in Iowa," *AJO-G*, 28 (1934), 299 (hospital births only).

1930–39

—See above Barrett, "Fifteen-Year Study," Daichman, "Cesarean Section," Dieckmann, "Cesarean Section," Monahan, "Johns Hopkins Hospital," and Plass, "129,539 Births;" in addition, Henry Buxbaum, "Obstetrics in the Home," *Surgical Clinics of North America,* February, 1943, p. 57 (for the Chicago Maternity Center); Robert DeNormandie, "Five-Year Study of Cesarean Sections in Massachusetts," *NEJM,* 8 October 1942, p. 533 (as a percent of hospital births); D. Anthony D'Esopo, "Trends in the Use of the Cesarean Section Operation," *AJO-G*, 58 (1949), 1121 (estimated from graph of rates for four large New York City hospitals); Clifford Lull, "A Survey of Cesarean Sections in Philadelphia," *AJO-G*, 46 (1943), 314 (data on forty-five hospitals for 1931); Roy W. Mohler, "A Report of the Cesarean Sections Done at the Philadelphia Lying-In Pennsylvania Hospital," *AJO-G*, 45 (1943), 467, 470 (for 1932–37); New York Academy of Medicine, Ransom S. Hooker, ed., *Maternal Mortality in New York City* (New York, 1933), p. 130 (hospitals only); James K. Quigley, "A Ten-Year Study of Cesarean Section in Rochester and Monroe County, 1937 to 1946," *AJO-G*, 58 (1949), 42 (data back to 1926); and Abraham B. Tamis, "A Critical Analysis of Cesarean Section in a Large Municipal Hospital," *AJO-G*, 40 (1940), 251 (for the Morrisania City Hospital of New York, which due to its policy of operating only on desperate cases, had a quite low rate of abdominal deliveries—8 per 100—and a quite high mortality rate—11 per 100 sections).

1940–49

—See above Dieckmann, "Cesarean Mortality," D'Esopo, "Trends," Lull, "Cesarean Sections," and Quigley, "Ten-Year Study;" in addition, R. D. Bryant's remarks on Cincinnati's seven hospitals in the discussion of Charles A. Gordon, "Cesarean Section Death,"

A/O-G, 63 (1952), 293; Nicholson Eastman, *Williams Obstetrics,* 11th ed. (New York: Appleton-Century-Crofts, 1956), p. 1137 (for data on Minneapolis in 1946; Ramsay County, Minn. in the 1940s; and Alabama, 1945–47); and O. Hunter Jones, "Cesarean Section in Present-Day Obstetrics," *A/O-G,* 126 (1976), 522 (on the Charlotte Memorial Hospital since 1940).

1950–59

—See above Jones, "Cesarean Section," (containing remarks by E. D. Colvin on Emory University's hospital) and Gordon, "Cesarean Section;" in addition, Nicholson Eastman and Louis Hellman, *Williams Obstetrics,* 13th ed. (New York: Appleton Century Crofts, 1966), p. 1126 (for data from the large teaching hospitals of the "Obstetrics Statistical Cooperative," 1951–62, and for seven other major hospitals in the late 1950s; and Nejdat Mulla and James Bates, "Cesarean Section in a General Community Hospital," *A/O-G,* 82 (1961), 669 (in Youngstown, Ohio).

1960–69

—American College of Obstetricians and Gynecologists, *National Study of Maternity Care: Survey of Obstetric Practice and Associated Services in Hospitals in the United States* (Chicago: ACOG, 1970), p. 17 (data on hospitals having in 1967 more than 2,000 births, and on smaller hospitals); John R. Evrard, et al., "Cesarean Section and Maternal Mortality in Rhode Island, 1965–1975," *Obstetrics and Gynecology,* 50 (1977), 595 (also has data on five New York City hospitals 1965–75); Fredric D. Frigoletto, et al., "Maternal Mortality Rate Associated with Cesarean Section," *A/O-G,* 136 (1980), 969 (The maternal mortality rate for 10,231 sections done in the Boston Hospital for Women in 1968–78 was zero.); Louis M. Hellman and Jack A. Pritchard, *Williams Obstetrics,* 14th ed. (New York: Appleton-Century-Crofts, 1971), p. 1168 (data from the Obstetrics Statistical Cooperative for 1965–68, for seven other large hospitals, and for Hartford, which had a section rate in 1964 of 9.7 per 100); and Diana Petitti, et al., "Cesarean Section in California, 1960 through 1975," *A/O-G,* 133 (1979), 392.

1970–78

—See Evrard, "Cesarean Section," Frigoletto, "Maternal Mortality," and Petitti, "Cesarean Section"; in addition, Sidney F. Bottoms, "The Increase in the Cesarean Birth Rate," *NEJM,* 6 March 1980, p. 559 (reporting a 1976 survey of sixty-four hospitals "throughout the United States"); and Jack A. Pritchard and Paul C. MacDonald, *Williams Obstetrics,* 16th ed. (New York: Appleton-Century-Crofts, 1980), p. 1082 (1978 statistics on various large hospitals)

Table 8.1 (page 192)

MALMÖ

—Erik Lindqvist, *Ueber die Aborte in Malmö, 1897–1928* (Helsinki, 1931), tabulated from data on p. 19.
All other statistics from E. Roesle, "Die Ergebnisse der Magdeburger Fehlgeburtenstatistik," *Statistisches Jahrbuch der Stadt Magdeburg,* 1927, p. 113.

Table 8.2 (page 194)

1901–09

—Bertel von Bonsdorff, *The History of Medicine in Finland, 1828–1918* (Helsinki: Finnish Society of Sciences, 1975), p. 219 (a Helsinki hospital, 1901, 10 percent); Erik Lindqvist, *Über die Aborte in Malmö, 1897–1928* (Helsinki, 1931), p. 121 (a Malmö hospital, 1903–

09, 25 percent); Paul Seegert, "Verlauf und Ausbreitung der Infektion beim septischen Abortus," *ZGH*, 67 (1906), 344 (a Berlin hospital, 1896–1906, 15 percent); and Paul Titus, "A Statistical Study of a Series of Abortions Occurring in the Obstetrical Department of the Johns Hopkins Hospital," *AJO*, 65 (1912), 962–67 (ca. 1900–10, 49 percent).

1910–19

Bonsdorff, *Medicine in Finland*, (38 percent); Lundqvist, *Aborte in Malmö*, (21 percent); Eida Aronson, *Contribution à l'étude . . . des avortements* (Paris: diss. med., 1914), pp. 19–20 (Paris-Pitié, 1911–13, 36 percent); Emil Bovin, "Die Resultate exspektativer Behandlung bei . . . Abortus," *Acta Gynecologica Scandinavica*, 3 (1924–25), 94 (a Stockholm hospital, 1914–19, 28 percent); Bleichröder, "Ueber die Zunahme der Fehlgeburten in den Berliner städtischen Krankenhäusern," *Berliner klinische Wochenschrift*, 9 March 1914, p. 452 (1912, 48 percent); Rudolf Commichau, "Ein Beitrag zur Abortfrage," *ZGH*, 94 (1929), 177 (a Nürnberg hospital, 1910, 15 percent); Max Gerstmann, "Statistisches über Aborte," *MGH*, 68 (1925), 225–27 (a Breslau hospital, 1912–19, 57 percent); Josef Halban, "Zur Behandlung der Fehlgeburten," *ZGB*, 45 (1921), 441 (a Vienna hospital, 1910–20, 29 percent); W. Latzko, "Die Behandlung des fieberhaften Abortus," *ZBG*, 45 (1921), 427 (Vienna-Bettina, 1911–19, 33 percent); and Ludwig Nebel, "Ueber das Verhältnis von Aborten zu Geburten in Mainz," *ZBG*, 45 (1921), 1659 (1910–19, 16 percent).

1920–29

Bovin, "Behandlung," 29 percent; Gerstmann, "Statistisches," 62 percent; Commichau, "Abortfrage," on Jena, 25; Lundqvist, *Malmö*, 22 percent; and Nebel, "Mainz," 21 percent; Atle Berg, "Statistische Untersuchungen der von 1920 bis 1929 im Städtischen Krankenhaus Ullevaal in Oslo behandelten Aborte," *Acta Obstetricia et Gynecologica Scandinavica*, 11 (1931), 73 (56 percent); Hugo Lappin, *Statistik der Aborte in den Jahren 1925–1926* (Munich: med. diss., 1927), p. 9 (48 percent); Henri Latargez, *Etude statistique de 588 cas d'avortements* (Lille: med. diss., 1938), p. 41 (Lille-Charité, 1924–36, 37 percent); Thomas V. Pearce, "Three Hundred Cases of Abortion," *JOB*, 37 (1930), 806 (a Camberwell hospital, 1923–29, 34 percent); Sigismund Peller, *Fehlgeburt und Bevölkerungsfrage* (Stuttgart, 1930), p. 143 (a Vienna hospital, 1925–27, 28 percent); Raymond E. Watkins, "A Five-Year Study of Abortion," *AJO-G*, 26 (1933), 164 (an Oregon hospital, 1927–32, 33 percent); Witherspoon, *AJO-G*, 26 (1933), 368 (a New Orleans hospital, 1924–32, 9 percent—"diagnosed microscopically"); and H. Wellington Yates, "Treatment of Abortion," *AJO-G*, 3 (1922), 45 (a Detroit hospital, 1921, 37 percent).

1930–39

T. K. Brown, "A Bacteriologic Study of 500 Consecutive Abortions," *AJO-G*, 32 (1936), 805 (a St. Louis hospital, mid-1930s, 60 percent had "positive uterine cultures"—not stated whether febrile); R. D. Dunn, "A Five-Year Study of Incomplete Abortions at the San Francisco Hospital," *AJO-G*, 33 (1937), 150 (1930–35, 85 percent infected "as evidenced by fever and leucocytosis"); Fuchs, summary of lecture, *ZBG*, 55 (1931), 1921 (Danzig, ca. 1930, 10 percent); Charles E. Galloway, "Treatment of Early Abortion," *AJO-G*, 38 (1939), 249 (Evanston hospital, 1930s, 12 percent); Virginia Clay Hamilton, "The Clinical and Laboratory Differentiation of Spontaneous and Induced Abortion," *AJO-G*, 41 (1941), 62 (New York-Bellevue, 1938–39, 20 percent); Harry P. Mencken and Henry H. Lansman, "The Results in Treatment of 600 Incomplete Abortions," *AJO-G*, 40 (1940), 1012 (a Queens hospital, 1935–40, 24 percent); Henry J. Olson, et al., "The Problem of Abortion," *AJO-G*, 45 (1943), 673 (a Milwaukee hospital, 1937–40, 17 percent); H. S. Pasmore, "A Clinical and Sociological Study of Abortion," *JOB*, 44 (1937), 456–57 (a London hospital, 1935, 69 percent); E. Philipp, "Der heutige Stand der Bekämpfung der Fehlgeburt," *ZBG*, 64 (1940), 227 (a Kiel hospital, 1933–38, 44 percent); and Jalmar H. Simons, "Statistical Analysis of One Thousand Abortions," *AJO-G*, 37 (1939), 843 (a Minneapolis hospital, 1930–33, 26 percent).

Table 9.1 (page 230)

FRANCE (1850–52)

—Jean Bourgeois-Pichat, "Évolution générale de la population française depuis le XVIIIᵉ siècle," *Population*, 6 (1951), 659–60; based on age-specific mortality rates per 10,000 population.

ENGLAND AND WALES (1851–55)

—Chester Beatty Research Institute, *Serial Abridged Life Tables, England and Wales, 1841–1965*, 2nd ed. (London: Royal Cancer Hospital, 1970), based on "Conventional Abridged Life Tables" (pp. 39–86), which go to 1970; data from "$5^q x$."

ITALY (1901–11)

—Associazione per lo Sviluppo Dell'Industria nel Mezzogiorno, *Un Secolo di Statistische Italiane Nord et Sud, 1861–1961* (Rome: Svimez, 1961), pp. 118–19; *probabilità di morte* computed from life tables.

Table 9.2 (page 232)

W. P. D. Logan, "Mortality in England and Wales from 1848–1947," *Population Studies*, 4 (1950–51), 138–65, tables 2A-9A. Male-females ratios based on mean annual death rates per million population.

Table 9.3 (page 235)

ENGLAND–WALES (1848–72)

—W. P. D. Logan, "Mortality in England and Wales from 1848 to 1947," *Population Studies*, 4 (1950–51), 138–65 ("Diseases of the digestive system").

DENMARK, TOWNS (1876–85)

—*Denmark. Its Medical Organization, Hygiene and Demography* (Copenhagen, 1891), p. 429 ("Diseases of alimentary organs").

NORWAY (1899–1902)

—*Dodeligheten og dens Arsaker i Norge, 1856–1955* (Oslo: Statistisk Sentralbyra, 1961), pp. 150, 180 ("intestinal diseases").

Table 9.4 (page 238)

OLDENBURG (1855–64).

Statistische Nachrichten über das Grossherzogthum Oldenburg, 11 (1870), 220.

DENMARK (1840–44).

Otto Andersen, *Regional Mortality Differences in Denmark around the Middle of the 19th Century* (Copenhagen: Universitetets Statistiske Institut, 1975), p. 11.

NORWAY (1899–1902).

Dodeligheten og dens Arsaker i Norge, 1856–1955 (Oslo: Statistisk Sentralbyra, 1961), p. 136.

Table 10.1 (page 278)

—Paul F. Mundé, "A Report of the Gynecological Service of Mount Sinai Hospital, New York, from January 1st, 1883, to December 31st, 1894," *AJO*, 32 (1895), table 1 on pp. 468–70.

INDEX